Pediatric incontinence

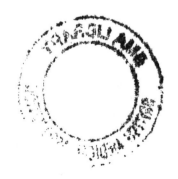

Pediatric incontinence

Evaluation and clinical management

EDITOR

Israel Franco, MD

Professor of Urology, New York Medical College, Director of Pediatric Urology, Maria Fareri Children's
Hospital, Valhalla, NY, USA

Paul F. Austin, MD

Professor of Urologic Surgery, Director of Pediatric Urology Research
Washington University in St. Louis School of Medicine, St. Louis, MO, USA

Stuart B. Bauer, MD

Senior Associate in Urology, Associate Director, Neurourology
Boston Children's Hospital, Boston, MA, USA

Alexander von Gontard, MD

Department of Child and Adolescent Psychiatry, Saarland University Hospital, Homburg, Germany

Yves Homsy, MD

Children's Urology Group, Clinical Professor, University of South Florida, All Children's Hospital/Johns
Hopkins Medicine, Saint-Joseph's Children's Hospital, Tampa/St. Petersburg, FL, USA

WILEY Blackwell

Library of Congress Cataloging-in-Publication Data

Pediatric incontinence : evaluation and clinical management / editor, Israel Franco, Paul F. Austin, Stuart B. Bauer, Alexander von Gontard, Yves Homsy.
    p. ; cm.
  Includes bibliographical references and index.
  ISBN 978-1-118-81479-6 (cloth)
I. Franco, Israel (Pediatric urologist), editor.   II. Austin, Paul F., editor.   III. Bauer, Stuart B. (Stuart Barry), 1943– , editor.   IV. Gontard, Alexander von, editor.   V. Homsy, Yves, editor.
[DNLM: 1. Child.   2. Fecal Incontinence.   3. Adolescent.   4. Infant.   5. Neurogenic Bowel.
6. Urinary Bladder, Neurogenic.   7. Urinary Incontinence.   WS 310]
  RC866.D43
  616.3′5–dc23
                                    2015017764
A catalogue record for this book is available from the British Library.

Set in 9.5/13pt Meridien by SPi Global, Pondicherry, India
Printed and bound in Malaysia by Vivar Printing Sdn Bhd

1 2015

The editors of this text would like to dedicate this book to two important groups of exceptional people in our lives, the first being our families and loved ones who endured with our absences while we were attending meetings, working during weekends, and preparing for courses at nights and formulating the manuscripts and lectures on the computer for countless hours to help educate others regarding the topics encompassed in this text.

We also dedicate this book to our second families, the children who have provided us with the opportunity to help them and at the same time learn from them the valuable skills and lessons to make advances in the field of bowel and bladder dysfunction.

Contents

Contributors

Paul F. Austin, MD, FAAP

Professor of Urologic Surgery, Director of Pediatric Urology Research, Division of Urologic Surgery, Washington University in St. Louis, School of Medicine, St. Louis Children's Hospital, St. Louis, MO, USA

Dieter Baeyens, PhD

Associate Professor, Psychology and Educational Sciences, Research Unit Parenting and Special Education, Leuven University, Leuven, Belgium

Ubirajara Barroso Jr., MD

Professor and Chief of Division of Urology, Federal University of Bahia and Professor of Pediatric Urology, Bahiana School of Medicine, Centro Médico Aliança, Salvador, Bahia, Brazil

Stuart B. Bauer, MD

Senior Associate in Urology, Associate Director, Neurourology, Department of Urology, Boston Children's Hospital, Harvard University, Boston, MA, USA

Marc A. Benninga, MD

Professor in Pediatrics, Department of Pediatric Gastroenterology and Nutrition, Emma Children's Hospital/Academic Medical Center, Amsterdam, The Netherlands

Wendy F. Bower, MD

Department of Epidemiology and Preventive Medicine, School of Public Health and Preventive Medicine, Health Services Unit, Monash University, Melbourne, Australia

Terry L. Buchmiller, MD, FAAP, FACS

Assistant Professor, Surgery Harvard Medical School, Department of Surgery, Associate in Surgery, Boston Children's Hospital, Boston, MA, USA

Mark P. Cain, MD

Department of Pediatric Urology, Riley Hospital for Children at IU Health, Indiana University School of Medicine, Indianapolis, IN, USA

Maria Luisa Capitanucci, MD

Urology Unit, Department of Nephrology and Urology, Children's Hospital Bambino Gesu', Rome, Italy

Alonso Carrasco Jr., MD

Department of Urology, Mayo Clinic Rochester, Rochester, MN, USA

Shang-Jen Chang, MD, MPH
Division of Urology, Taipei Tzu Chi Hospital, The Buddhist Medical Foundation,Tzu Chi University, New Taipei, and Buddhist Tzu Chi University, Hualien, Taiwan

Janet W. Chase, MD
Victorian Children's Continence Clinic, Cabrini Hospital, Melbourne, Australia

Rafal Chrzan
University Children's Hospitals UMC Utrecht and AMC Amsterdam, Utrecht, The Netherlands

Pieter Dik
University Children's Hospitals UMC Utrecht and AMC Amsterdam, Utrecht, the Netherlands

Beth A. Drzewiecki, MD
Assistant Professor of Urology, Department of Urology, Children's Hospital at Montefiore, Bronx, NY, USA

Moira E. Dwyer, MD
Department of Urology, Mayo Clinic Rochester, Rochester, MN, USA

Cecilie Ejerskov, MD
Gastroenterology Unit, Department of Pediatrics, Aarhus University Hospital, Aarhus, Denmark

Monika Equit, PhD
Clinical and Research Psychologist, Psychotherapist, Department of Clinical Psychology and Psychotherapy, University of Saarland, Saarbrücken, Germany

Eliane Garcez da Fonseca, MD, PhD
Associate Professor of Pediatrics, Pediatric Urodynamic & Continence Unit, Department of Pediatrics, The School of Medical Sciences, The University of the State of Rio de Janeiro & Souza Marques Medical School, Rio de Janeiro, Brazil

Israel Franco, MD FAAP, FACS
Professor of Urology, New York Medical College, Director of Pediatric Urology, Maria Fareri Children's Hospital, Valhalla, NY, USA

Mario De Gennaro, MD
Urology Unit, Department of Nephrology and Urology, Children's Hospital Bambino Gesu', Rome, Italy

Alexander von Gontard, MD
Department of Child and Adolescent Psychiatry, Saarland University Hospital, Homburg, Germany

Luitzen-Albert Groen, MD
Department of Pediatric and Reconstructive Urology, Ghent University Hospital, Ghent, Belgium

Piet Hoebeke, MD, PhD
Department of Paediatric and Reconstructive Urology, Ghent University Hospital, Ghent, Belgium

Yves Homsy, MD, FAAP, FRCSC
Children's Urology Group, Clinical Professor, University of South Florida, All Children's Hospital/Johns Hopkins Medicine, Saint Joseph's Children's Hospital, Tampa/St. Petersburg, FL, USA

Tom P.V.M. de Jong, MD
University Children's Hospitals UMC Utrecht and AMC Amsterdam, Utrecht, The Netherlands

Konstantinos Kamperis, MD
Department of Pediatrics, Aarhus University Hospital, Aarhus, Denmark

William E. Kaplan, MD
Professor of Urology, Division of Pediatric Urology, Northwestern University Feinberg School of Medicine, Ann and Robert H. Lurie Children's Hospital of Chicago, Chicago, IL, USA

Antoine E. Khoury, MD, FRCSC, FAAP
Department of Urology, Children's Hospital of Orange County, University of California in Irvine, Irvine, CA, USA

Aart J. Klijn, MD
University Children's Hospitals UMC Utrecht and AMC Amsterdam, Utrecht, The Netherlands

Vera Loening-Baucke, MD
Professor Emerita, Pediatrics Department, General Pediatric Division, University of Iowa, Iowa City, IA, USA

Tryggve Nevéus, MD, PhD
Associate Professor, Senior Consultant, Pediatric Nephrology Unit, Department of Women's and Children's Health, Uppsala University, Uppsala University Children's Hospital, Uppsala, Sweden

Oreoluwa Ogunyemi, MD
Fellow in Pediatric Urology, Stanford University School of Medicine, Lucile Packard Children's Hospital, Stanford, CA, USA

Michael S. Park, MD
Department of Neurosurgery & Brain Repair, Morsani College of Medicine, University of South Florida, Tampa, FL, USA

Prof Dr Ann Raes
Department of Pediatric Nephrology, Ghent University Hospital, Ghent, Belgium

Catherine Renson
Department of Pediatric Nephrology, Ghent University Hospital, Ghent, Belgium

Yuri E. Reinberg, MD, MBA
Associate Professor of Urology, Department of Urological Surgery, Children's Hospitals & Clinics of Minnesota, Pediatric Surgical Associates Ltd., Minneapolis, MN, USA and Mayo Clinic Medical School, Rochester, MN, USA

Søren Rittig, MD, PhD
Department of Pediatrics, Aarhus University Hospital, Aarhus, Denmark

Charlotte Siggaard Rittig
Gastroenterology Unit, Department of Pediatrics, Aarhus University Hospital, Aarhus, Denmark

Alexander Swidsinski, MD
Medizinische Klinik und Poliklinik, Gastroenterologie, Hepatologie and Endokrinologie, Charité, Universitaetsmedizin Berlin, Campus Charite Mitte, Berlin, Germany

Gerald F. Tuite, MD
Pediatric Neurosurgeon, All Children's Hospital/Johns Hopkins Medicine, Saint Petersburg, FL, USA

Johan Vande Walle, MD, PhD
Professor in Pediatric Nephrology, University Hospital, Ghent, Belgium

Elias Wehbi, MD, FRCSC
Department of Urology, Children's Hospital of Orange County, University of California in Irvine, Irvine, CA, USA

Anne J. Wright, MBBCH, RCPCH
Consultant Paediatrician in charge of Children's Bladder Clinic, Paediatric Nephro-Urology Department, Evelina Children's Hospital, Guy's and St Thomas' NHS Foundation Trust, London, UK

Hsi-Yang Wu, MD
Associate Professor of Urology, Stanford University Medical Center Pediatric Urology Fellowship Program Director, Lucile Packard Children's Hospital, Stanford, CA, USA

Stephen Shei-Dei Yang, MD, PhD
Division of Urology, Taipei Tzu Chi Hospital, The Buddhist Medical Foundation,Tzu Chi University, New Taipei, and Buddhist Tzu Chi University, Hualien, Taiwan

Elizabeth B. Yerkes, MD
Associate Professor of Urology, Division of Pediatric Urology, Northwestern University Feinberg School of Medicine, Ann and Robert H. Lurie Children's Hospital of Chicago, Chicago, IL, USA

Preface

Treatment of children with urinary and bowel problems requires special people who are driven to help them achieve continence and reduce distress. The management of these children has often been neglected in the past although effective therapeutic approaches are available. It takes a very dedicated person to do this work. A group of such like-minded individuals was formed to foster progress in the care of the child with bowel and bladder issues. The end result was the International Children's Continence Society, with its multidisciplinary mentality to address this problem. This organization has brought together specialists from many disciplines including pediatricians, nephrologists, pediatric urologists, urotherapists, nurses, child psychiatrists, and psychologists in order to help establish guidelines and teaching tools so that others interested in taking care of children with incontinence will have a rational and workable blueprint for investigation and care.

Looking at the presently available literature, we saw the need for a book that addressed the issues of bowel and bladder incontinence in a comprehensive manner. Most texts rarely cover more than one or two of the topics that we touch upon in this volume, whether they are urologic, nephrologic pediatric, child psychiatric, or neurologic books. It was the vision of the editors to develop a textbook that covers all aspects of bowel and bladder incontinence in children within one volume and utilize the expertise that is available in the International Children's Continence Society to put together what we feel is a truly comprehensive tome on the topic.

There has been increasing interest in the field and a drive to help these children with more practitioners entering into the discipline daily. A concise and directed document would be beneficial to all of them, whether they are experts or novices in the field. There have been other textbooks on urinary incontinence in children but none cover the breadth of information that is conveyed in this volume. We chose to make this a text that is useful to all who treat children with incontinence, whether it is due to neurogenic causes or functional problems.

The editors asked all the authors to provide the reader with a practical, evidence-based "how I do it" guide to managing problems in children, which should allow the reader to replicate assessment and treatment procedures easily, without having to go to multiple sources. We felt that this should be a guidebook and a complementary compendium to the various ICCS courses that have been and are being given worldwide. We feel that we have accomplished this task and hope that the reader feels the same way so that ultimately children and families will benefit from this book.

The Editors

Israel Franco, MD

Stuart B. Bauer, MD

Paul Austin, MD

Yves Homsy, MD

Alexander von Gontard, MD

SECTION 1

Pathophysiology of bowel and bladder dysfunction

Israel Franco

Introduction

> Francis Bacon wrote, "Knowledge is power.—Nam et ipsa scientia potestas est."
>
> *Meditationes Sacræ. De Hæresibus.*

To be able to understand the child with urinary and fecal incontinence, it is critical that we have the knowledge on how the systems function individually and interact with each other and the brain. There have been tremendous advances in the fields of neuroscience and neurophysiology that have opened up the doors to new treatments and mechanisms that explain how the systems function.

Without this power, we relied primarily on old models that excluded the higher cortical centers and trusted heavily on vesicocentric models to explain lower urinary tract symptoms as bladder or bowel only problems. These vesicocentric concepts have been proven wrong, and it has become apparent that the system of bowel and bladder control is evermore complex than we imagined. We understand now that the bladder mucosa is a sensory organ in direct communication with the CNS and the bladder and bowel communicate with each other through connections in the spinal cord and other centers. These changes in how we perceive the neurophysiology of bowel and bladder control will help us understand better what is needed to better treat our patients in the future.

In Chapter 1, Drs. Wu and Ogunyemi have condensed decades of work on the neurophysiology of voiding. They help us understand where we are today regarding this topic in a concise and logical manner. Without this foundation, the reader is apt to be at a disadvantage when it comes to managing the treatment of patients with bowel and bladder dysfunction.

Pediatric Incontinence: Evaluation and Clinical Management, First Edition. Edited by Israel Franco, Paul F. Austin, Stuart B. Bauer, Alexander von Gontard and Yves Homsy.
© 2015 John Wiley & Sons, Ltd. Published 2015 by John Wiley & Sons, Ltd.

In Chapter 2, Drs. Ejerskov and Siggard have gone about the business of explaining bowel physiology and functional anatomy. Again, understandings of these processes are essential for any practitioner who is actively taking care of children with BBD. Most of the readers will not have a background in this topic since the majority of us who take care of these children with BBD are in the fields that are directly related to the urologic and nephrologic management of these children. In this chapter, we see the overlap with the autonomic nervous system and the role that serotonin may play in these children affecting both systems.

In Chapter 3, I (Franco) have put together what we have available on the central control and processing of bladder signals. This is based on work in the field of neuroscience that has expanded in a geometric fashion from its early reports in 1997 to a multitude of publications in the last few years with more publications each year giving us more insight into the process. I have relied heavily on the work of Griffith and Fowler since they have contributed a tremendous amount to the literature helping explain the sensory processes that are taking place during micturition and bladder filling. There are numerous others who have contributed to this field and the synthesis of all these works has given us a better understanding of bladder control and voiding. It was the gastroenterologists who were prescient enough to begin to use functional MRI technology to evaluate functional bowel issues before it was on the urologic radar and we look at their data as well to better understand children with BBD.

CHAPTER 1

Neurophysiology of voiding

Oreoluwa Ogunyemi and Hsi-Yang Wu

Lucile Packard Children's Hospital, Stanford, CA, USA

Anatomy of the lower urinary tract

The three main components of the bladder are the detrusor smooth muscle, connective tissue, and urothelium. The detrusor constitutes the bulk of the bladder and is arranged into inner longitudinal, middle circular, and outer longitudinal layers [1]. Elastin and collagen make up the connective tissue, which determines passive bladder compliance [2]. Elevated type III collagen and decreased elastin are associated with poorly compliant bladders [2]. Active compliance is determined by the detrusor, which is able to change its length over a wider range than skeletal muscle, allowing for a wide variation in bladder volume while maintaining a low pressure [2]. The detrusor maintains a baseline tension, which is modulated by hormones, local neurotransmitters, and the autonomic nervous system. Impedance studies reveal that compared to other smooth muscles, the detrusor is not electrically well coupled. This decreases the likelihood of detrusor overactivity (DO) during filling [2].

The urothelium has multiple layers, consisting of basal cells, intermediate cells, and luminal umbrella cells. The umbrella cells have tight junction complexes, lipid molecules, and uroplakin proteins that contribute to barrier function. A sulfated polysaccharide glycosaminoglycan layer covers the lumen of the bladder and defends against bacterial infection. Although the urothelium was previously thought to be an inert barrier, we now know that urothelial cells participate in afferent signaling. Bladder nerves terminate close to, as well as on urothelial cells. Urothelial cells have pain receptors and mechanoreceptors, which can be modulated by ATP to activate or inhibit sensory neurons. Abnormal activation of these channels by inflammation can lead to pain responses to

Pediatric Incontinence: Evaluation and Clinical Management, First Edition. Edited by Israel Franco,
Paul F. Austin, Stuart B. Bauer, Alexander von Gontard and Yves Homsy.
© 2015 John Wiley & Sons, Ltd. Published 2015 by John Wiley & Sons, Ltd.

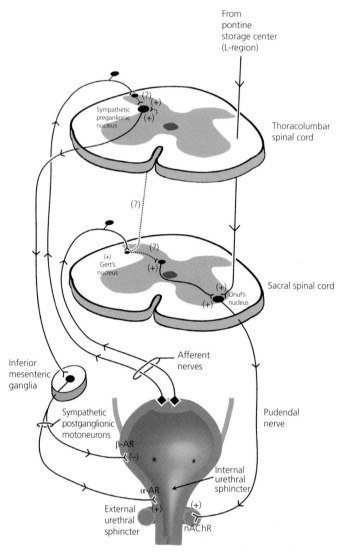

Figure 1.1 Storage function. α-AR, α adrenergic receptor; β-AR, β adrenergic receptor; nAChR, nicotinic acetylcholine receptor. Source: Beckel and Holstege [4]. Reproduced with permission from Springer.

normally nonnoxious stimuli. Urothelial cells release factors such as acetylcholine, ATP, prostaglandins, and nitric oxide that affect sensory nerves [3].

The internal and external urethral sphincters (EUS) are vital for urinary continence. The internal urethral sphincter functions as a unit with the bladder base and trigone to store urine. The EUS is comprised of inner smooth muscle surrounded by outer skeletal muscle. It is omega shaped, with the majority of its muscle anterior to the urethra, and the opening of the omega sitting posteriorly. The smooth muscle is comprised of a thick longitudinal layer and an outer circular layer. The smooth muscle of the female EUS has less sympathetic innervation than that of the male, and the male EUS is larger in size. The skeletal muscle of the EUS has both slow and fast twitch fibers, of which the slow twitch fibers are more important in maintaining tonic force in the urethra. Contraction of the EUS, coaptation of the mucosa, as well as engorgement of blood vessels in the lamina propria contribute to urinary continence [2].

The lower urinary tract (LUT) is innervated by both the autonomic and somatic nervous systems. Sympathetic nervous system control of the LUT travels via the hypogastric nerve (T_{10}-L_2) (Figure 1.1, sympathetic preganglionic nucleus in thoracolumbar spinal cord), while parasympathetic control travels via the pelvic nerve (S_{2-4}) (Figure 1.1, Gert's nucleus in sacral spinal cord) [4, 5]. The somatic motor neurons control the skeletal muscle of the EUS via the pudendal nerve (S_{2-4}) [4]. Its motor neurons are found in Onuf's nucleus (Figure 1.1, sacral spinal cord). The sympathetic and somatic nervous systems promote storage, while the parasympathetic system promotes emptying.

Afferent mechanisms

The sensation of bladder fullness is carried by two types of afferent fibers via the pelvic, hypogastric, and pudendal nerves. A-delta (Aδ) fibers, which are activated at low thresholds, are myelinated large diameter nerves that conduct action potentials quickly [3]. C-fibers are high threshold, unmyelinated nerves that conduct signals more slowly, and usually transmit pain sensations. Normal bladder sensations are carried by Aδ fibers, whereas C-fibers become more important in diseased bladders [3]. In humans, C-fibers are found in the urothelial and suburothelial layers, whereas Aδ fibers are found in the smooth muscle [6]. A certain population of C-fibers is called silent afferents, because they normally respond to chemical or irritative stimuli. While these stimuli are uncommon in the bladder, chemical irritation can sensitize the bladder, to cause abnormal responses to normal stretch [3]. The transient receptor potential vanilloid type 1 (TRPV$_1$) receptor responds to pain, heat and acidity. Vanilloids, such as resiniferatoxin, desensitize C-fibers and suppress painful sensation [7]. Although initial studies suggested that resiniferatoxin may improve neurogenic DO, it is currently being studied as a treatment for cancer related pain [8], rather than as a treatment of DO.

Although we have long known that acetylcholine (muscarinic agonist) and ATP (purinergic agonist) act via the parasympathetic nervous system to cause bladder contraction, they have been shown to play a role in afferent sensation as well. Muscarinic acetylcholine receptors are found on urothelial cells, suburothelial interstitial cells of Cajal, and on afferent nerves. The urothelium releases acetylcholine and ATP in response to stretch, both of which enhance spontaneous activity in interstitial cells of Cajal, to cause bladder smooth muscle contractions.

This enhancement of spontaneous contractions may cause an increase in "afferent noise" that may be interpreted as urgency [9]. In spinalized rats, botulinum toxin lowers ATP release from the urothelium and blocks detrusor contraction [2]. Another mechanism of botulinum toxin's action is by decreasing afferent firing from the bladder [10].

Adjacent pelvic organs such as the colon and uterus can affect urinary continence [2]. This may be due to a common afferent system via the hypogastric nerve, or intermediary neurons allowing for cross talk between pelvic organs [3]. Distension of the colon from constipation is a well-recognized cause of urinary incontinence in children. This is likely due to changes in bladder afferent signaling arising from a chronically distended colon, which prevents the child from recognizing a full bladder [11].

Spinal cord and brainstem

During bladder storage, afferent signals from the hypogastric nerve and pelvic nerve travel to the thoracolumbar and sacral spinal cord, respectively (Figure 1.1). The hypogastric nerve sends signals via the sympathetic nervous system to block bladder contraction and contact the internal urethral sphincter. Onuf's nucleus maintains contraction of the EUS, which is coordinated with bladder storage by the pontine micturition center (PMC) in the medial pons (Figure 1.1, L-region).

Once the bladder pressure threshold is exceeded, afferent signals travel via the pelvic nerve to synapse on interneurons in Gert's nucleus in the S_{1-2} spinal cord [4] (Figure 1.2). These interneurons send projections up to the periaqueductal gray (PAG) in the midbrain to initiate voiding, which occurs if the cerebral cortex determines that it is appropriate to void. The PAG sends caudal projections to the PMC, which is the final efferent center of the LUT. The PMC sends projections caudally to the sacral parasympathetic nucleus, activating the neurons, which cause bladder contraction and EUS relaxation [4] (Figure 1.2).

Although the mechanism of sacral or pudendal neuromodulation remains unclear, the two likely locations would be the peripheral nervous system (including the autonomic nervous system efferents) or the brainstem (PAG and PMC) and cortex [12, 13]. Positron emission tomography imaging shows that sacral neuromodulation restores normal afferent midbrain activity in women with Fowler's syndrome, which is characterized by EUS overactivity. Prior to neuromodulation, they exhibit continuous EUS activity and lack of bladder afferent activity reaching the PAG or PMC. After neuromodulation and reestablishment of normal bladder afferent activity, they regain control of EUS activity [14]. Functional MRI evaluation confirms that neuromodulation reduced deactivation in the PAG, suggesting that exaggerated EUS

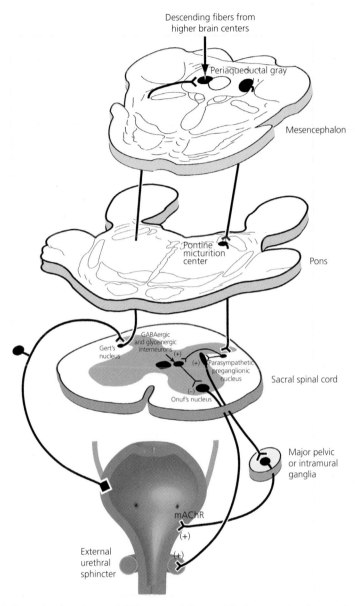

Descending fibers from
higher brain centers

Periaqueductal gray

Mesencephalon

Pontine
micturition
center

Pons

GABAergic
and glycinergic
interneurons

Gert's
nucleus

(+)

(+)

Parasympathetic
preganglionic
nucleus

Sacral spinal cord

(-)

Onuf's nucleus

Major pelvic
or intramural
ganglia

mAChR

(+)

External
urethral
sphincter

(+)

Figure 1.2 Emptying function. mAChR, muscarinic acetylcholine receptor. Source: Beckel and Holstege [4]. Reproduced with permission from Springer.

afferent activity is capable of blocking normal bladder afferent sensation from reaching the cortex [15]. Inhibition of DO is also believed to result from inhibition of abnormal afferent activity. Pudendal nerve neuromodulation represents a more peripheral means to stimulate S_{2-4} and inhibit the voiding reflex, decreasing uninhibited detrusor contractions and increasing bladder capacity [12].

Cortex

The role of the cerebral cortex in controlling voiding function has recently been described using PET scanning and functional MRI, to reveal differences in patients with normal LUT function, and those with DO. The PAG gathers information from the median prefrontal cortex, anterior cingulate gyrus, and insula. It is unclear whether these connections function as a looped relay system to the PAG or if they individually connect to the PAG. The median prefrontal cortex is a decision-making area, taking into account emotions and social context. The anterior cingulate gyrus generates autonomic response to stress and conflict, and the insula processes visceral sensations. Patients with DO show decreased MRI response at small bladder volumes, but have exaggerated responses in the anterior cingulate gyrus at large bladder volumes. When leakage occurs, deactivation of the anterior cingulate gyrus occurs. One hypothesis states that this is a learned response to imminent urinary leakage, which requires increased monitoring by the anterior cingulate gyrus in order to maintain continence [16–18].

Efferent mechanisms, peripheral

The hypogastric nerve causes detrusor relaxation via β-adrenergic receptors and internal urethral sphincter contraction via α-adrenergic receptors [4] (Figure 1.1). Both of these effects enhance storage function. α_1 Antagonists are used off-label to treat children with obstructive voiding patterns. β_3 Adrenergic agonists increase bladder capacity without increasing voiding pressure or post void residual volume [19]. They are approved for treatment of DO in adults, but are not yet approved for children. In male rats, hypogastric nerve stimulation releases norepinephrine and raises urethral pressure, while in female rats the release of nitric oxide predominates over norepinephrine, resulting in a decrease in urethral pressure [20]. If this sex difference is present in humans, this would suggest that electrical stimulation of the hypogastric nerve to enhance internal urethral sphincter contraction would be more effective in males.

The axons of the pelvic nerve travel to two groups of postganglionic neurons in the detrusor and pelvic plexus [2]. The first group causes detrusor contraction by releasing acetylcholine and ATP, while the second group causes internal urethral sphincter relaxation by releasing nitric oxide [2, 4, 7] (Figure 1.2).

Muscarinic antagonists such as oxybutynin block muscarinic receptors. As previously discussed under afferent mechanisms, it is believed that muscarinic antagonists are effective at treating urgency during the storage phase by blocking the enhancement of afferent noise, which may be responsible for spontaneous contractions. M_3 receptors cause detrusor contraction, while M_2 receptors enhance M_3 activity. Despite the relative abundance of $M_2:M_3$ receptors in the bladder (3:1), M_2 receptors play a secondary role in modulating M_3 receptor response. Although there is always a concern with causing urinary retention in patients when using muscarinic antagonists, there is a therapeutic window in which afferent signals can be blocked without affecting bladder contractility [7, 9]. There is one clinical scenario in which completely blocking bladder contractility is useful: neurogenic bladder patients who are already using clean intermittent catheterization to drain their bladders. In these cases, high doses of muscarinic antagonists or botulinum toxin can prevent bladder contractility. Botulinum toxin increases bladder capacity and decreases maximal detrusor pressure by preventing acetylcholine release [21].

ATP stimulates atropine-resistant, noncholinergic, nonadrenergic detrusor contraction, modulates urothelial signaling, and regulates afferent nerve activity. Despite these multiple mechanisms, which would predict that purinergic (P2 × 3) antagonists would be effective in the treatment of DO, they are currently being developed as treatments for pain. The main obstacle for developing a safe and tolerable purinergic antagonist is the fact that ATP is an important molecule in every organ system in the body, so developing a bladder-specific molecule has been difficult. It is proposed that purinergic signaling becomes more important in obstructed bladders [7, 22].

Prostaglandins facilitate voiding by altering neurotransmitter release or by inhibiting the breakdown of acetylcholine [2]. While there are multiple prostaglandins, it is believed that prostaglandin E2 (PGE2) interacts with EP1 receptors to drive DO [23]. Urinary levels of PGE2 were found to be elevated in both men and women with OAB compared to controls [24, 25]. Nonsteroidal anti-inflammatory drugs, which block prostaglandins, are commonly used after surgery to decrease bladder spasms in children.

Efferent mechanisms, central

The pudendal nerve has small neurons with both somatic and autonomic components. The skeletal muscle component of the EUS is regulated by GABA, the major inhibitory neurotransmitter in the spinal cord [7]. Baclofen (GABA agonist) can be used to treat detrusor sphincter dyssynergia, although it is more often used to treat limb spasticity via an intrathecal route [7, 26]. Injection of botulinum toxin into the EUS decreases its contractility, and is another means to temporarily block EUS contractility.

Imipramine, a tricyclic antidepressant drug, has been used for refractory nocturnal enuresis [27]. However, its mechanism of action in treatment of DO remains unclear. It may enhance serotonin and norepinephrine (NE) reuptake inhibition, directly relax smooth muscle, or increase urethral resistance [5, 28].

Serotonin (5-HT) modulates the afferent system and may affect the bladder and EUS by supraspinal enhancement of bladder storage as well as EUS tonic activity at Onuf's nucleus (Figure 1.3a) [2, 30, 31]. Glutamate is the major spinal

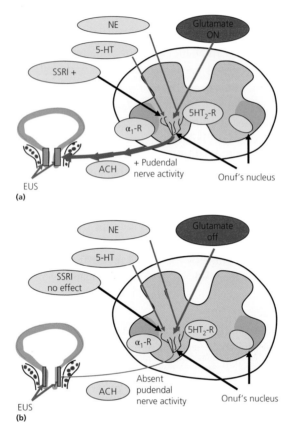

Figure 1.3 (a) Serotonin and storage function. **(b)** Serotonin and emptying function. 5-HT, serotonin; 5HT$_2$-R, serotonin type 2 receptor; Ach, acetylcholine; NE, norepinephrine; SSRI, selective serotonin reuptake inhibitor; α_1-R, alpha 1 adrenergic receptor. Source: Adapted from Franco [29]. © Elsevier.

cord regulator of the EUS [32] (Figure 1.3a). In the presence of glutamate, both 5-HT and NE can enhance its contraction of the EUS. However, if glutamate is absent, neither 5-HT nor NE can independently cause the EUS to relax (Figure 1.3b). Glutamate can be considered the on/off switch, while 5-HT and NE adjust the gain in the system [31]. The major problem with developing glutamate agonists to enhance continence by increasing EUS activity is that they do not penetrate the blood–brain barrier; therefore, glutamate agonists require intrathecal administration [33]. Duloxetine (a combined serotonin and norepinephrine reuptake inhibitor) decreases voiding frequency and incontinent episodes. Duloxetine reduced the motor threshold for EUS contraction and increased urethral phasic contractions in healthy women without affecting urethral resting pressure, suggesting that it both enhanced the afferent urethral response and increased signaling from the cortex to the EUS [34]. It is approved for stress incontinence in Europe, but not the United States.

Development of urinary continence

The human neonate initially voids hourly [35], developing an increased bladder capacity in two phases: at birth and then at 3 years of age [36]. Since neonates do not have voluntary control of urination, it was believed that a local sacral reflex was responsible for emptying the bladder without involving the brain. However, electroencephalography suggests that most neonates experience cortical arousal and awaken before voiding, so the brain is always involved with voiding [37]. The interrupted infant voiding pattern results from a lack of coordination between the bladder and the external sphincter, which causes elevated voiding pressures until the child reaches the age of 18 months. One-week-old boys void with detrusor pressures of 117 cm H_2O, and girls with pressures of 75 cm H_2O [36, 38]. Overactive contractions are rarely seen during urodynamic studies carried out in asymptomatic infant [38, 39], indicating that the urinary frequency is due to a small bladder capacity rather than OAB.

Our understanding of neural control and smooth muscle function of the neonatal bladder is derived from animal models. Neonatal rats are unable to void spontaneously [40] and are dependent on their mother to lick the perigenital area to cause bladder emptying. By 3 weeks of age (the age of weaning), neonatal rats are able to void spontaneously in response to bladder filling [41]. At first glance, this might suggest that the neonatal nervous system is not mature, and additional maturation of the hypogastric, pelvic, or pudendal nerves needs to occur. However, this is not consistent with the fact that human and rat fetuses start to urinate by the second trimester, so the voiding reflex needs to be functional during prenatal life. What actually happens in rats is that the perigenital reflex inhibits the mature bladder emptying reflex at the sacral level, and this inhibition is removed at weaning [42, 43]. Experimental bladder distension does not change the onset of spontaneous voiding at 3 weeks, but prolongs the perigenital reflex for another 2 weeks [44]. Surgical reduction of bladder volume causes the immediate onset of spontaneous voiding in neonatal rats [45]. These findings suggest that maturation from immature and mature voiding reflexes requires central neural control, despite having afferent and efferent connections, which are ready for use at birth.

Animal studies show that the neonatal bladder smooth muscle produces more pressure per gram of tissue and is more dependent on local calcium levels than adult bladder smooth muscle [46–49]. Neonatal bladders also have large-amplitude spontaneous contractions, which are downregulated with maturation [50, 51]. The elevated voiding pressures seen in infants may represent immature smooth muscle function. Once the detrusor becomes more mature and less overactive, it becomes easier for the brain to control. Since the brain makes the decision to void by integrating emotions, social context, stress, and visceral sensation, toilet training can be derailed by multiple factors, resulting in persistent urinary incontinence.

Conclusion

While the neurophysiology of voiding is based on a relatively simple circuit, our ability to improve the treatment of pediatric urinary incontinence will depend on finding more focused methods of regulating bladder sensation and coordinating bladder and EUS function. While there are many possible targets, most of our current therapies are aimed at peripheral efferent systems, and we are only beginning to understand and develop treatments aimed at the afferent system, such as neuromodulation. The challenges of developing treatments aimed at the cerebral cortex and central efferent systems are the next frontier for physicians and researchers treating pediatric urinary incontinence.

References

1 Chung B, Sommer G, Brooks JD. Anatomy of the lower urinary tract and male genitalia. In: Wein A, Kavoussi L, Novick A, Partin A, Peters C, editors. *Campbell-Walsh Urology*. 10th ed. Philadelphia: Elsevier Saunders; 2011. p. 33–70.

2 Yoshimura N, Chancellor M. Physiology and pharmacology of the bladder and urethra. In: Wein A, Kavoussi L, Novick A, Partin A, Peters C, editors. *Campbell-Walsh Urology*. 10th ed. Philadelphia: Elsevier Saunders; 2011. p. 1786–833.

3 Birder L, de Groat W, Mills I, Morrison J, Thor K, Drake M. Neural control of the lower urinary tract: Peripheral and spinal mechanisms. *Neurourol Urodyn*. 2010;**29**:128–39.

4 Beckel J, Holstege G. Neurophysiology of the lower urinary tract. In: Andersson K, Michel M, editors. *Urinary Tract* (Handbook of Experimental Pharmacology). Vol. **202**. Berlin: Springer; 2011.

5 Yeung CK, Sihoe JD. Non-neuropathic dysfunction of the lower urinary tract in children. In: Wein A, Kavoussi L, Novick A, Partin A, Peters C, editors. *Campbell-Walsh Urology*. 10th ed. Philadelphia: Elsevier Saunders; 2011. p. 3411–30.

6 Wiseman OJ, Brady CM, Hussain IF, Dasgupta P, Watt H, Fowler CJ, et al. The ultrastructure of bladder lamina propria nerves in healthy subjects and patients with detrusor hyperreflexia. *J Urol*. 2002;**168**:2040–5.

7 de Groat WC, Yoshimura N. Pharmacology of the lower urinary tract. *Annu Rev Pharmacol Toxicol*. 2001;**41**:691–721.

8 http://clinicaltrials.gov/ct2/show/NCT00804154 (accessed February 12, 2015).

9 Andersson KE. Antimuscarinic mechanisms and the overactive detrusor: An update. *Eur Urol*. 2011;**59**:377–86.

10 Ikeda Y, Zabbarova IV, Birder LA, de Groat WC, McCarthy CJ, Hanna-Mitchell AT, et al. Botulinum neurotoxin serotype A suppresses neurotransmitter release from afferent as well as efferent nerves in the urinary bladder. *Eur Urol*. 2012;**62**:1157–64.

11 Wyndaele M, De Wachter S, De Man J, Minagawa T, Wyndaele JJ, Pelckmans PA, et al. Mechanisms of pelvic organ crosstalk: 1. Peripheral modulation of bladder inhibition by colorectal distention in rats. *J Urol*. 2013;**190**:765–71.

12 Vasavada S, Rackley R. Electrical simulation and neuromodulation in storage and emptying failure. In: Wein A, Kavoussi L, Novick A, Partin A, Peters C, editors. *Campbell-Walsh Urology*. 10th ed. Philadelphia: Elsevier Saunders; 2011. p. 2026–46.

13 Amend B, Matzel KE, Abrams P, de Groat WC, Sievert KD. How does neuromodulation work. *Neurourol Urodyn*. 2011;**30**:762–5.

14 Dasgupta R, Critchley HD, Dolan RJ, Fowler CJ. Changes in brain activity following sacral neuromodulation for urinary retention. *J Urol.* 2005;**174**(6):2268–72.

15 Kavia R, DasGupta R, Critchley H, Fowler C, Griffiths D. A functional magnetic resonance imaging study of the effect of sacral neuromodulation on brain responses in women with Fowler's syndrome. *BJU Int.* 2010;**105**:366–72.

16 Griffiths D, Derbyshire S, Stenger A, Resnick N. Brain control of normal and overactive bladder. *J Urol.* 2005;**174**:1862–7.

17 Griffiths D, Tadic SD. Bladder control, urgency, and urge incontinence: Evidence from functional brain imaging. *Neurourol Urodynam.* 2008;**27**:446–74.

18 Drake MJ, Fowler CJ, Griffiths D, Mayer E, Paton JFR, Birder L. Neural control of the lower urinary and gastrointestinal tracts: Supraspinal CNS mechanisms. *Neurourol Urodyn.* 2010; **29**:119–27.

19 Andersson K, Chapple C, Cardozo L, Cruz F, Hashim H, Michel M, et al. Pharmacological treatment of urinary incontinence. In: Abrams P, Cardozo L, Khoury S, Wein A, editors. *Incontinence.* 4th ed. Paris: Health Publications Ltd; 2009. p. 631–700.

20 Kontani H, Shiraoya C. Sex differences in urethral pressure response to electrical stimulation of the hypogastric nerves in rats. *J Urol.* 2000;**163**:1364–8.

21 Schulte-Baukloh H, Priefert J, Knispel HH, Lawrence GW, Miller K, Neuhaus J. Botulinum toxin A detrusor injections reduce postsynaptic muscular M2, M3, P2X2, and P2X3 receptors in children and adolescents who have neurogenic detrusor overactivity: A single-blind study. *Urology.* 2013;**81**(5):1052–7.

22 Ford APDW, Cockayne DA. ATP and P2x purinoreceptors in urinary tract disorders. In: Andersson K, Michel M, editors. *Urinary Tract* (Handbook of Experimental Pharmacology). Vol. **202**. Berlin: Springer; 2011.

23 Andersson KE. Prostanoid receptor subtypes: New targets for OAB drugs? *J Urol.* 2009; **182**:2099–100.

24 Kim JC, Park EY, Hong SH, Seo SI, Park YH, Hwang TK. Changes in urinary nerve growth factor and prostaglandins in male patients with overactive bladder symptom. *Int J Urol.* 2005;**12**:875–80.

25 Kim JC, Park EY, Seo SI, Park YH, Hwang TK. Nerve growth factor and prostaglandins in the urine of female patients with overactive bladder. *J Urol.* 2006;**175**:1773–6.

26 Steers WD, Meythaler JM, Haworth C, Herrell D, Park TS. Effects of acute bolus and chronic intrathecal baclofen on genitourinary dysfunction due to spinal cord pathology. *J Urol.* 1992;**148**(6):1849–55.

27 Neveus T, Tullus K. Tolterodine and imipramine in refractory enuresis; a placebo-controlled crossover study. *Pediatr Nephrol.* 2008;**23**:263–7.

28 Hunsballe JM, Djurhuus JC. Clinical options for imipramine in the management of urinary incontinence. *Urol Res.* 2001;**29**:118–25.

29 Franco I. Overactive bladder in children: Part 1. Pathophysiology. *J Urol.* 2007;**178**:761–8.

30 Cheng CL, de Groat WC. Role of 5-HT1A receptors in control of lower urinary function in anesthetized rats. *Am J Physiol Renal Physiol.* 2010;**298**:F771–8.

31 Thor KB. Serotonin and norepinephrine involvement in efferent pathways to the urethral rhabdosphincter: Implications for treating stress urinary incontinence. *Urology.* 2003;**62** (S4A):3–9.

32 Furuta A, Asano K, Egawa S, de Groat WC, Chancellor MB, Yoshimura N. Role of α2-adrenoceptors and glutamate mechanisms in the external urethral sphincter continence reflex in rats. *J Urol.* 2009;**181**:1467–73.

33 Hawkins RA. The blood-brain barrier and glutamate. *Am J Clin Nutr.* 2009;**90**:867S–74.

34 Boy S, Reitz A, Wirth B, Knapp PA, Braun PM, Haferkamp A, et al. Facilitatory neuromodulative effect of duloxetine on pudendal motor neurons controlling the urethral pressure: A functional urodynamic study in healthy women. *Eur Urol.* 2006;**50**:119–25.

35 Gladh G, Persson D, Mattson S, Lindstrom S. Voiding patterns in healthy newborns. *Neurourol Urodyn.* 2000;**19**:177–84.

36 Sillen U. Bladder function in healthy neonates and its development during infancy. *J Urol.* 2001;**166**:2376–81.

37 Yeung CK, Godley ML, Ho CK, Ransley PG, Duffy PG, Chen CN, et al. Some new insights into bladder function in infancy. *Br J Urol.* 1995;**76**:235–40.

38 Yeung CK, Godley ML, Dhillon HK, Duffy PG, Ransley PG. Urodynamic patterns in infants with normal lower urinary tracts of primary vesico-ureteric reflux. *Br J Urol.* 1998;**81**:461–7.

39 Bachelard M, Sillen U, Hansson S, Hermansson G, Jodal U, Jacobsson B. Urodynamic pattern in asymptomatic infants: Siblings of children with vesicoureteral reflux. *J Urol.* 1999;**162**:1733–8.

40 Capek K, Jelinek J. The development of the control of water metabolism: I. The excretion of urine in young rats. *Physiol Bohemoslov.* 1956;**5**:91–6.

41 Maggi CA, Santicioli P, Meli A. Postnatal development of micturition reflux in rats. *Am J Physiol.* 1986;**250**:R926–31.

42 Araki I, de Groat WC. Developmental synaptic depression underlying reorganization of visceral reflex pathways in the spinal cord. *J Neurosci.* 1997;**17**:8402–7.

43 de Groat WC. Plasticity of bladder reflex pathways during postnatal development. *Physiol Behav.* 2002;**77**:689–92.

44 Wu HY, de Groat WC. Maternal separation uncouples reflex from spontaneous voiding in rat pups. *J Urol.* 2006;**175**:1148–51.

45 Ng YK, Wu HY, Lee KH, Yeung CK. Bladder reduction surgery accelerates the appearance of spontaneous voiding in neonatal rats. *J Urol.* 2010;**183**:370–7.

46 Zderic SA, Hypolite J, Duckett JW, Snyder HM 3rd, Wein AJ, Levin RM. Developmental aspects of bladder contractile function: Sensitivity to extracellular calcium. *Pharmacology.* 1991;**43**:61–8.

47 Zderic SA, Sillen U, Liu GH, Snyder H 3rd, Duckett JW, Wein AJ, et al. Developmental aspects of bladder contractile function: Evidence for an intracellular calcium pool. *J Urol.* 1993;**150**:623–5.

48 Zderic SA, Sillen U, Liu GH, Snyder HM 3rd, Duckett JW, Gong C, et al. Developmental aspects of excitation contraction coupling of rabbit bladder smooth muscle. *J Urol.* 1994;**152**:679–81.

49 Wu HY, Zderic SA, Wein AJ, Chacko S. Decrease in maximal force generation in the neonatal mouse bladder corresponds to shift in myosin heavy chain isoform composition. *J Urol.* 2004;**171**:841–4.

50 Szell EA, Somogyi GT, de Groat WC, Szigeti GP. Developmental changes in spontaneous smooth muscle activity in the neonatal rat urinary bladder. *Am J Physiol Regul Integr Comp Physiol.* 2003;**285**:R809–16.

51 Ng YK, de Groat WC, Wu HY. Smooth muscle and neural mechanisms contributing to the down-regulation of neonatal rat spontaneous bladder contractions during postnatal development. *Am J Physiol Regul Integr Comp Physiol.* 2007;**292**:R2100–12.

CHAPTER 2

Neurophysiology of defecation

Cecilie Ejerskov and Charlotte Siggaard Rittig

Gastroenterology Unit, Department of Pediatrics Aarhus University Hospital, Aarhus, Denmark

Normal defecation patterns

Defecation pattern in childhood differs with age and is determined by the change from breastfeeding to solid foods. At infancy when breast fed, defecation occurs from six to seven times a day to once every seventh day, which is considered the norm, in average three times daily. At 6–12 months, the average defecation rate is just below two times per day, and at 1–3 years, the average defecation rate is one and a half times per day. At 3–12 years, the defecation rate settles at once daily. There is no difference in gender until puberty. During puberty and adulthood, the defecation rate among females is less than among males.

To appreciate colorectal motility of defecation, neurophysiology, and the various pathological changes related hereto, it is important to understand the functional anatomy and neurophysiology of colon, rectum, and anus [1–3].

Functional anatomy of colon, rectum, and anus

The main functions of **the large intestine** are intraluminal bacterial fermentation of nutrients resistant to digestive enzymes (e.g., short-chain fatty acids), to reabsorb water and electrolytes, and to transport and store feces until it can be discharged from the body. The large intestine is composed of the cecum; the ascending, the transverse, the descending, and the sigmoid segments of the colon; the rectum; and the anus. Main function of the right side of the colon is absorption of water and electrolytes, whereas the main function of the left side of the colon is storage and evacuation of feces.

Pediatric Incontinence: Evaluation and Clinical Management, First Edition. Edited by Israel Franco, Paul F. Austin, Stuart B. Bauer, Alexander von Gontard and Yves Homsy.
© 2015 John Wiley & Sons, Ltd. Published 2015 by John Wiley & Sons, Ltd.

Histologically, the wall of the large intestine is made up of mucosa, submucosa, tunica muscularis, and serosa. The **mucosa** consists of an inner layer epithelium, underlying lamina propria, and muscularis mucosae. Distributed within the columnar epithelium are absorptive cells, goblet cells, and enteroendocrine cells. The lamina propria is a connective tissue rich in cells. It includes immunocompetent cells, nerve fibers, fibroblasts, lymphatic vessels, and capillaries. The muscularis mucosae is a thin layer of intestinal smooth muscle. The **submucosa** consists of loose connective tissue and substantial fatty tissue and here lies the **submucosal plexus (Meissner's plexus)**, one of the plexuses of the enteric nerve system (ENS), together with larger nerves, blood and lymph vessels. The **tunica muscularis** consists of the inner complete circular layer, which during contraction divides the colon into segments, the characteristic haustra, and an outer incomplete longitudinal layer, which is made up by three flat longitudinal bands, teniae coli. In the rectum, the teniae disappear and the longitudinal muscle layer becomes complete. Feces is transported as a result of contractions in the muscle layer containing the **myenteric plexus (Auerbach's plexus)**, the other plexus of the ENS located between the circular and the longitudinal layers. The **serosa** consists of a mesothelial lining resembling the visceral peritoneal

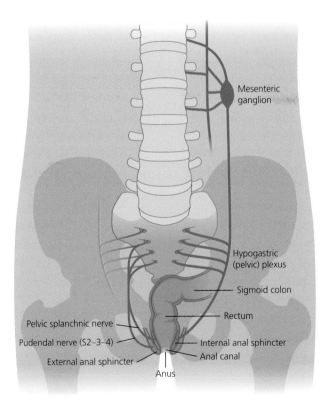

Figure 2.1 Anatomy of the rectum and nerves.

surface. Some parts of colon and rectum and the distal one-third part of rectum are located outside the peritoneum, and those parts are adherent to their surroundings by the **tunica adventitia**. The **rectum** initially runs distally and posteriorly, then directly downward, and finally anteriorly and ends as the anus in the perineum. The rectum is closely related to the bladder. The rectum is divided into two segments: the rectal ampulla and the anal canal. As a reservoir for storage of feces, the function of the rectum is to maintain fecal continence and allow defecation at an appropriate time and place. The upper and the lower parts of the anal canal are separated by a mucocutaneous zone. The lower squamous epithelium is rich in somatosensory fibers and highly sensitive to temperature, touch, movement, and pain. The **anal canal** in children is estimated to be between 2.5 and 3 cm long. At the anorectal junction, the puborectalis muscle creates an angle of approximately 80°, which is considered to contribute to anal continence. The continuation of the circular smooth muscle layer constitutes the internal anal sphincter (IAS), whereas the external anal sphincter (EAS) consists of striated muscle and hence partly under voluntary control. With the support from the pelvic floor, the levator ani muscle, the IAS and EAS maintain a higher pressure in the anal canal than in the rectal ampulla (Figure 2.1) [4, 5].

Colorectal motility and defecation

There are at least three regulatory mechanisms in the gastrointestinal tract: endocrine, paracrine, and the enteric nervous system (ENS). The scope of this paragraph is the ENS, its modulators and colorectal motility.

Overall, neural control of colorectal motility is provided by the **ENS, the intrinsic nervous system**, modulated through the **extrinsic nervous system; the lumbar sympathetic nerves; sacral parasympathetic nerves; and extrinsic sensory innervations.**

The intrinsic nervous system

The majority of the neural control of colorectal motility is meditated by the ENS. Auerbach's plexus mainly controls the motility and Meissner's plexus mainly controls the secretion and blood flow. Generally, the ENS consists of sensory neurons, interneurons, and both excitatory and inhibitory motor neurons. Different neurotransmitters, neuropeptides, and other molecules either inhibit (e.g., noradrenalin, dopamine, somatostatin) or increase (e.g., acetylcholine, serotonin, histamine) motility.

The extrinsic nervous system

Indirectly, by modulating the ENS via the interneurons, the sacral parasympathetic nerves increase digestion and motility while the lumbar sympathetic nerves decrease digestion and motility. This is caused by, respectively, an increase/decrease of vasodilation, secretion, and peristaltic activity and relaxation/constriction of the sphincters. The colorectal extrinsic sensory innervation is provided by spinal afferent neurons, and a subpopulation of these, mechanosensitive afferents, which are highly sensitive to intestinal distension by feces, can consequently be an important factor of conscious awareness of rectal filling, continence, and in initiating defecation. The somatic innervation of the extrinsic anal sphincter is via a perineal branch of the S4 nerve and the pudendal nerve.

Muscle contractions and colorectal motility

The contraction of the smooth muscle cells is initiated by slow waves generated by the intestinal cells of Cajal, pacemaker cells. Not all slow waves cause contraction but are influenced by the stretch of the muscle cells and the ENS. The categorization of contractions is phasic or tonic. **Phasic contractions** are short lasting (seconds) and cause elevated intraluminal pressure. **Tonic contractions** are less well defined and last longer and may not necessarily cause an increase in intraluminal pressure. **Phasic colonic high-amplitude propagating contractions** are responsible for propulsion of feces and often occur after awakening and after a meal. These contractions may continue as colonic mass movements into the rectum and cause defecation. Rectal motor complexes (RMC) are bursts of strong phasic contractions lasting minutes and with contraction frequencies of 3–10/min. Since RMC activity is more prominent during sleep/in the night, the function of RMC is speculated to have a role in the maintenance of continence. Current promising pediatric anorectal investigations are manometry, measuring contractility in the anus and rectum and impedance planimetry, studies of rectal compliance.

Defecation, to void feces from the distal colon and rectum, is a complex process involving the previously described ENS, autonomic nervous system, and smooth and striated muscles. It is initiated when a colonic mass movement continues to rectum generating a slow distension of the rectal wall. As the distension proceeds, the filling of rectum stimulates the rectoanal inhibitory reflex (RAIR), mediated by ENS, and causes relaxation of the IAS. Additionally, the rectum now serves as a conduit and the RAIR stimulates the filling of the upper anal canal. The upper anal canal's sensory innervations make it possible to detect consistency and thereby distinguish between air, solid, and liquid. The filling creates the urge to defecate. Defecation will proceed with the voluntary relaxation of the puborectal muscle, straightening of the anorectal angle, and relaxation of the EAS. Defecation is normally improved by the Valsalva maneuver. As wall tension relaxes, the defecation reflex subsides and rectal compliance increases, which leads to a resting pressure of the anal canal higher than in rectum, thereby reaching continence (Figure 2.2).

In the research of the neurotransmitter serotonin (5-HT)'s influence on the gastrointestinal canal, the most consistent findings are that more than 90% of the body's 5-HT is found in the enterochromaffin cells in the gastrointestinal

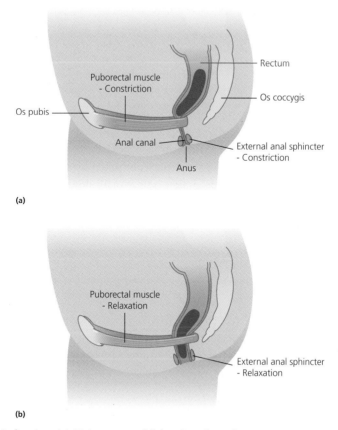

Figure 2.2 Defecation. **(a)** Maintenance of defecation. **(b)** Defecation.

canal and that plasma 5-HT has been found increased in diarrheal diseases and decreased in constipation. Overall, the 5-HT$_4$ agonist prucalopride in the treatment of chronic constipation among adults if laxatives prove insufficient has showed promising results but still research among children is lacking.

Clinical trial research in the treatment of functional gastrointestinal disorders and irritable bowel syndrome (IBS) with 5-HT is still small, mostly in adults but ongoing and has generally shown that it is effective. Higher brain centers that influence and control defecation are the frontal cortex and the emotional motor system, the amygdala, the stria terminalis, and the hypothalamus. In humans, response to external stressors is mediated through the coordinated action of the hypothalamic–pituitary–adrenal (HPA) axis and the sympathetic branch of the autonomic nervous system. With this in mind, a novel etiopathological model for IBS proposing altered central stress circuits has been introduced. It is hypothesized that triggering of these circuits by external stressors results in the development of gut and extraintestinal symptoms in predisposed individuals. Research in treatment with 5-HT$_3$-antagonist in IBS among adults found decrease in brain activity in the emotional motor systems with correlates to a decrease in gastrointestinal symptoms [4–12].

References

1 Bekkali N, Moesker FM, Van Toledo L, et al. Bowel habits in the first 24 months of life: preterm-versus term-born infants. *J Pediatr Gastroenterol Nutr* 2010;**51**(6):753–758.

2 Corazziari E, Staiano A, Miele E, et al. Italian Society of Pediatric Gastroenterology, Hepatology, and Nutrition. Bowel frequency and defecatory patterns in children: a prospective nationwide survey. *Clin Gastroenterol Hepatol* 2005;**3**(11):1101–1106.

3 Steer CD, Emond AM, Golding J, et al. The variation in stool patterns from 1 to 42 months: a population-based observational study. *Arch Dis Child* 2009;**94**(3):231–233.

4 Herold A, Lehur P-A, Matzel KE, O'Connell PR, editors. *Coloproctology (European Manual of Medicine)*. Berlin/Heidelberg: Springer-Verlag/GmbH & Co.K; 2008.

5 Koeppen BM, Stanton BA. *Berne and Levy Physiology*, 6th edition. Philadelphia: Mosby Elsevier; 2008.

6 Brookes SJ, Dinning PG, Gladman MA. Neuroanatomy and physiology of colorectal function and defaecation: from basic science to human clinical studies. *Neurogastroenterol Motil* 2009;**21**(Suppl 2):9–19.

7 Joensson IM, Hagstroem S, Fynne L, et al. Rectal motility in pediatric constipation. *J Pediatr Gastroenterol Nutr* 2014;**58**(3):292–296.

8 Joensson IM. *Childhood Constipation*. Aarhus, Denmark: Aarhus University; 2011.

9 Fassov J. *Sacral Nerve Stimulation for Irritable Bowel Syndrome*. Aarhus, Denmark: Aarhus University; 2013.

10 Camilleri M. Serotonin in the gastrointestinal tract. *Curr Opin Endocrinol Diabetes Obes* 2009;**16**(1):53–59.

11 Camilleri M, Deiteren A. Prucalopride for constipation. *Expert Opin Pharmacother* 2010;**11**(3):451–461.

12 Spiller R, Aziz Q, Creed F, et al. Guidelines on the irritable bowel syndrome: mechanisms and practical management. *Gut* 2007;**56**(12):1770–1798.

CHAPTER 3

Functional brain imaging in bowel and bladder control

Israel Franco

Maria Fareri Children's Hospital, Valhalla, NY, USA

Introduction

The elucidation of the control of micturition has had a remarkable renaissance with the introduction of functional brain imaging. Its introduction in the early 1990s has added a tremendous amount of knowledge to a field that was relegated to information garnered from vertebrate animal studies and patients with specific lesions that could be studied clinically. Over the last decade, we have seen remarkable changes in the development of a model of brain activity based on numerous clinical studies in both humans and animals. Among these, a considerable number of functional brain imaging studies have been published. These functional imaging studies provide evidence that the prefrontal cortex (PFC), and other supraspinal regions (periaqueductal gray (PAG), insula, thalamus, hypothalamus, anterior cingulate cortex (ACC)) are metabolically active during bladder filling and emptying. Unfortunately, all these studies have been done in adults and we must extrapolate these findings to children. We will look to define the role of these portions of the brain during micturition in this chapter. Having this information will allow us to better understand how dysfunction in these portions of the brain may interact with other disorders that are commonly associated with dysfunction in these sites such as chronic pain syndromes, irritable bowel syndrome, and neuropsychiatric problems. Chapter 7 in his textbook will discuss neuropsychiatric disorders, and look at functional MRI data that is available from that specialty. Once these two realms are examined and compared side by side, we see that there is a remarkable overlap in the two fields.

Pediatric Incontinence: Evaluation and Clinical Management, First Edition. Edited by Israel Franco,
Paul F. Austin, Stuart B. Bauer, Alexander von Gontard and Yves Homsy.
© 2015 John Wiley & Sons, Ltd. Published 2015 by John Wiley & Sons, Ltd.

Background

Up until the early 1990s, the only way to know what was going on in the brain was through clinical evaluation of patients with neurologic exams and examining patients with specific brain lesions. It was the advent of improved scanning of whole brain images and powerful computer tomographic analysis that marshaled in the era of functional brain imaging. Functional brain imaging is the use of neuroimaging technology to evaluate brain function with the idea of trying to understand the relationship between activity in certain brain areas and specific functions. Single photon computerized tomography (SPECT), which used gamma-ray photons, and subsequently positron emission tomography (PET), which relies on the fact that a positron is emitted when isotopes decay, were used initially. The spatial resolution of PET was twice that of SPECT and furthermore its temporal resolution was superior, so that this method proved very valuable and it was with PET that much of the early functional brain imaging discoveries were made. Both of these techniques rely on injection of a radioactive substance, which can be concentrated in a metabolically active brain region and subsequently picked up by the scanner. A means of obtaining information without radiation was devised with the advent of functional MR. The signal-to-noise ratio (SN) is low; therefore, subjects undergoing fMRI need to do repeated contractions of the pelvic floor or multiple fill–empty cycles of the bladder to capture the data that are needed.

The science of functional brain imaging has grown explosively in the last decade but the complete literature on the topic of brain control of bladder function is limited to about 50 articles, exclusive of reviews. This small number of articles has begun to shape and alter dramatically our view of bladder control.

The first attempt to use functional brain imaging to examine neurologic control of the bladder was by Fukuyama et al. [1] in 1996. They performed SPECT imaging and showed areas of brain activation during micturition in healthy normal volunteers. Despite poor spatial resolution, activity was seen in the pons, the left sensorimotor cortex, the right frontal cortex, and bilateral supplementary motor areas. In the same year, Holstege's published their first micturition-related study, looking at PET in 17 male subjects [2]. This study was remarkable in that there was sufficient spatial resolution to show that the pontine micturition center (PMC) or Barrington's nucleus was activated in the subjects who were able to void in the scanner while those who were unable to void showed more lateral activation in a region that was thought to be important in storage [3]. Subsequent human imaging studies have not visualized this lateral region when it might have been expected to be activated. The current thinking is that the PMC is active in both storage and voiding, being actively inhibited during storage and activated by input from the PAG area. (It is important to note that functional imaging may not be able to distinguish between activation and inhibition (Figure 3.1).

Before the introduction of functional neuroimaging, work by Holstege in the cat had identified that the major destination of bladder-related afferents from

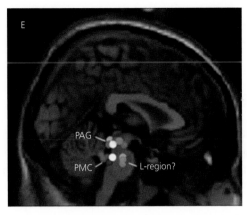

Figure 3.1 Reported locations of peak activation and (deactivation in a few cases) of brainstem areas activated during withholding of urine or full bladder or during voiding, projected on a medial section of the brain (based on PET, fMRI, and SPECT studies in healthy controls). Source: Reproduced with permission from Wiley. From Ref. [4].

the sacral region was the PAG. Holstege had termed this the "emotional motor system." He felt that this center was critical to the maintenance of homeostasis and reproductive function [5]. The demonstration of PAG activation on bladder filling and with micturition in their PET imaging experiments confirmed that group's scientific predictions and showed a similarity between the neural control of the bladder in cats and humans. Subsequent studies, which focused on brain activation and bladder filling, by both Athwal et al. [6] and Matsuura et al. [7], showed prominent activation of the PAG on bladder filling further confirming the role of the PAG in micturition control.

Functional brain imaging has contributed vastly to our understanding of the nature of human "enteroception." Enteroception can be defined as "the sense of the physiological condition of the entire body." Pain and temperature have been reassigned to enteroception so that not only visceral sensations are part of enteroception. The cardinal feature of enteroceptive system is that the afferent input is from small diameter (Aδ and C) fibers [8].

Homeostatic afferents are now regarded as the "missing" sensory limb of the efferent autonomic nervous system. These afferents project via the spinothalamic tracts to subcortical homeostatic centers including the hypothalamus and PAG. In humans, they relay in the thalamus and converge on the nondominant anterior insula. The insula, an island of cortex, lies buried deep to the lateral sulcus, which separates the temporal lobe from the frontoparietal cortices. The insula has come to be regarded as the homeostatic afferent cortex and has been shown to be activated by a range of modalities associated with visceral sensation. Insula activation was seen in PET studies by Blok et al. [2] but recently has been more extensively studied in the fMRI experiments carried out by the Pittsburgh group [4, 9, 10]. They have been able to show a correlation between the degree of bladder filling and insula activation in healthy controls, with an exaggerated increase in activation at high volumes in a group composed of almost entirely of older women with urgency (Figure 3.2).

Anterior cingulate cortex

A key feature of bodily or enteroceptive sensations is their association with an affective, motivational aspect and hence their value in homeostasis. The anterior cingulate cortex (ACC) is the cortical region associated with motivation. If the insula is regarded as the limbic sensory cortex, the ACC can be considered as the limbic motor cortex [12], the two being frequently seen to be coactivated in functional brain imaging studies [13]. A wide range of cerebral functions have been attributed to the ACC over the years as its activation is seen with many different executive tasks but the demonstration that output was correlated with sympathetic activation leads to the hypothesis that the ACC "mediates context-driven modulation of bodily arousal states" [13]. Furthermore, there is a suggestion that the location of activation in the ACC, a widely distributed area, depends on the nature of the task to be performed: stimuli with a largely emotional content activate the ventral ACC, while tasks involving cognitive processing activate a more dorsal region [14]. ACC activation has been demonstrated in all functional imaging bladder experiments.

The ACC is also the site where pain is processed [15]. The proximity of the nociceptive, motor, and attentional regions of ACC [16] suggests possible local interconnections that might allow the output of the ACC pain area to command immediate behavioral reactions. Similarly, the ACC pain area might participate in the substantial interconnections between the ACC and the "fight or flight" regions of the midbrain, the PAG matter [17]. The anatomical connections between ACC, IC (rostral insula), SI, and SII (primary and secondary somatosensory cortices) [18] suggest that these regions do not function independently in encoding different aspects of pain but are highly interactive.

Another key feature of the ACC is the role it plays in autonomic control. Critchley et al. [19] have shown through fMRI and neuropsychological and physiological observations that a direct link exists between ACC activity and modulation of cardiac function via sympathetic output. Their observations argue for control of the ACC in the production and control of behaviorally integrated patterns of autonomic activity.

The ACC also plays a major role in the field of gastroenterology. Studies have shown that the ACC is activated in its dorsal subdivision and there is decreased activation in the ventral subdivision in response to visceral stimulus. While the dorsal ACC is associated with cognitive and attentional aspects of stimulus response, the ventral components are associated with affective and autonomic responses. The finding of greater dorsal activation by visceral stimulus in IBS is consistent with

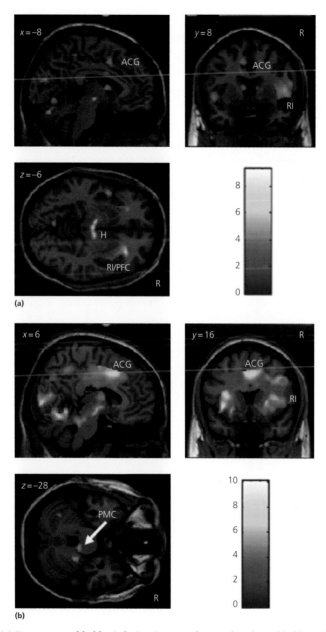

Figure 3.2 (a) Responses to bladder infusion in normal controls at large bladder volumes: Insular response is greater on the right. **(b)** Responses to bladder infusion in subjects with urge incontinence at large bladder volumes. RI, right insula; ACG, anterior cingulate gyrus (aka ACC); H, hypothalamus; RI/PFC, right anterior insula and or lateral prefrontal cortex; R, right. Color bar shows scale of student's *t* values. Source: Griffiths et al. [11]. Reproduced with permission from Elsevier.

findings on fMRI and the concept of greater attentional attribution to visceral stimulus in IBS. On the other hand, the decreased activation of the ventral ACC and medial prefrontal cortex in IBS is suggestive of possible deficiencies in the activation of the endogenous pain inhibition systems [20]. Autonomic function abnormalities have also been documented in patients with functional gastrointestinal disorders. Bharucha et al. found a frequent association of motility disorder with autonomic dysfunction in 27–29% of the patients with motility disorders [17].

Work by Millan [21] has shown that several supraspinal areas can directly and indirectly affect the nociceptive processing that occurs in the dorsal horn via descending pain modulating system. The system includes the anterior midcingulate cortex (aMCC) working together with other subcortical areas such as the hypothalamus and the PAG. When needed, this system modulates nociceptive information at the

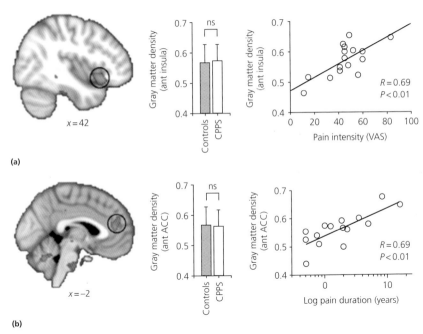

Figure 3.3 CP/CPPS brain mapping. Whole brain covariate map of voxel-wise gray matter density and pain intensity in patients with CP/CPPS shows positively correlated regions. **(a)** Right anterior insula was main region identified (ant insula, blue circle) and further analyzed (bar graph and scatterplot). Peak right anterior insula gray matter density shows no difference between patients with CP/CPPS and healthy controls (bar graph), and significant positive correlation between density and pain intensity in patients with CP/CPPS (scatterplot). VAS, visual analog scale; ns, not significant. **(b)** Whole brain covariate map of voxel-wise gray matter density and pain duration (in log units) shows regions positively correlated with pain chronicity, identifying mainly anterior cingulate cortex (blue circle). Bar graph shows no difference for peak ACC gray matter density between patients with CP/CPPS and healthy controls. Scatterplot depicts significant positive correlation between ACC density and pain chronicity in patients with CP/CPPS. Source: Farmer et al. [23]. Reproduced with permission from Elsevier.

dorsal horn and thus controls the amount of pain perceived. There is evidence of cortical thinning in the aMCC, which may account for the functional attenuation and potentially serve in any impairment in the pain inhibition that the descending modulation system and endogenous pain processes exert [22].

The ACC appears to be involved in the processes involved in CP/CPPS: recent work by Farmer et al. [23] reveals that the ACC gray matter volume is significantly correlated in a positive manner with the longer duration of pelvic pain in patients with CP/CPPS. Thus, patients with longer pain duration are likely to have increased ACC gray matter. The implications of this are yet to be sorted out (Figure 3.3).

Prefrontal cortex

The prefrontal cortex (PFC) is that part of the frontal cortex anterior to the motor strip and supplementary motor areas (Figure 3.4). It is the part of the brain that separates humans from subprimates. The ventral regions are involved in aspects of cognition and the inferior lateral parts, emotions. The orbitofrontal

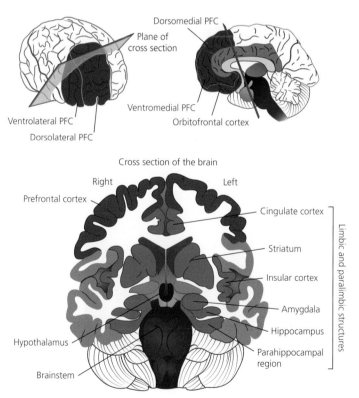

Figure 3.4 Anatomical structures involved in regulation of food intake. Adapted from Alonso-Alonso and Pascual-Leone [24].

or prefrontal lateral cortex (PFLC) has extensive interconnections with the limbic system—the hypothalamus, amygdala, insula, and ACC. Subjective evaluation of gustatory, thermal, and pain stimuli is thought to depend on sequential processing in the insula and orbitofrontal cortex, the latter providing feelings of pleasantness or unpleasantness according to the body's homeostatic needs while intensity correlates with amygdala activation [25]. The importance of the prefrontal cortex in bladder control was established from clinical studies both by Ueki [26] and subsequently by Andrew and Nathan [27]. The Andrew and Nathan paper shows that the location of lesions that were clinically demonstrated to have long-term effects on bladder function was in white matter tracts (connecting pathways consisting of myelinated axons) in the medial frontal regions (Figure 3.5). Functional imaging of brain activation echoing neuronal

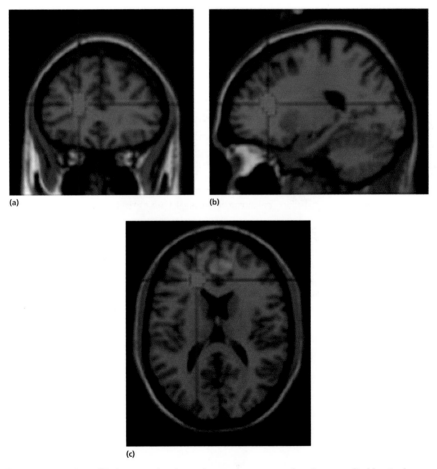

(a)   (b)

(c)

Figure 3.5 Location of lesions causing incontinence in a group of patients studied by Andrew and Nathan [27]. The red ellipse shows where white matter lesions caused lasting urinary tract dysfunction. The Cyan ellipse shows the location of gray matter lesions that caused transient dysfunction. Source: Fowler and Griffiths [25]. Reproduced with permission from Wiley.

metabolic activity inevitably detects only gray matter (containing neural cell bodies). This led to some difficulty reconciling the reported clinical and imaging data, which only recently has been clarified. In the original PET experiments by Blok et al. [2], the medial prefrontal area was seen to be activated in those who could successfully void in the scanner. It was hypothesized that this is the region that is "involved in making the decision whether or not micturition should take place." Many subsequent experiments have shown lateral prefrontal areas of activation during withholding of urine or a full bladder. It is known that reciprocal activation and deactivation of the medial and lateral PFC can be seen in certain psychiatric disorders as well as in response selection and monitoring, indicating that there is a link between these two sites.

Cortical areas such as the prefrontal cortex have the ability to inhibit limbic system activation and have been implicated in the therapeutic effects of distraction techniques, such as hypnosis therapy and the use of placebo [28].

In a work by Tadic et al. [29] in patients with white matter hyperintensities, with increasing bladder filling, as the threat of the possible incontinence increased, there was an increase in the activity of the medial/superior frontal gyrus adjacent to the dorsal ACC. Concomitantly, there was deactivation of the perigenual ACC adjacent to the ventromedial prefrontal cortex. This deactivation suggests that this is a response to threatened incontinence aimed at suppressing it. The authors also conclude that the anterior thalamic radiation (ATR) is a critical white matter pathway involved in continence. This pathway accounts for 55% of the global white matter and its anterior terminus is the medial prefrontal cortex, an area that has been identified in numerous stroke and trauma studies as critical to long-term continence. The anatomical connections of this pathway connect to several regions that are deactivated by bladder filling. Therefore, the ATR seems to carry a signal to or from all these regions that is associated with their deactivation and presumably maintains continence by inhibiting the PAG and PMC.

A common observation in children with OAB is that many can be obese [30]. A link between obesity and the PFC has been proposed by Alonso-Alonso and Pascual-Leone, both from Harvard [24]. They suggest that a reduction in activity in the PFC is associated with overeating and reduced physical activity. In the PFC, cortisol modulates dopaminergic projections with a remarkable degree of lateralization. Dopaminergic projections to the right hemisphere display an enhanced sensitivity to stressors that are perceived as severe and uncontrollable such as those that arise from social conflict [31]. Thus, chronic psychological stress can disinhibit reflexive circuits through a cortisol-induced right PFC dysfunction that is caused by a prolonged activation of the hypothalamic–pituitary–adrenal axis. This reduction in activity in the PFC can lead to the inability to inhibit the urge to urinate and in many instances leads to urge incontinence as well as fecal incontinence. It is known that there is also an increased association with fecal incontinence and obesity. This may also provide theoretical support for our ideas of stress-related OAB.

PAG and PMC

The PAG is involved in neurobiological functions that include the control and expression of pain, analgesia, fear, anxiety, vocalization, lordosis, cardiovascular function, and reproductive behavior. The lateral PAG appears to coordinate active defensive behaviors and nonopioid analgesia, and it also has a hypertensive effect. The ventrolateral PAG appears to coordinate passive defensive behaviors and opioid analgesia, and it also has a hypotensive effect. Some of these functions, for example, descending modulation of pain, have been more clearly defined by than others, but the putative functions all seem to play a role in protection of the individual by integrating afferent information from the periphery and information from higher centers. These functions may be segregated within the PAG (e.g., anxiety and pain based on current understandings of its anatomical subdivisions). Conceptually, the structure may be involved in balancing or segueing information related to survival [32].

Forebrain projections to the PAG arise mainly from the prefrontal cortex, the insular cortex, and the amygdala. Further, the PAG receives highly organized projections from the central nucleus of the amygdala and, in turn, has reciprocal connections with the central nucleus. The PAG also projects to the thalamus, hypothalamus, brainstem, and deep layers of the spinal cord with some somatotopic organization, but projections to cortical regions have not been identified [32].

The central role of the PAG is evident, as it both receives sacral afferents and transmits efferent signals (via the PMC) to the sacral spinal cord. During storage, it is chronically suppressed by a net inhibition from the many other regions shown in Figure 3.6a. These include prefrontal cortex and hypothalamus, as well as insula and anterior cingulate cortex. Inhibition of the PAG by the prefrontal cortex may be particularly [33] important, because lesions in this pathway lead to incontinence, as shown by Andrew and Nathan [27] (Figure 3.5). The PAG has multiple connections that enable it to coordinate and control all essential bodily functions, not just voiding [34] and it appears to perform much of the required signal processing. The PMC however is the ultimate arbiter of lower urinary tract function, acting as a switch between the storage and voiding phases. It is believed that, for voiding to occur, the PMC requires both an excitatory signal from the PAG and a "safe" signal from the hypothalamus as suggested by Figure 3.6b. In accordance with neuroanatomical observations in the cat, Figures 3.6a and 3.7 suggest that the PAG (rather than the PMC) receives sacral afferent input. Correspondingly, in humans, neuroimaging studies show increasing activation on bladder filling in PAG but not in PMC [6, 9, 35]. Other regions shown in Figure 3.7 include basal ganglia and cerebellum. Activation of the cerebellum and the basal ganglia (especially putamen) is often reported in imaging studies but has not been systematically studied. Transposing the data from Figure 3.7 back to a structural brain,

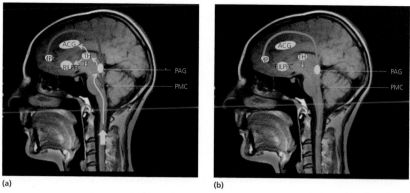

(a)   (b)

Figure 3.6 A preliminary working model of lower urinary tract control by higher brain centers. **(a)** During storage, ascending afferents (yellow) synapse on the midbrain periaqueductal gray (PAG); they are relayed via the hypothalamus (H) and thalamus (TH) to the dorsal anterior cingulate cortex (ACC) and to the right insula (RI) and to the lateral prefrontal cortex (LPFC); in the storage phase, they pass to the medial PFC (MPFC, red arrow) where the decision to void or not maybe made. In this phase, the decision is not to void, and this situation is maintained by chronic inhibition of the PAG via a long pathway (red arrows) from the MPFC; consequently, the pontine micturition center (PMC) is also suppressed, and voiding does not occur. **(b)** When the decision to void is made, the MPFC relaxes its inhibition of the PAG (green arrow) and the hypothalamus (H) also provides a "safe" signal; consequently, the PAG excites the PMC, which in turn sends descending motor output (green arrow) to the sacral spinal cord that ultimately relaxes the urethral sphincter and contracts the detrusor, so that voiding occurs. Voiding is continued to completion by continuing afferent input, probably to the PAG. Source: Fowler and Griffiths [25]. Reproduced with permission from Wiley.

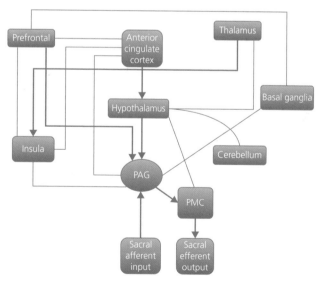

Figure 3.7 Using the PPI data from the Pittsburgh group [10], it was possible to show probable connections between forebrain and brainstem structures that are involved in the control of micturition. Arrows show probable directions of connectivity but do not preclude movement in the opposite direction. Source: Fowler and Griffiths [25]. Reproduced with permission from Wiley.

Figure 3.6a and b has been proposed as a summary illustration of current thinking about brain control of the bladder during filling and emptying, respectively.

Conclusion

Throughout this chapter, we have seen that the PFC, ACC, PAG, and PMC play critical roles in the control of micturition. Unfortunately, we have little data regarding these processes in children. We can only extrapolate from the information that is available to us that these processes are not different in children. It is possible that children with their greater ability to exhibit neuroplasticity can change more readily than adults, but this is yet to be defined. We do know that maturational changes due occur in the child and that these changes are more likely to come to bear at the PFC since it is well known that this site continues to mature till the mid-20s. Regardless of these shortcomings, the work that is now readily available is starting to point to the brain as the critical site in many of our most pernicious problems that face physicians who treat children with bowel and bladder dysfunction. A better understanding of these mechanisms will allow us to treat these issues with more refined medications and techniques than ever before.

Acknowledgments

The editors of this book sought out the two most notable authorities on this subject to write this chapter. Dr Clare Fowler was invited, but she is now retired and enjoying her gardening and gracefully declined. Dr Derek Griffiths was the other person that we designated to author this chapter but due to numerous other commitments he could not find enough time to write this chapter. He graciously agreed to review the manuscript and evaluate its factual content. He also kindly provided us with some of the images within the chapter. The work herein is based primarily on an exhaustive review that Dr Griffiths and Fowler wrote in 2010 and with new data that has been added to the literature since that publication.

References

1 Fukuyama H, Matsuzaki S, Ouchi Y, Yamauchi H, Nagahama Y, Kimura J, et al. Neural control of micturition in man examined with single photon emission computed tomography using 99mTc-HMPAO. *Neuroreport.* 1996;**7**(18):3009–12.
2 Blok BF, Willemsen AT, Holstege G. A PET study on brain control of micturition in humans. *Brain.* 1997;**120**(Pt 1):111–21.

3 Holstege G, Griffiths D, de Wall H, Dalm E. Anatomical and physiological observations on supraspinal control of bladder and urethral sphincter muscles in the cat. *J Comp Neurol.* 1986;**250**(4):449–61.

4 Griffiths D, Tadic SD. Bladder control, urgency, and urge incontinence: evidence from functional brain imaging. *Neurourol Urodyn.* 2008;**27**(6):466–74.

5 Holstege G, Bandler R, Saper CB. The emotional motor system. *Prog Brain Res.* 1996;**107**:3–6.

6 Athwal BS, Berkley KJ, Hussain I, Brennan A, Craggs M, Sakakibara R, et al. Brain responses to changes in bladder volume and urge to void in healthy men. *Brain.* 2001;**124**(Pt 2):369–77.

7 Matsuura S, Kakizaki H, Mitsui T, Shiga T, Tamaki N, Koyanagi T. Human brain region response to distention or cold stimulation of the bladder: a positron emission tomography study. *J Urol.* 2002;**168**(5):2035–9.

8 Craig AD. Interoception: the sense of the physiological condition of the body. *Curr Opin Neurobiol.* 2003;**13**(4):500–5.

9 Griffiths D, Derbyshire S, Stenger A, Resnick N. Brain control of normal and overactive bladder. *J Urol.* 2005;**174**(5):1862–7.

10 Tadic SD, Griffiths D, Schaefer W, Resnick NM. Abnormal connections in the supraspinal bladder control network in women with urge urinary incontinence. *Neuroimage.* 2008;**39**(4):1647–53.

11 Griffiths D, Tadic SD, Schaefer W, Resnick NM. Cerebral control of the bladder in normal and urge-incontinent women. *Neuroimage.* 2007;**37**(1):1–7.

12 Devinsky O, Morrell MJ, Vogt BA. Contributions of anterior cingulate cortex to behaviour. *Brain.* 1995;**118**(Pt 1):279–306.

13 Critchley HD, Wiens S, Rotshtein P, Ohman A, Dolan RJ. Neural systems supporting interoceptive awareness. *Nat Neurosci.* 2004;**7**(2):189–95.

14 Bush G, Luu P, Posner MI. Cognitive and emotional influences in anterior cingulate cortex. *Trends Cogn Sci.* 2000;**4**(6):215–22.

15 Rainville P, Duncan GH, Price DD, Carrier B, Bushnell MC. Pain affect encoded in human anterior cingulate but not somatosensory cortex. *Science.* 1997;**277**(5328):968–71.

16 Corbetta M, Miezin FM, Shulman GL, Petersen SE. Selective attention modulates extrastriate visual regions in humans during visual feature discrimination and recognition. *Ciba Found Symp.* 1991;**163**:165–75; discussion 75–80.

17 Bharucha AE, Isowa H, Hiro S, Guan Z. Differential effects of selective and non-selective muscarinic antagonists on gastrointestinal transit and bowel function in healthy women. *Neurogastroenterol Motil.* 2013;**25**(1):e35–43.

18 Friedman DP, Murray EA, O'Neill JB, Mishkin M. Cortical connections of the somatosensory fields of the lateral sulcus of macaques: evidence for a corticolimbic pathway for touch. *J Comp Neurol.* 1986;**252**(3):323–47.

19 Critchley HD, Mathias CJ, Josephs O, O'Doherty J, Zanini S, Dewar BK, et al. Human cingulate cortex and autonomic control: converging neuroimaging and clinical evidence. *Brain.* 2003;**126**(Pt 10):2139–52.

20 Tillisch K, Mayer EA. Pain perception in irritable bowel syndrome. *CNS Spectr.* 2005;**10**(11):877–82.

21 Millan MJ. Descending control of pain. *Prog Neurobiol.* 2002;**66**(6):355–474.

22 Blankstein U, Chen J, Diamant NE, Davis KD. Altered brain structure in irritable bowel syndrome: potential contributions of pre-existing and disease-driven factors. *Gastroenterology.* 2010;**138**(5):1783–9.

23 Farmer MA, Chanda ML, Parks EL, Baliki MN, Apkarian AV, Schaeffer AJ. Brain functional and anatomical changes in chronic prostatitis/chronic pelvic pain syndrome. *J Urol.* 2011;**186**(1):117–24.

24 Alonso-Alonso M, Pascual-Leone A. The right brain hypothesis for obesity. *JAMA*. 2007;**297**(16):1819–22.

25 Fowler CJ, Griffiths DJ. A decade of functional brain imaging applied to bladder control. *Neurourol Urodyn*. 2010;**29**(1):49–55.

26 Ueki K. Disturbances of micturition observed in some patients with brain tumours. *Neurol Med Chir*. 1960;**2**:25–33.

27 Andrew J, Nathan PW. Lesions on the anterior frontal lobes and disturbances of micturition and defaecation. *Brain*. 1964;**87**:233–62.

28 Mayer EA, Naliboff BD, Craig AD. Neuroimaging of the brain-gut axis: from basic understanding to treatment of functional GI disorders. *Gastroenterology*. 2006;**131**(6):1925–42.

29 Tadic SD, Griffiths D, Murrin A, Schaefer W, Aizenstein HJ, Resnick NM. Brain activity during bladder filling is related to white matter structural changes in older women with urinary incontinence. *Neuroimage*. 2010;**51**(4):1294–302.

30 Oliver JL, Campigotto MJ, Coplen DE, Traxel EJ, Austin PF. Psychosocial comorbidities and obesity are associated with lower urinary tract symptoms in children with voiding dysfunction. *J Urol*. 2013;**190**(4 Suppl):1511–5.

31 Berridge CW, Espana RA, Stalnaker TA. Stress and coping: asymmetry of dopamine efferents within the prefrontal cortex. In: Hugdahl K, editor. *The Asymmetrical Brain*. Cambridge, MA: MIT Press; 2003.

32 Linnman C, Moulton EA, Barmettler G, Becerra L, Borsook D. Neuroimaging of the periaqueductal gray: state of the field. *Neuroimage*. 2012;**60**(1):505–22.

33 Rowe JB, Toni I, Josephs O, Frackowiak RS, Passingham RE. The prefrontal cortex: response selection or maintenance within working memory? *Science*. 2000;**288**(5471):1656–60.

34 Holstege G. Micturition and the soul. *J Comp Neurol*. 2005;**493**(1):15–20.

35 Blok BF, Sturms LM, Holstege G. Brain activation during micturition in women. *Brain*. 1998;**121**(Pt 11):2033–42.

SECTION 2

Epidemiological aspects of bowel and bladder dysfunction

Alexander von Gontard

Introduction

Epidemiology deals with the prevalence and patterns of conditions in defined populations. Nonselected, population-based studies provide representative data showing that BBD comprises a heterogeneous group of disorders that are very common in childhood. In the first chapter of this section, Anne Wright provides a comprehensive overview of international studies on nocturnal enuresis, daytime urinary incontinence, and fecal incontinence and associated factors.

Not only is BBD as a disorder very common, but so are co-occurring subjective symptoms. Health-related quality of life is an umbrella construct encompassing a wide spectrum of domains. Children with BBD experience on a whole a lower quality of life than continent children—comparable to children with other chronic physical illnesses. Eliana Fonseca provides an overview on studies on children with functional, as well as neurogenic BBD and aptly illustrates the effects on quality of life with quotations of patients.

Children with BBD are also affected by comorbid emotional and behavioral symptoms and disorders, as Alexander von Gontard shows in Chapter 6. Thirty to fifty percent of children with fecal incontinence, 20–40% with daytime urinary incontinence, and 20–30% with nocturnal enuresis have clinically relevant disorders according to standardized classification systems such as the DSM-5. These disorders not only cause distress and incapacitation, but will also interfere negatively with the treatment of incontinence if not addressed.

But what is the cause for the common association of BBD and accompanying neuropsychiatric disorders? Many studies point toward shared neurobiolgical

Pediatric Incontinence: Evaluation and Clinical Management, First Edition. Edited by Israel Franco,
Paul F. Austin, Stuart B. Bauer, Alexander von Gontard and Yves Homsy.
© 2015 John Wiley & Sons, Ltd. Published 2015 by John Wiley & Sons, Ltd.

and genetic etiologies, as Israel Franco's Chapter 7 elucidates. This means that behavioral disorders are often not a consequence of BBD but that, to the contrary, inherent neurobiological factors are responsible for both—BBD and associated neuropsychiatric disorders. This may be the reason for persisting BBD in some of the affected patients.

CHAPTER 4

The epidemiology of childhood incontinence

Anne J. Wright

Paediatric Nephro-Urology Department, Evelina Children's Hospital, Guy's and St Thomas' NHS Foundation Trust, London, UK

Introduction

The attainment of bladder and bowel control is a normal and important developmental milestone in children. Episodes of incontinence in the preschool age group are common, but epidemiological studies show that bowel and daytime bladder control are achieved before nighttime control with the former attained in the majority of children at 3–4 years of age and the latter between 3½ and 5 years. In general, girls achieve continence earlier than boys. This is despite cultural and social differences in toilet training.

Some children have a delay in achieving bladder and/or bowel control, some achieve control and then relapse and some have persistent ongoing incontinence. A minority of children will have organic or underlying pathology responsible for their incontinence, but the majority have functional incontinence to which this chapter is confined.

The definitions of day- and nighttime urinary and fecal incontinence have been variously described with general consensus as to what constitutes an episode but variable or no definition of frequency and severity which makes comparison and meta-analysis of studies difficult (see Table 4.1).

For the child who suffers from daytime urinary incontinence (DI) or fecal incontinence (FI), their problem is very public being evident within school, home, and leisure environments making them prone to embarrassment and ridicule. Removal of the child to address the incontinence, hopefully by tolerant carers, reduces their participation in day-to-day activities. The impact of nocturnal enuresis (NE) occurs predominantly within the family setting but has increasing social impact as the child gets older and wants to stay away from home at night. The associations of incontinence with emotional/

Pediatric Incontinence: Evaluation and Clinical Management, First Edition. Edited by Israel Franco,
Paul F. Austin, Stuart B. Bauer, Alexander von Gontard and Yves Homsy.
© 2015 John Wiley & Sons, Ltd. Published 2015 by John Wiley & Sons, Ltd.

Table 4.1 Definitions of childhood incontinence.

	Source	Definition
Nocturnal enuresis	DSM-III [1]	The involuntary voiding of urine at least twice a month for children between the ages of 5 and 6 years and once a month for older children
	DSM-IV [2]	Involuntary or voluntary, repeated voiding into the bed or clothes in the absence of medical conditions or substance effect in a child of at least 5 years of age (or equivalent developmental level) at least twice a week for 3 consecutive months or causing clinically significant distress or impairment in social, academic, or other important areas of function
	DSM-5 [3]	As DSM-IV. Subtype: Nocturnal only; passage of urine only during nighttime sleep
	ICD-10 [4]	Involuntary urinary voiding at night for at least 3 months, at a mental age where wetting is unacceptable, at least twice a month in patients younger than 7 years and at least monthly in those older than 7 and not a consequence of a neurological disorder, seizures, or structural urinary tract abnormalities
	ICCS 2006 [5]	Intermittent incontinence (urinary leakage in discrete amounts) while or during sleeping
	ICCS-2014 [6]	Intermittent incontinence (leakage of urine that occurs in discrete amounts) occurring during sleep in a child ≥5 years at least once/month for 3 months. Frequent enuresis is ≥4/week; infrequent is <4×/week
	Primary [2, 5, 6]	The child has never achieved continence or has been dry for <6 months
	Secondary [2, 5, 6]	The child has relapsed and started wetting after a dry period of at least 6 months
	Monosymptomatic [5, 6]	Enuresis in children without any other lower urinary tract symptoms or bladder dysfunction (excluding nocturia)
	Non-monosymptomatic [5, 6]	Enuresis in children with any lower urinary tract symptoms including increased/decreased voiding frequency, daytime incontinence, urgency, hesitancy, straining, a weak stream, intermittency, holding maneuvers, a feeling of incomplete emptying, postmicturition dribble and genital or LUT pain
Daytime urinary incontinence	DSM-IV [2]	Involuntary or voluntary repeated voiding into the bed or clothes in the absence of medical conditions or substance effect in a child of at least 5 years of age (or equivalent developmental level) at least twice a week for 3 consecutive months or causing clinically significant distress or impairment in social academic or other important areas of function
	DSM-5 [3]	As DSM-IV. Subtype: Diurnal only; passage of urine during waking hours
	ICCS 2006 [5]	Daytime incontinence is any wetting episode occurring in discrete amounts during the daytime from at least 5 years of age
	ICCS-2014 [6]	The leakage of urine in discrete amounts while awake in a child of ≥5 years at least once/month for 3 months
	ICD-10 [4]	Involuntary urinary voiding during the day for at least 3 months, at a mental age where wetting is unacceptable, at least twice a month in patients younger than 7 years and at least monthly in those older than 7 and not a consequence of a neurological disorder, seizures, or structural urinary tract abnormalities

Table 4.1 (*Continued*)

	Source	Definition
Fecal incontinence	ROME III [7]	The voluntary or involuntary passage of feces into the underwear or in socially inappropriate places, in a child with a developmental age of at least 4 years
	ICCS 2006 [5]	Fecal incontinence is an umbrella term encompassing any sort of deposition of feces in inappropriate places, functional and organic
		Functional fecal incontinence can be used as a synonym for encopresis
Encopresis	DSM-IV [2]	The voluntary or involuntary passage of feces in inappropriate places in a child 4 years or older after organic causes have been ruled out. It must occur at least once/month for 3 months
	DSM-5 [3]	As DSM-IV
	ICD-10 [4]	The voluntary or involuntary passage of feces in inappropriate places in a child 4 years or older after organic causes have been ruled out. It must occur at least once monthly for a duration of 6 months
Constipation	ROME III [7]	Two or more of the ff in a child with a developmental age of at least 4 years at least 1×/week for 2/12 : ≤2 defecations/week, FI at least 1×/week, history of retentive posturing or excessive volitional stool retention, history of painful or hard bowel movements, presence of large fecal mass in the rectum, history of large diameter stools that block toilet
	PACCT [8]	Two or more of ff in previous 8 weeks from age ≥2 years : <3 bowel movements/week, ≥1 episode of FI/week, large stool in rectum or on abdominal exam, large stools that block toilet, retentive posturing, and painful defecation
	ROME II [9]	In infants and preschool children at least 2 weeks of scybalous pebble-like stools for a majority of stools *or* firm stools ≤2×/week *and* no evidence of structural, endocrine, or metabolic disorders

behavioral problems for the child as well as psychosocial and financial issues for the family are well established.

Thus, quantification of the problem and understanding of risk factors are important for service provision, treatment, and impact for adult life particularly as evidence increases that childhood incontinence continues into adult life [10, 11].

The data presented in this chapter shows prevalence rates for NE, DI, and FI in children and young people derived from large, population-based cohorts published in the English language. A search of the electronic database PubMed and hand-search of references for earlier publications was performed and includes information from 1950 to 2014. The majority of studies use a cross-sectional design utilizing questionnaires completed by parents (and/or children) based on qualitative impressions of eliminatory behaviors. Ascertainment of incontinence prevalence was not always the primary goal of the study.

Nocturnal enuresis

Prevalence

The largest number of epidemiological studies is available for NE with 45 studies included (see Table 4.2).

Up until 1995, 15 studies were confined to developed countries with the notable exception of Sudan in 1986. The lowest reported prevalence rates were

Table 4.2 The prevalence of childhood nocturnal enuresis.

Author	Country	Study date*	Study type	n	Response rate, %	Definition
Blomfield and Douglas [12]	UK	1953	Longitudinal cohort b 1946	4,294	80	<Several nights/week
Croudace et al. [13]	UK	1950–1961	Longitudinal cohort b 1946[†]	3,272	60.5	1×/month
Rutter et al. [14]	UK Isle of Wight	1965, 1968/1969	Cross-section	359	88.7	<1×/week
				1,814	88.5	
				1,913	82.8	
Essen and Peckham [15]	UK	1965 and 1969	Longitudinal cohort b 1958	12,232	75	Ever wet >5 years
						1×/month
Foxman et al. [16]	USA	1975, 1976	Cross-section	1,724	98	×1 in 3/12
Fergusson et al. [17]	New Zealand	1977–1985	Longitudinal cohort b 1977	1,092	86.3	Any
Byrd et al. [18]	USA	1981	Cross-section	10,960		1/year
Hellstrom et al. [19]	Sweden Goteborg	1982	Cross-section	3,556	98.5	×1 in 3/12
Verhulst et al. [20]	Netherlands South	1983	Cross-section	2,070	79.6	DSM III
Jarvelin et al. [21]	Finland	1984	Cross-section	3,206	92	>1×6/12
Rahim and Cederblad [22]	Sudan	1986*	Cross-section	8,462		<2/week
Devlin [23]	Ireland	1991*	Cross-section	1,760	98	1×/month
Spee-van der Wekke et al.[†] [24]	Netherlands	1992–1993	Cross-section	5,360	96	DSM III-R
						DSM IV
Watanabe et al. [25]	Japan	1994*	Cross-section	2,033		None

from two studies in the Netherlands with good concordance: 6.2% [24] and 6.47% [20] with a similar definition of once/month. The highest rate was 18.9% in Australia [26] (definition of <1/month), which reduced to 7.8% using a definition of once/month. Sudan appears to have a genuinely higher prevalence of 17.4% (<several times/week) [22], which may partly be accounted for by inclusion of a low age limit of 3 years. The United States [18] uses a definition of any wetting over 1 year giving a high prevalence that halves when

Age range/ mean, years	Overall prevalence, %	M, %	F, %	1°, %	2°, %	MNE, %	NMNE, %	Associated significant factors
7.75	7.3	8.1	6.4					
4–15	16							
7		15.2	12.2					Age at 14 years
9/10		6.1	3.5					
14		1.9	1.2					
7	10.7	11.6	9.7					SES, sibrank, DD, Ht, CLA
11	4.8	6.0	3.5					
5–13	14	16	12					Age, G
2–8	7.4 at 8 years							FH, DD, SD
5–17	11							Age, G, BI
7	9.6	11.9	7.1			52	47.9	G (MNE)
4–16	6.47	8.8	5.4					G
7	9.8	8.6	3.9	41.7	58.3	65.3	34.7	G (MNE), FH, DD, LBW
3–15	17.4	16.2	18.7					
4–14	13	15	12	71	29			Age, SES, DI, FI, BI, Str
5–15	6.2	8.1	4.2					Age, G, DD
	3.4	4.4	2.3					
		15	5					

(Continued)

Table 4.1 (*Continued*)

Author	Country	Study date*	Study type	n	Response rate, %	Definition
Bower et al. [26]	Australia Sydney	1995	Cross-section	2,292	74	≥1×/month
Kalo and Bella [27]	Saudi Arabia	1996*	Cross-section	740		1×/month
Liu et al. [28]	China Shandong	1997	Cross section	3,344	93	Somewhat
Lee et al. [29]	Korea	1997	Cross section	7,012	55	1×/month
Hansen et al. [30]	Denmark	1997*	Cross-section	1,557	56	<1×/week
Rona et al. [31]	UK England Scotland	1997*	Cross-section	14,674	87.2	<1×/week
Serel et al. [32]	Turkey Isparta	1997*	Cross-section	5,523	96	Several ×/year
Soderstrom et al. [33]	Sweden	1997	Cross-section	1,478	67	1×/month
Sureshkumar et al. [34]	Australia	1998	Cross-section	1,419	70	1×/week
Chiozza et al. [35]	Italy	1998*	Cross-section	7,012	77.2	DSM III
						DSM IV
Butler et al. [36]	UK ALSPAC	1998–2000	Longitudinal cohort b 1991/1992	8,145	72.4	<2×/week
						DSM IV
Gur et al. [37]	Turkey Istanbul	1999	Cross-section	1,576	98.5	>1×/month
Hansakunachai et al. [38]	Thailand	2001	Cross-section	3,453	70.1	DSM IV
Kanaheswari [39]	Malaysia	2001	Cross-section	2,487	73.8	1×/month
Chang et al. [40]	Taiwan	2001*	Cross-section	1,176	70	1×6/12
Kajiwara et al. [41]	Japan	2002	Cross-section	5,282	76.4	>1×/month
Bakker et al. [42]	Belgium	2002*	Cross-section	4,332	77.0	<1×/month
Cher et al. [43]	Taiwan	2002*	Cross-section	7,225	80.3	1×/month
Ozkan et al. [44]	Turkey	2003	Cross-section	14,060	93.1	MNE only
Mota et al. [45]	Brazil	2003–2004	Cross-section	580	98.3	1×/month

Age range/ mean, years	Overall prevalence, %	M, %	F, %	1°, %	2°, %	MNE, %	NMNE, %	Associated significant factors
5–12	18.9							G (MNE)
6–16/9.9		10	14					
6–16/11.1	4.3	5.5	3.0					G
7–12/9.2	10.7	14.2	7.1			87.9	12.1§	
6–9/7	17.7	22.3	13.6					
5–11	9.7	11.7	7.9					Age, G, birth rank, sleep
7–12	11.5	14.3	7.6					Age, FH, G
7.35	6.97	8.4	4.4					Age, DI
10.4	2.61	5.5	0.9					
4–6	15.3					71.9	28.1§	FH, Str
6–14	3.8	4.2	3.4	52.8				G, FH, SES, BW, Str, FI
6–14	1.7	2.1	1.3	68.8				
7.5	15.5	20.2	10.5					G, DI, UF, DU
7.5	2.6	3.6	1.6					
6–16/10.5	12.4	12.2	12.7					G (MNE), age, LFS
5–15/9.6	3.9	3.7	4.07					FH, FI
7–12	8	8.9	7.3	77.5	22.5			Age, G, ethnic group
6–11	8.9			87.6	11.4			G, FH, sleep, Str
7–12	5.9	7.5	4.1			59.4	40.6	G, Const
10–14/11.5	5.6	7.2	3.9	77		37.6	62.4	
6–12	5.5	7.4	4.31					Age, G, LFS, PE, PS
5–11	9							
6–9	17.5	20.1	15.1			3.6		Age, SES

(Continued)

Table 4.1 (Continued)

Author	Country	Study date*	Study type	n	Response rate, %	Definition
Wen et al. [46]	China Henan	2003–2004	Cross-section	10,088	85.5	×1/month¶
Inan et al. [47]	Turkey Edirne	2005	Cross-section	1,694	84.7	DSM III
						DSM IV
von Gontard et al. [48]	Germany	2006	Cross-section	1,379	99.1	<1×/month
Chung et al. [49]	Korea	2006	Cross-section	16,516	85.8	1×/month
Yeung et al. [50]	Hong Kong	2006*	Cross-section	16,512	78.6	1×3/12
Safarinejad [51]	Iran	2007*	Cross-section	6,889	91.1	ICD-10
Aljefri et al. [52]	Yemen Al-Mukalla	2007–2008	Cross-section	832	93.4	2×/week
Yousef et al. [53]	Yemen Aden	2007–2009	Cross-section	656	73.7	1×6/12
Kyrklund et al. [54]	Finland	2012*	Cross-section	594	32	<1×/week
Fockema et al. [55]	South Africa	2012*	Cross-section	3,389	72.1	ICCS 2006
Srivastava et al. [56]	India	2013*	Cross-section	1,212	80.8	ICCS 2006 MNE only

the definition is reduced to ≥6 episodes in last 12 months with similar rates to other developed countries.

After 1995, 30 studies have demonstrated variable prevalence from around the globe (see Figures 4.1 and 4.2).

With regard to studies that have a frequency of wetting once/month, Italy [35] has the lowest prevalence (3.8%) and Brazil [45] the highest (17.5%). For twice/week, Italy [35] is once again the lowest (1.7%) and Turkey [47] the highest (6.4%). A previously performed meta-analysis [57] gives a rate of 10% at 7 years (once or more/1–3 months in nine studies), 3.1% at 11–12 years (once or more/month in seven studies), and 0.5–1.7% at 16–17 years (three studies).

Four studies were longitudinal cohorts—three from the United Kingdom (the Medical Research Council 1946 [12], the National Child Development Study 1958 [15], and the Avon Longitudinal Study (ALSPAC) 1991/1992 [36]) and one from New Zealand (the Christchurch Child Development Study

Age range/ mean, years	Overall prevalence, %	M, %	F, %	1°, %	2°, %	MNE, %	NMNE, %	Associated significant factors
5–18	4.07	4.57	3.56			78.83		
7–11/9.2	9.8	10.1	9.4					Const, uti, Str, LFS
6	6.4 9.9	12.9	6.4					G
5–13	5.6	6.2	4.9					Uti, PE, SES
5–19/13.68	3.1	4.05	2.31				20.7§	Age, severity
5–18/11.2	5.7	5.9	5.4	74.5	25.5		13.2§	Age, FH, LFS, PE, PS
6–15/11.5	28.6	21.2	35.1					Age, G, FH, LFS, Str, sleep
6–15+	17.2	17.4	17.1	76.1	23.9			Age, FH, Str, PE, DI
4–26/15.0	4.0	6.5	2.1					
5–10	16	10.28	5.71			14.4	1.6	G, FH, Const
6–12	12.6	16.3	10.7					Age, G

1°, primary; 2°, secondary; BI, behavioural issues; BW, birth weight; CLA, child in care; Const, constipation; DD, developmental delay; DI, daytime urinary incontinence; DU, daytime urgency; F, female; FH, family history; FI, fecal incontinence; G, gender; ht, height; LBW, low birth weight; LFS, large family size; M, male; MNE, monosymptomatic nocturnal enuresis; NMNE, nonmonosymptomatic nocturnal enuresis; PE, parent education; PS, parenting style; SD, sleep duration; SES, socioeconomic status; Sibrank, sibling rank; Str, stress (variably defined); UF, urinary frequency; UI, urge incontinence; UTI, urinary tract infection.
*Publication date if study date not available.
†Same cohort as Blomfield and Douglas [12].
‡Large cohort of children with special needs not included in figures.
§NE + DI.
¶Primary NE only.

1977 [17]). Longitudinal studies allow identification of clusters of individuals following trajectories of typical and atypical development using powerful statistical modeling called longitudinal latent class analysis (LLAC). Croudace and colleagues [13] used these methods for nighttime bladder control in the 1946 MRC Health and Development cohort with complete data available from

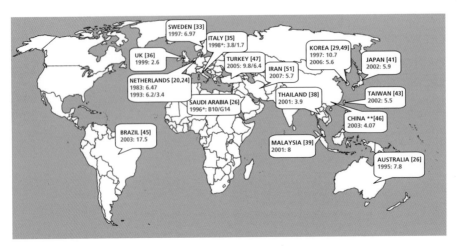

Figure 4.1 Global prevalence of nocturnal enuresis with severity frequency of 1×/month or 2×/week. ■, frequency of 1×/month; ■ , frequency of 2×/week; B, boys; G, girls; *Date is the date of ascertainment or publication if not available. **PNE only.

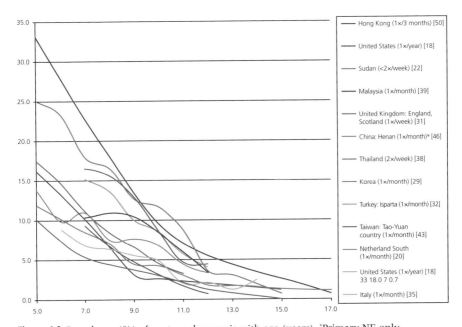

Figure 4.2 Prevalence (%) of nocturnal enuresis with age (years). *Primary NE only.

62.5% (*n* = 3252) and incomplete data from 90.9% (*n* = 4755) revealing four trajectories over the age range 4–15 years:

1 Normal (84%); dry at night between 4 and 6 years.
2 Delayed acquisition of nighttime control (primary enuresis) with two sub-groups; a transient group (8.7%) with resolution of probability of enuresis from approximately 55% at 4 years of age to less than 10% by 8 years, and a

persistent group (1.8%) with 100% probability of enuresis at 6 years resolving steadily and completely by 15 years.

3 Chronic group (2.6%); increased probability of wetting from 75% at 4 years of age to 100% at 8 years of age and some decline from 11 years to just above 50% at 15 years.

4 Relapsing group or secondary enuresis (2.9%); steady increase in probability of wetting from approximately 15% wet at 4 years to nearly 60% at 11 years with some reduction thereafter to just above 10% at 15 years.

Overrepresentation of the relapsing group may explain findings that enuresis prevalence can increase after 5 years of age or fail to spontaneously resolve in several cross-sectional studies [20, 39, 47].

Importantly, Joinson and colleagues used LLAC to analyze the larger ALSPAC cohort [58] from 4.5 to 9.5 years finding broadly similar trajectories to Croudace despite a time lapse of 45 years.

Factors associated with nocturnal enuresis
Age

The prevalence of enuresis decreases with age with an annual spontaneous resolution rate of 15–21%/year [28, 29]. Five studies give a prevalence of approximately 9.7% at 7 years and 5.5% at 10 years of age (frequency 1×/month) [20, 41, 43, 46, 47] (see Table 4.3). Adult rates of enuresis are 0.5% [59] (see Figure 4.2).

Table 4.3 Prevalence of enuresis at 7 and 10 years of age.

Author	Country	Definition	Prevalence at 7 years, %	Prevalence at 10 years, %
Soderstrom et al. [33]	Sweden	Any	7	2.6
Serel et al. [32]	Turkey	Several ×/year	15.1	8.5
Chang et al. [40]	Taiwan	1×6/12	12	3
Yeung et al. [50]	Hong Kong	1×3/12	10.1	2.6
Lee et al. [29]	Korea	<1/month	16.5	8.6
Verhulst et al. [20]	Netherlands South	1×/month	10.9	6.8
Kajiwara et al. [41]	Japan	1×/month	8.8	—
Cher et al. [43]	Taiwan	1×/month	9.3	3.1
Wen et al. [46]	China	1×/month*	8.4	4.2
Inan et al. [47]	Turkey	1×/month	11.3	7.9
Rahim and Cederblad [22]	Sudan	<2×/week	17.9	11.6
Rona et al. [31]	England and Scotland	1×/week	5.1	1.8
Hansakunachai et al. [38]	Thailand	2×/week	5.3	3

*PNE only.

Gender

The majority of studies show that enuresis is more common in boys than in girls (almost 2:1 in Western countries) and this appears particularly true at younger age groups, in milder severity wetting and MNE [19, 21, 32, 37] suggesting a maturational component. Other studies show an equal prevalence in Brazil [45], Turkey [47], Iran [51], Thailand [38], and the Yemen [52].

Frequency severity

Most children with enuresis wet the bed less than once a week. In the English ALSPAC cohort, 12.8% bedwet no more than once/week, 2.4% wet 2×/week, and 0.2% at least once/night at 7.5 years of age [36]. In the ALSPAC LLAC trajectories, there was a strong relationship with wetting more than 2×/week and the chronic group at 4.5–9.5 years [58]. In Japan, the prevalence rates for enuresis at least once/month, more than 1×/week, and nightly were 5.9, 3.7, and 0.9% of total cohort (7–12 years), respectively [41].

Primary/secondary enuresis

Nine studies give prevalence rates of primary versus secondary enuresis and these vary from 41.7 to 87.6%, although four of these studies show rates between 74.5 and 77.5%. Overall, primary enuresis is more common than secondary and accounts for three quarters of enuresis.

MNE/NMNE

Five studies differentiate between MNE and NMNE. Two Swedish studies show an MNE prevalence rate of 6.4% [21] and 7.4% [19] at 7 years of age, a UK study [36] shows 11% at 7.5 years of age, and a Belgium study shows 2.1% between 10 and 14 years [42]. Japan and China show generally lower but similar rates at 3.5% [41] and 3.2% [46], respectively. At 7 years of age, MNE accounted for 52–78.9% of the total cohorts. The Japanese and Chinese studies had age ranges of 7–12 and 5–18 and 59.4 and 78.9% had MNE. In the older Belgian cohort (10–14 years), MNE accounted for a lesser proportion of 37.6%.

Culture and time

The evidence for ethnic or cultural differences in NE is inconclusive. With regard to cultural differences, there appears to be a lower rate of enuresis in Chinese children and Chinese authors postulate that this is due to earlier toilet training, cosleeping with the parents, and small family size [46]. Yeung however found an increase in reported enuresis rates in Hong Kong Chinese following a public education program [50]. Sudan [22] appears to have higher rates than elsewhere which is in keeping with high rates in the Yemen but not Saudi Arabia or Iran. Four Turkish studies show broadly similar rates (9–12.4%).

There are three longitudinal population cohorts in the United Kingdom that compare NE in the seventh year of life with broadly similar definitions and evidence of increasing prevalence with time: 7.3% [12] in 1953 (M 8.1/F 6.4), 10.7% [15] in 1965 (M 11.6/F9.7), and 15.5% [36] in 1998–2000 (M20.2/F10.5). This is an interesting trend with reasons that can only be speculative.

Family factors

There is strong evidence that family history is associated with enuresis and lesser but significant evidence that larger family size, birth order, parental education level, and parenting style also play a role [15, 17, 21, 31, 32, 34, 35, 43, 49, 51, 53, 55]. Poorer socioeconomic status (SES) has also been associated with enuresis although a large population study (ALSPAC) found none.

Emotional factors

Several studies have shown that the presence of stress factors (variably defined) is associated with enuresis as well as behavioral problems [15, 18, 23, 34, 35, 47, 51, 53].

Child factors

Developmental delay [15, 17, 21, 24] and sleep factors [17, 31, 51] have also been associated.

Daytime urinary incontinence

Prevalence

There are fewer studies documenting the prevalence of DI in children—five studies from 1952 to 1995 and seventeen thereafter (see Table 4.4). There is a tendency toward a higher prevalence rate in the newer studies with possible increasing awareness with time (see Figure 4.3). The rates for DI have a wide variation but in studies that have ascertained both NE and DI, DI rates are lower than NE in 12 out of 15 [12, 19, 21, 26, 29, 30, 32–34, 36, 48, 51]. In five studies, DI prevalence is higher than NE but in two comparison is not possible because of definition and age range incompatibility [45, 54]. DI appears to be more prevalent than NE in Japan (6.3 vs 5.9%) [62], Korea (11.2 vs 5.6%) [49], and Belgium (7.9 vs 5.6%) [42].

At 7 years of age, the prevalence rate for DI ranges between 4.9% [19] and 11.7% [30] with three studies in between giving rates of 6.3% [33], 6.9% [29], and 7.9% [60]. At 11–12 years of age, the prevalence rate ranges between 0.8 and 12.5% [29, 49, 51, 61, 63]; meta-analysis of three studies was possible giving an overall prevalence of 6.4% (535/8323) [29, 61, 63]. At 16–17 years of age, one study gives a prevalence rate of 0.5% [51]. There are remarkable similarities between the curves for the United Kingdom [60] and Korea [49] with an increase in DI seen at 6.5 years and at 9 years, respectively, which may represent secondary onset wetting although this is not recorded in either of these studies.

Table 4.4 Prevalence of daytime urinary incontinence.

Author	Country	Study date*	Study type	n	Response rate, %	Definition	Age range/mean, years	Overall prevalence, %	M, %	F, %	Isolated DI, %	Associated significant factors
Blomfield et al. [12]	UK	1952	Longitudinal cohort b 1946	4,351	92.0		6	2.9	1.8	4.1	0.9	
Hellstrom et al. [19]	Sweden	1982	Cross-section	3,556	98.5	1 x 3/12–<1x/week	7	4.9	3.8	6.0	0.7	G, DU
Jarvelin et al.[†] [21]	Finland	1984	Cross-section	2,892	93.5	>1x/6 months	7/7.2	3.3	2.8	3.7	1.8	G
Devlin [23]	Ireland	1991*	Cross-section	1,746	98.0		4–14	5.7			4.0	
Bower et al. [26]	Australia	1995	Cross-section	2,292	74.0	<1x/month	5–12	5.5			2.0	
						1x/month		0.4				
						2x/week		0.8				
Swithinbank et al. [60]	UK	1995–2002	Longitudinal cohort b 1991/1992	10,819	55.5–69.2	<2x/week	4.5	13.6			6.5	Age
Soderstrom et al. [33]	Sweden	1997	Cross-section	1,478	67.0	1x/month	9.5	4.4				NE, FI
							7	6.3	6.8	5.8		
Lee et al. [29]	Korea	1997	Cross-section	7,012	55	>1x/month	10	4.3	4.1	4.3		
Serel et al. [32]	Turkey	1997*	Cross-section	5,523	96.0		7–12	3.4	4.4	2.5	2.1	Age
Hansen et al. [30]	Denmark	1997*	Cross-section	1,557	56.0	<1x/week	7–12	0.5	0.7	0.2		
Sureshkumar et al. [34]	Australia	1998	Cross-section	1,419	70.0	1x/6 months	6–9/7	11.7	9.9	13.3		G, FH, Str
							4–6/5.9	8.8	7.4	9.3		
						1x/month		1.2	1.1	1.3		
						2x/week		2.0	1.9	2.0		
Swithinbank et al. [61]	UK	1998*	Longitudinal	1,176	79.9	Some regularity	11–12	12.5	7.2	16.6		Age, G
							15–16	3.0	1.0	4.7		

Study	Country	Year	Design	N	%	Definition	Age					Associated factors
Kajiwara et al. [62]	Japan	2002	Cross-section	5,282	76.4	≥1×/month prev 6/12	7–12/9.3	6.3	6.2	6.3	4.6	Age, UF, cystitis, infreq BM
Kajiwara et al. [41]	Japan	2002	Cross-section	5,282	76.4	OAB=↑UF and/or UI 1×/month	7–12/9.3	17.8	19.1	16.6		Age, cystitis
Bakker et al. [42]	Belgium	2002*	Cross-section	4,332	77.0	<1×/month	10–14/11.5	7.9	7.1	8.8	4.4	33.2% wet, 1/month
Yousef et al. [63]	Yemen	2003	Cross-section	1,061	62.3	2×/6 months	4–6	3.2	2.8	3.7		Birth order, working mother, Str
Mota et al. [45]	Brazil	2003–2004	Cross-section	580	98.3	≥2×/week	3–9/6.1	2.7	2.4	3.1		SES
						1×/2 weeks>3 years age		20.2	18.2	21.9		
Sureshkumar et al. [64]	Australia	2003–2005	Cross-section	2,856	35.0	<1×/month	4.8–12.8/7.3	16.9			10.0	Age, G,NE, BI, Uti, FI, UF
von Gontard et al. [48]	Germany	2006	Cross-section	1,379	99.1	≥1×/month		6.1				
						≥2×/week		3.6				
						<1×/month	6	3.6	4.1	2.9		ADHD
Chung et al. [49]	Korea	2006	Cross-section	16,516	85.8	≥1×/month	5–13	2.0	2.5	1.4		NE, Uti, FI, Const, delayed toilet train, poor toilets
						≥1–3×/week		1.4	1.8	0.9		
						1×/month		11.2	10.6	11.9		
Safarinejad [51]	Iran	2007*	Cross section	6,889	91.1	Yes/no	5–18	2.0	2.1	2.0		
Kyrklund et al. [54]	Finland	2012*	Cross-section	410	32.0‡	≥Seldom	4–17	25.6	22.2	29.1		F > 12 years

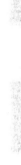

BI, behavioural issues; BM, bowel movements; DI, daytime urinary incontinence; DU, daytime urgency; F, female; FH, family history; FI, fecal incontinence; G, gender; M, male; NE, nocturnal enuresis; SES, socioeconomic status; Str, stress (variably defined); UF, urinary frequency; UTI, urinary tract infection.

*Publication date if study date not available.

†Excludes late school starters and mentally retarded children.

‡Overall cohort.

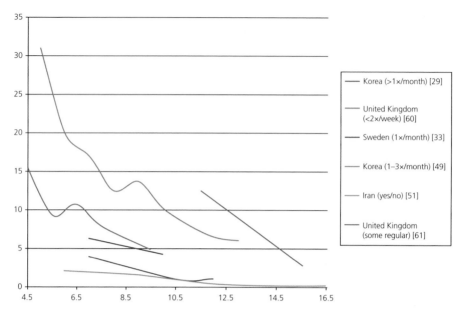

Figure 4.3 Prevalence of daytime urinary incontinence.

The English ALSPAC longitudinal study [65] found the following trajectories for DI over the age range 4.5–9.5 years:

1 Normative(86.2%); dry by 4.5 years
2 Delayed (6.9%); steadily decreasing probability of DI from 80% at 4.5 years of age to less than 10% at 9.5 years of age
3 Persistent (3.7%); probability of DI greater than 80% until 7.5 years of age with steady reduction to 60% at 9.5 years of age
4 Relapsing (3.2%); probability of DI less than 10% at 5.5 years of age increasing to 60% at 6.5 years with slow decline thereafter

There was no gender difference in the delayed group but girls outnumbered boys in the persistent and relapsing groups.

Factors associated with DI
Age
The prevalence of DI decreases with age; three studies allow calculation of an annual spontaneous cure rate with a range very similar to NE of 14.4% [29] to 22.2% [60]. A third study from Korea [49] is in between: 18.8% (see Figure 4.3).

Gender
Studies generally show a higher prevalence in girls than in boys and this ratio increases with age in contrast to NE [19, 34, 54, 60, 64].

Severity
At 4–10 years of age, studies show that prevalence drops with increased frequency of wetting and only a small number of children wet daily: 0.4–0.8% [19, 33, 34, 60].

Other risk factors

In addition to the aforementioned factors, the following factors have also been identified: family history [34], NE [64], FI/constipation [33, 62, 64], cystitis/urinary tract infection [62, 64], urinary frequency [62, 64], emotional stress [34], ADHD [48], and poor toilet facilities [63].

Fecal incontinence

Prevalence

Most FI is secondary to overflow from constipation but it can also occur without evidence of fecal retention in a group classified as functional nonretentive fecal incontinence [7]. Previous terms of fecal soiling and encopresis are common, but these have different meanings/definitions.

While there are quite a few studies reporting FI in community, hospital, and specialty clinics, there are few population-based epidemiological studies with only 12 studies identified in the literature with two preceding 1995. Prevalence rates are variable with a range of 0.6–6.9% between 5–7 years and 0.7–1.6% at 10–12 years (see Table 4.5). One of the issues may be interpretation of the terms FI by respondents. Two studies distinguish between staining and fecal accidents demonstrating that staining is fairly common (potentially in keeping with poor wiping or postponing issues) whereas FI is much less common [33, 73].

Six out of eight studies that assess NE ± DI as well as FI show it is the least prevalent of the incontinence disorders [14, 30, 36, 42, 48, 49]. Two studies from Sweden [33, 73] report a higher prevalence of FI than urinary incontinence but the definitions and age ranges are not comparable. Four of the studies also report the prevalence of constipation in the same cohorts using varying definitions [48, 49, 72, 73]: two studies showing that constipation rates are higher than FI rates [72, 73], one that is similar [48], and one where FI was more common than constipation [49].

The English longitudinal ALSPAC study found four trajectories with normal (89%), delayed (4.1%), persistent (2.7%), and relapsing (4.1%) patterns between the ages of 4.5 and 9.5 years [65]. Boys outnumbered girls in the delayed, persistent, and relapsing groups.

Risk factors for FI
Age

In keeping with NE and DI, FI diminishes with age in Korea [49], Sweden [73], and Sri Lanka [69]; there is no significant pattern in UK ALSPAC cohort.

Gender

Seven studies show increased prevalence of FI in males compared to females [14, 33, 36, 66, 69, 73].

Table 4.5 Prevalence of fecal incontinence and constipation.

Author	Country	Study date*	Study type	n	Response rate, %	Definition	Age range/mean, years	Overall prevalence, %	M, %	F, %	1°, %	2°, %	Associated significant factors
Faecal incontinence													
Bellman [66]	Sweden	1963	Cross-section	8,683		≥1/month	4	2.8					G
							5	2.2					G
Rutter et al. [14]	UK	1965	Cross-section	3,064		1x/month	10–12	0.8					G
Soderstrom et al. [33]	Sweden	1997	Cross-section	1,478	67.0	Any	7	9.8	13.1	6.3			G, hard/loose stools, DI
						FI	10	5.6	7	4.1			
							7	0.6					
							10	0.7					
Hansen et al. [30]	Denmark	1997*	Cross-section	1,557	56.0	<1x/week	6–9/7	6.9	8.3	5.6			G, DD, MA, DT
Butler et al. [36]	UK ALSPAC	1998–2000	Longitudinal cohort b 1991/1992	8,145	72.4	≥2x/week	7.5	0.9					
						≤1x/week–≥2x/week		6.6					
Miele et al. [67]	Italy	1999	Cross-section	9,660	87	Encopresis	0–12	0.14					
van der Wal et al. [68]	Netherlands	2000–2003	Cross-section	13,111	71	1x/month	5–6	4.1					
Bakker et al. [42]	Belgium	2002*	Cross-section	4,332	77.0	<1x/week	11–12	1.6					
							10–14/11.5	3.0	2.1	3.6	4.4		
von Gontard et al. [48]	Germany	2006	Cross-section	1,379	99.1	<1x/month	6	1.4	1.4	1.4			
						≥1x/month		0.9	0.8	1.1			
						≥1–3x/week		0.8	0.7	0.9			
Chung et al. [49]	Korea	2006	Cross-section	16,516	85.8	1x/month	5–13	7.8	9.8	5.8			

Study	Country	Year	Design	N	%	Definition	Age				Risk factors
Rajindrajith et al. [69]	Sri Lanka	2007	Cross-section	2,686	97	<1/week	10–16/13.2	2	1.56	0.44	Age, G, Str, SES, Const
Kyrklund et al. [70]	Finland	2012*	Cross-section	416	32.0†	Faecal accident	4–17	6.0			G
						Staining	4–17	37.5			Age
Constipation											
Miele et al. [67]	Italy	1999	Cross-section	9,660	87	Rome II	0–12	0.68			G, low maternal education, birth rank
Ludvigsson [71]	Sweden	2000–2002	Longitudinal cohort b 1997–1999	8,341	51.2	Constipation	2.5	6.5			
Mota et al. [45]	Brazil	2003–2004	Cross-section	580	98.3	>72 h between BM	3–9/6.1	3.1	3.3	3.0	SES
Inan et al. [72]	Turkey	2005	Cross-section	1,694	89.1	PACCT	7–12	7.2	7.3	7.2	FH, activity, school toilet refusal, bowel control >2 years
von Gontard et al. [48]	Germany	2006	Cross-section	1,379	99.1	1–3 BM/week	6	1.0	1.2	0.8	
Chung et al. [49]	Korea	2006	Cross-section	16,516	85.8	<3 BM/week	5–13	6.7	5.7	7.7	
Rajindrajith et al. [73]	Sri Lanka	2007	Cross-section	2,694	97.3	Rome III	10–16/13.2	15.4		14	Age, FH, war affected area, urban area
						Bristol stool type 1/2		11.8	9.5		
Kyrklund et al. [70]	Finland	2012*	Cross-section	416	32.0†	Constipation‡	4–17	9.4			G

1°, primary; 2°, secondary; BM, bowel movements; Const, constipation; DD, developmental delay; DI, daytime urinary incontinence; DT, difficult temperament; F, female; FH, family history; G, gender; M, male; MA, maternal anxiety; SES, socioeconomic status; Str, stress (variably defined).

*Publication date if study date not available.

†Overall response rate.

‡As interpreted by responders.

Others

Hard stool and constipation, developmental delay, maternal anxiety, stress, difficult temperament in the child, SES, and DI are all factors associated with FI [33, 36, 69].

Conclusion

Childhood incontinence is common with decreasing prevalence according to type (NE > DI > FI), age, and frequency severity. Only small numbers wet or soil daily. Associations include gender (boys for NE/FI and girls for DI), family history, stress, emotional/behavioral factors, and other incontinence types.

Longitudinal studies allow trajectory analysis revealing delayed, relapsing, and persistent patterns of incontinence for all types. Delayed attainment shows an annual spontaneous improvement that is reassuring for children, families, and clinicians. The relapsing and persistent groups (called chronic in NE) are more severe in nature with little spontaneous improvement. Based on these studies, the chances of spontaneous improvement for NE, DI, and FI are 66, 50, and 38%, respectively (the proportion of incontinent children that are in the delayed group/s). Research has not yet identified associations that would enable us to identify if a particular child falls into a particular trajectory allowing an answer to the most commonly asked parental question "Is my child going to grow out of this and by when?" This would also allow health services to more appropriately target the persistently affected child and alter the outcome for the individual and adult incontinence rates.

We now have numerous global cross-sectional studies on enuresis which far outweigh those on DI and FI. Future research needs to be targeted toward gathering further cross-sectional population information on DI and FI using rigorous application of definitions and research methods in order to be able to perform meta-analyses and compare trends. Longitudinal population studies are required for all three groups with particular attention paid to associated identifier factors including type of enuresis, DI, FI, and frequency severity. Only then will the crystal ball start to become clearer in relation to supporting efforts to alleviate the burden of incontinence for individuals and their families.

References

1 American Psychiatric Association. Diagnostic and Statistical Manual of Mental Disorders. 3rd ed. Washington, DC: American Psychiatric Association; 1980.
2 American Psychiatric Association. Diagnostic and Statistical Manual of Mental Disorders. 4th ed. Washington, DC: American Psychiatric Association; 1994.
3 American Psychiatric Association. Diagnostic and Statistical Manual of Mental Disorders. 5th ed. Arlington, VA: American Psychiatric Publishing; 2013.

4 World Health Organisation. The ICD-10 Classification of Mental and Behavioural Disorders: Diagnostic Criteria for Research. Geneva: World Health Organisation; 1993.

5 Neveus T, von Gontard A, Hoebeke P, Hjalmas K, Bauer S, Bower W, et al. The standardization of terminology of lower urinary tract function in children and adolescents: report from the Standardisation Committee of the International Children's Continence Society. J Urol 2006;176(1):314–324.

6 Austin PF, Bauer SB, Bower WF, Chase J, Franco I, Hoebeke P, et al. The standardization of terminology of lower urinary tract function in children and adolescents: update report from the Standardization Committee of the International Children's Continence Society. J Urol 2014;191(6):1863–1865.e13.

7 Rasquin A, Di Lorenzo C, Forbes D, Guiraldes E, Hyams JS, Staiano A, et al. Childhood functional gastrointestinal disorders: child/adolescent. Gastroenterology 2006;130(5): 1527–1537.

8 Benninga M, Candy DC, Catto-Smith AG, Clayden G, Loening-Baucke V, Di Lorenzo C, et al. The Paris Consensus on Childhood Constipation Terminology (PACCT) Group. J Pediatr Gastroenterol Nutr 2005;40(3):273–275.

9 Rasquin-Weber A, Hyman PE, Cucchiara S, Fleisher DR, Hyams JS, Milla PJ, et al. Childhood functional gastrointestinal disorders. Gut 1999;45(Suppl 2):II60–II68.

10 Salvatore S, Serati M, Origoni M, Candiani M. Is overactive bladder in children and adults the same condition? ICI-RS 2011. Neurourol Urodyn 2012;31(3):349–351.

11 Bongers ME, van Wijk MP, Reitsma JB, Benninga MA. Long-term prognosis for childhood constipation: clinical outcomes in adulthood. Pediatrics 2010;126(1):e156–e162.

12 Blomfield JM, Douglas JW. Bedwetting; prevalence among children aged 4–7 years. Lancet 1956;270(6927):850–852.

13 Croudace TJ, Jarvelin MR, Wadsworth ME, Jones PB. Developmental typology of trajectories to nighttime bladder control: epidemiologic application of longitudinal latent class analysis. Am J Epidemiol 2003;157(9):834–842.

14 Rutter M, Tizard J, Whitmore K. Education, Health and Behaviour. London: Longmans; 1970.

15 Essen J, Peckham C. Nocturnal enuresis in childhood. Dev Med Child Neurol 1976; 18:577–589.

16 Foxman B, Valdez RB, Brook RH. Childhood enuresis: prevalence, perceived impact, and prescribed treatments. Pediatrics 1986;77(4):482–487.

17 Fergusson DM, Horwood LJ, Shannon FT. Factors related to the age of attainment of nocturnal bladder control: an 8-year longitudinal study. Pediatrics 1986;78(5):884–890.

18 Byrd RS, Weitzman M, Lanphear NE, Auinger P. Bed-wetting in US children: epidemiology and related behavior problems. Pediatrics 1996;98(3 Pt 1):414–419.

19 Hellstrom AL, Hanson E, Hansson S, Hjalmas K, Jodal U. Micturition habits and incontinence in 7-year-old Swedish school entrants. Eur J Pediatr 1990;149(6):434–437.

20 Verhulst FC, van der Lee JH, Akkerhuis GW, Sanders-Woudstra JA, Timmer FC, Donkhorst ID. The prevalence of nocturnal enuresis: do DSM III criteria need to be changed? A brief research report. J Child Psychol Psychiatry 1985;26(6):989–993.

21 Jarvelin MR, Vikevainen-Tervonen L, Moilanen I, Huttunen NP. Enuresis in seven-year-old children. Acta Paediatr Scand 1988;77(1):148–153.

22 Rahim SI, Cederblad M. Epidemiology of nocturnal enuresis in a part of Khartoum, Sudan. I. The extensive study. Acta Paediatr Scand 1986;75(6):1017–1020.

23 Devlin JB. Prevalence and risk factors for childhood nocturnal enuresis. Ir Med J 1991–1992;84(4):118–120.

24 Spee-van der Wekke J, Hirasing RA, Meulmeester JF, Radder JJ. Childhood nocturnal enuresis in The Netherlands. Urology 1998;51(6):1022–1026.

25 Watanabe H, Kawauchi A, Kitamori T, Azuma Y. Treatment system for nocturnal enuresis according to an original classification system. Eur Urol 1994;25(1):43–50.

26 Bower WF, Moore KH, Shepherd RB, Adams RD. The epidemiology of childhood enuresis in Australia. Br J Urol 1996;78(4):602–606.

27 Kalo BB, Bella H. Enuresis: prevalence and associated factors among primary school children in Saudi Arabia. Acta Paediatr 1996;85(10):1217–1222.

28 Liu X, Sun Z, Uchiyama M, Li Y, Okawa M. Attaining nocturnal urinary control, nocturnal enuresis, and behavioral problems in Chinese children aged 6 through 16 years. J Am Acad Child Adolesc Psychiatry 2000;39(12):1557–1564.

29 Lee SD, Sohn DW, Lee JZ, Park NC, Chung MK. An epidemiological study of enuresis in Korean children. BJU Int 2000;85(7):869–873.

30 Hansen A, Hansen B, Dahm TL. Urinary tract infection, day wetting and other voiding symptoms in seven- to eight-year-old Danish children. Acta Paediatr 1997;86(12): 1345–1349.

31 Rona RJ, Li L, Chinn S. Determinants of nocturnal enuresis in England and Scotland in the '90s. Dev Med Child Neurol 1997;39(10):677–681.

32 Serel TA, Akhan G, Koyuncuoglu HR, Ozturk A, Dogruer K, Unal S, et al. Epidemiology of enuresis in Turkish children. Scand J Urol Nephrol 1997;31(6):537–539.

33 Soderstrom U, Hoelcke M, Alenius L, Soderling AC, Hjern A. Urinary and faecal incontinence: a population-based study. Acta Paediatr 2004;93(3):386–389.

34 Sureshkumar P, Craig JC, Roy LP, Knight JF. Daytime urinary incontinence in primary school children: a population-based survey. J Pediatr 2000;137(6):814–818.

35 Chiozza ML, Bernardinelli L, Caione P, Del Gado R, Ferrara P, Giorgi PL, et al. An Italian epidemiological multicentre study of nocturnal enuresis. Br J Urol 1998;81 Suppl 3:86–89.

36 Butler RJ, Golding J, Northstone K, ALSPAC Study Team. Nocturnal enuresis at 7.5 years old: prevalence and analysis of clinical signs. BJU Int 2005;96(3):404–410.

37 Gur E, Turhan P, Can G, Akkus S, Sever L, Guzeloz S, et al. Enuresis: prevalence, risk factors and urinary pathology among school children in Istanbul, Turk Pediatr Int 2004;46(1):58–63.

38 Hansakunachai T, Ruangdaraganon N, Udomsubpayakul U, Sombuntham T, Kotchabhakdi N. Epidemiology of enuresis among school-age children in Thailand. J Dev Behav Pediatr 2005;26(5):356–360.

39 Kanaheswari Y. Epidemiology of childhood nocturnal enuresis in Malaysia. J Paediatr Child Health 2003;39(2):118–123.

40 Chang P, Chen WJ, Tsai WY, Chiu YN. An epidemiological study of nocturnal enuresis in Taiwanese children. BJU Int 2001;87(7):678–681.

41 Kajiwara M, Inoue K, Kato M, Usui A, Kurihara M, Usui T. Nocturnal enuresis and overactive bladder in children: an epidemiological study. Int J Urol 2006;13(1):36–41.

42 Bakker E, van Sprundel M, van der Auwera JC, van Gool JD, Wyndaele JJ. Voiding habits and wetting in a population of 4,332 Belgian schoolchildren aged between 10 and 14 years. Scand J Urol Nephrol 2002;36(5):354–362.

43 Cher TW, Lin GJ, Hsu KH. Prevalence of nocturnal enuresis and associated familial factors in primary school children in Taiwan. J Urol 2002;168(3):1142–1146.

44 Ozkan S, Durukan E, Iseri E, Gurocak S, Maral I, Ali Bumin M. Prevalence and risk factors of monosymptomatic nocturnal enuresis in Turkish children. Indian J Urol 2010;26(2):200–205.

45 Mota DM, Victora CG, Hallal PC. Investigation of voiding dysfunction in a population-based sample of children aged 3 to 9 years. J Pediatr (Rio J) 2005;81(3):225–232.

46 Wen JG, Wang QW, Chen Y, Wen JJ, Liu K. An epidemiological study of primary nocturnal enuresis in Chinese children and adolescents. Eur Urol 2006;49(6):1107–1113.

47 Inan M, Tokuc B, Aydiner CY, Aksu B, Oner N, Basaran UN. Personal characteristics of enuretic children: an epidemiological study from South-East Europe. Urol Int 2008;81(1):47–53.

48 von Gontard A, Moritz AM, Thome-Granz S, Freitag C. Association of attention deficit and elimination disorders at school entry: a population based study. J Urol 2011;186(5):2027–2032.

49 Chung JM, Lee SD, Kang DI, Kwon DD, Kim KS, Kim SY, et al. An epidemiologic study of voiding and bowel habits in Korean children: a nationwide multicenter study. Urology 2010;76(1):215–219.

50 Yeung CK, Sreedhar B, Sihoe JD, Sit FK, Lau J. Differences in characteristics of nocturnal enuresis between children and adolescents: a critical appraisal from a large epidemiological study. BJU Int 2006;97(5):1069–1073.

51 Safarinejad MR. Prevalence of nocturnal enuresis, risk factors, associated familial factors and urinary pathology among school children in Iran. J Pediatr Urol 2007;3(6):443–452.

52 Aljefri HM, Basurreh OA, Yunus F, Bawazir AA. Nocturnal enuresis among primary school children. Saudi J Kidney Dis Transpl 2013;24(6):1233–1241.

53 Yousef KA, Basaleem HO, bin Yahiya MT. Epidemiology of nocturnal enuresis in basic schoolchildren in Aden Governorate, Yemen. Saudi J Kidney Dis Transpl 2011;22(1):167–173.

54 Kyrklund K, Taskinen S, Rintala RJ, Pakarinen MP. Lower urinary tract symptoms from childhood to adulthood: a population based study of 594 Finnish individuals 4 to 26 years old. J Urol 2012;188(2):588–593.

55 Fockema MW, Candy GP, Kruger D, Haffejee M. Enuresis in South African children: prevalence, associated factors and parental perception of treatment. BJU Int 2012;110(11 Pt C):E1114–E1120.

56 Srivastava S, Srivastava KL, Shingla S. Prevalence of monosymptomatic nocturnal enuresis and its correlates in school going children of Lucknow. Indian J Pediatr 2013;80(6): 488–491.

57 Buckley BS, Lapitan MC, Epidemiology Committee of the Fourth International Consultation on Incontinence, Paris, 2008. Prevalence of urinary incontinence in men, women, and children—current evidence: findings of the Fourth International Consultation on Incontinence. Urology 2010;76(2):265–270.

58 Joinson C, Heron J, Butler R, Croudace T. Development of nighttime bladder control from 4–9 years: association with dimensions of parent rated child maturational level, child temperament and maternal psychopathology. Longitudinal Life Course Stud 2009;1(1):73–94.

59 Hirasing RA, van Leerdam FJ, Bolk-Bennink L, Janknegt RA. Enuresis nocturna in adults. Scand J Urol Nephrol 1997;31(6):533–536.

60 Swithinbank LV, Heron J, von Gontard A, Abrams P. The natural history of daytime urinary incontinence in children: a large British cohort. Acta Paediatr 2010;99(7):1031–1036.

61 Swithinbank LV, Brookes ST, Shepherd AM, Abrams P. The natural history of urinary symptoms during adolescence. Br J Urol 1998;81 Suppl 3:90–93.

62 Kajiwara M, Inoue K, Usui A, Kurihara M, Usui T. The micturition habits and prevalence of daytime urinary incontinence in Japanese primary school children. J Urol 2004;171(1):403–407.

63 Yousef KA, Basaleem HO, Al-Sakkaf KA. Daytime urinary incontinence among kindergarten children in Aden Governorate, 2003. Saudi J Kidney Dis Transpl 2010;21(6):1092–1099.

64 Sureshkumar P, Jones M, Cumming R, Craig J. A population based study of 2,856 school-age children with urinary incontinence. J Urol 2009;181(2):808–815; discussion 815–816.

65 Heron J, Joinson C, Croudace T, von Gontard A. Trajectories of daytime wetting and soiling in a United Kingdom 4 to 9-year-old population birth cohort study. J Urol 2008;179(5):1970–1975.

66 Bellman M. Studies on encopresis. Acta Paediatr Scand 1966;Suppl 170:1+.

67 Miele E, Simeone D, Marino A, Greco L, Auricchio R, Novek SJ, et al. Functional gastrointestinal disorders in children: an Italian prospective survey. Pediatrics 2004;114(1):73–78.

68 van der Wal MF, Benninga MA, Hirasing RA. The prevalence of encopresis in a multicultural population. J Pediatr Gastroenterol Nutr 2005;40(3):345–348.

69 Rajindrajith S, Devanarayana NM, Benninga MA. Constipation-associated and nonretentive fecal incontinence in children and adolescents: an epidemiological survey in Sri Lanka. J Pediatr Gastroenterol Nutr 2010;51(4):472–476.

70 Kyrklund K, Koivusalo A, Rintala RJ, Pakarinen MP. Evaluation of bowel function and fecal continence in 594 Finnish individuals aged 4 to 26 years. Dis Colon Rectum 2012;55(6):671–676.

71 Ludvigsson JF, Abis Study Group. Epidemiological study of constipation and other gastrointestinal symptoms in 8000 children. Acta Paediatr 2006;95(5):573–580.

72 Inan M, Aydiner CY, Tokuc B, Aksu B, Ayvaz S, Ayhan S, et al. Factors associated with childhood constipation. J Paediatr Child Health 2007;43(10):700–706.

73 Rajindrajith S, Devanarayana NM, Adhikari C, Pannala W, Benninga MA. Constipation in children: an epidemiological study in Sri Lanka using Rome III criteria. Arch Dis Child 2012;97(1):43–45.

CHAPTER 5

Quality of life factors in bladder and bowel dysfunction

Eliane Garcez da Fonseca

Pediatric Urodynamic & Continence Unit, Department of Pediatrics, The School of Medical Sciences, The University of the State of Rio de Janeiro & Souza Marques Medical School, Rio de Janeiro, Brazil

Quality of life factors in BBD

For a long time, the evaluation of patients with bladder and bowel dysfunction (BBD) relied exclusively on measures of severity and clinical scores. However, there is a progressive acknowledgment that medical interventions should also aim at improving the quality of life.

Quality of life (QoL) is the "the individual's perception of their position in life in the context of their culture and value systems in which they live and in relation to their expectations, their standards and concerns" [1]. The evaluation of quality of life is subjective; it tells about the patient's perception of the disease and is not directly related to the severity of the disease [2]. Often, assessments of clinical and physiological parameters have low correlation with self-reported quality of life assessments; the latter may be independent predictors of unfavorable outcomes [3].

Studies carried out with children and adolescents with enuresis, urinary incontinence, chronic constipation, and fecal incontinence have pointed out the impact of these disorders on their lives and their families [4–9] (Figure 5.1). This impact in QoL has been demonstrated to be comparable to that seen in other chronic disorders [7].

> They are shameless…are playing, playing and then they pee in their panties… that is not a disease [4].
>
> It's hard…I hit him, I catch the wet bed-sheets and rub them on him…I say that he is a man now…to embarrass him I tell all his friends [4].

Loss of self-esteem, social isolation, poor school performance, psychological impairment, and intrahousehold violence have been described [4–10]. Lack of understanding of enuresis and incontinence as a symptom make

---

Pediatric Incontinence: Evaluation and Clinical Management, First Edition. Edited by Israel Franco,
Paul F. Austin, Stuart B. Bauer, Alexander von Gontard and Yves Homsy.
© 2015 John Wiley & Sons, Ltd. Published 2015 by John Wiley & Sons, Ltd.

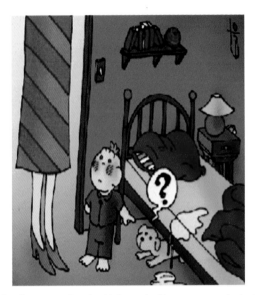

Figure 5.1 Enuresis has been associated with loss of self-esteem, psychological impairment, and intrahousehold violence. Source: Illustration by Guto Mesquita. Reproduced with permission from Guto Mesquita.

several children get punished and denied treatment. In a population-based study, 46% of enuretic children informed that had already been punished because of the enuresis and urinary incontinence but only one family had looked for treatment [6].

Gladh et al compared the QoL of a group of neurologically healthy children with urinary incontinence with the QoL scores of a control group of school children. The patient group had a significantly lower index than the control group both with and without items related to incontinence, with significant differences concerning the total index, social network, friends, support, and motor control. The greatest difference in QoL was among the youngest group (aged 6–8 years) with lower score in basic and intellectual functions, social relations as well as actual well-being and self-esteem. Interestingly, 13% of control group reported incontinence and did not score as well as their continent peers but better than the study patients, which is in accordance with the concept that the perception of negative impact of a condition on QoL is a determinant of health-care system use [5].

Natale et al. studied groups of children with urinary incontinence (UI) and voiding postponement (VP). Children with UI had a lower QoL than controls, and children with VP had a lower QoL and a higher rate of behavioral disorders than those with UI. QoL was highly associated with mental health problems in general, social isolation, anxiety, and depression [8].

Constipation and fecal incontinence (FI) are also source of distress for a child and family. Bongers et al. studied health-related QoL (HRQoL) demonstrated that frequent episodes of fecal incontinence are associated with lower HRQoL regarding emotional and social functioning in children with constipation. Emotional concerns were more predominant than social consequences: 78% of the children abhorred having feces in their underwear, 50% reported being ashamed of their FI, 80% of the children were worried about the odor arising from their FI, two thirds of the children were afraid that FI happens during school time, and 40% try to hide their defecation problem. It is important to note that 23% of children reported regular bullying by other children because of their defecation problem [9] (Figure 5.2).

Furthermore, fecal incontinence was demonstrated to be associated with internalizing (social withdrawal, anxiety, and depression) and externalizing (delinquent behavior and aggression) behavior problems [10].

Although not largely studied in children, several studies with adults indicate that successful treatment of constipation has a favorable effect on QoL [11]. When childhood BBD continues into adulthood, it influences HRQoL negatively with psychosocial consequences [12, 13]. These results highlight the importance of valuing these complaints, removing the child's guilt and not delaying the start of treatment.

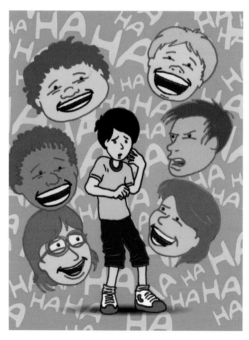

Figure 5.2 Twenty-three percent of children with constipation and fecal incontinence reported regular bullying by other children because of their defecation problem. Source: Illustration by Guto Mesquita. Reproduced with permission from Guto Mesquita.

Neurogenic BBD

Myelomeningocele (MMC) is the commonest cause of neurogenic BBD (NBBD) in children. The complexity of MMC malformation, which involves multiple organs, will influence not only in the survival but also in QoL [14].

Continence is related to psychosocial development and QoL of children with MMC and NBBD. It increases social acceptance, school development, acceptance of physical appearance and behavior, resulting in increased self-esteem of these children. Proper management of bladder and bowel should be established in childhood promoting not only the preservation of renal function but also social continence [14].

Another important aspect in these children's childhood is the preparation for adult life with autonomy. Studies have shown that adolescents and young adults with spina bifida have a lower rate of independence, education, employment, relationships, and social interaction [14, 15].

Children with MMC should be encouraged to participate in self-care, in household chores and family events since an early age. The academic and social life should be valued as well as the acquisition of skills needed in everyday life. When there is failure in this process, it will be more difficult to achieve independence in adult life [14–16]. On the other hand, the participation of the family encouraging the overcoming of barriers imposed by MMC, results in an improvement of about 25% in the QoL of these children [16] (Figure 5.3).

Children who are born with congenital anomalies have the desire to be normal and to be treated as such. When children are brought up in mainstream education and are integrated in school socially this results in self-image improvements, except for the dimension of sexuality [17].

> I would like to be very happy, find a husband, a boyfriend....I have a question: This problem I have may hinder my having children? (Mariana, girl, 18 years old, with myelomeningocele) [18].
> I hope to have a family, if all these things, that is, if these guys (doctors) get something to help me. They have to ensure that everything works. Basically so I can have sex (Sam, boy, 20 years old, with myelomeningocele) [18].

With the arrival of adolescence, there is not only the maturation and development of the body but also the psychosocial emotional development and sexual maturation. For young patients with MMC, these processes become a challenge considering their mobility restrictions, which often worsen with age and obesity. Moreover, aspects related to urinary and fecal continence may keep them dependent on other people's care and thus limit their social life [14, 18, 19].

Moreover, restrictions and physical stigmas can be used by society in general and family members in building overprotected and infantilized individuals, which may lead to bringing about a barrier in social relationships, including

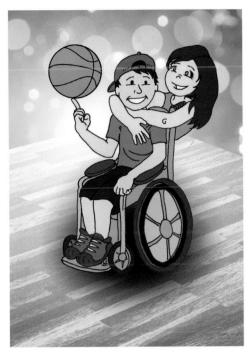

Figure 5.3 The social life should also be valued when dealing with patients with myelomeningocele. Source: Illustration by Guto Mesquita. Reproduced with permission from Guto Mesquita.

emotional and sexual ones [15]. The difficulty of society to notice possibilities of emotional and sexual attachment in these individuals limits their life chances. Studies with adolescents with MMC and NBBD reveal the existence of a lack of information regarding sexuality and physical disability both within families and on the part of health services [17, 18].

A good QoL is present when the hopes and expectations of an individual are met through experience [20]. Thus, getting to know the expectations of patients and working them through in a realistic way are essential to promote improved QoL. Clinical management of these patients has advanced considerably in recent decades. Pursuit of QoL, the rescue of these patients' self-esteem and preparing them for an independent adulthood represent new challenges.

References

1 WHOQOL GROUP. The World Health Organization Quality of Life Assessment: position paper from the world health organization. *Soc Sci Med* 1995; **41**:1403–9.
2 Carr AJ, Gibson B, Robinson PG. Is quality of life determined by expectations or experience? *BMJ* 2001; **322**:1240.

3 Mapes DL, Lopes AA, Satayathum S, McCullough KP, Goodkin DA, et al. Health-related quality of life as a predictor of mortality and hospitalization: the dialysis outcomes and practice patterns study (DOPPS). *Kidney Int* 2003; **64**(1):339–49.

4 Soares AHR, Moreira MCN, Monteiro LMC, Fonseca EMGO. Child enuresis and parental meanings: a qualitative perspective for healthcare professional. *Rev Bras Saude Mater Infant* 2005; **5**(3):301–11.

5 Gladh G, Eldh M, Mattsson S. Quality of life in neurologically healthy children with urinary incontinence. *Acta Paediatr* 2006; **95**:1648–52.

6 Fonseca EG, Bordallo AP, Garcia PK, Munhoz C, et al. Lower urinary tract symptoms in enuretic and nonenuretic children. *J Urol* 2009; **182**(4 Suppl):1978–83.

7 Bachmann C, Lehr D, Janhsen E, Sambach H, et al. Health related quality of life of a tertiary referral center population with urinary incontinence using the DCGM-10 questionnaire. *J Urol* 2009; **182**:2000–6.

8 Natale N, Kuhn S, Siemer S, Stockle M, von Gotard A. Quality of life and self-esteem for children with urinary urge incontinence and voiding postponement. *J Urol* 2009; **182**:692–8.

9 Bongers ME, van Dijk M, Benninga MA, Grootenhuis MA. Health related quality of life in children with constipation-associated fecal incontinence. *J Pediatr* 2009; **154**(5):749–53.

10 Von Gotard A, Baeyens D, Hoecke EV, Warzak WJ, et al. Psychological and psychiatric issues in urinary and fecal incontinence. *J Urol* 2011; **185**:1432–7.

11 Wald A, Sigurdsson L. Quality of life in children and adults with constipation. *Best Pract Res Clin Gastroenterol* 2011; **25**:19–27.

12 Bongers MEJ, Benninga MA, Maurice-Stam H, Grootenhuis MA. Health-related quality of life in young adults with symptoms of constipation continuing from childhood into adulthood. *Health Qual Life Outcomes* 2009; **7**:20.

13 Tubaro A. Defining overactive bladder: epidemiology and burden of disease. *Urology* 2004; **64**:2–6.

14 Woodhouse CR. Myelomeningocele: neglected aspects. *Pediatr Nephrol* 2008; **23**:1223–31.

15 Liptak GS, Kennedy JA, Dosa NP. Youth with spina bifida and transitions: health and social participation in a nationally represented sample. *J Pediatr* 2010; **157**(4):584–8.

16 Kirpalani HM, Parkin PC, Willan AR, Fehlings D, et al. Quality of life in spina bifida: importance of parental hope. *Arch Dis Child* 2000; **83**:293–7.

17 Cartwright DB, Joseph AS, Grenier CE. A self-image profile analysis of spina bifida adolescents in Louisiana. *J La State Med Soc* 1993; **145**:394–6.

18 Soares AHR, Moreira MCN, Monteiro LMC. Disabled adolescents: sexuality and stigma. *Cien Saude Colet* 2008; **13**(1):185–94.

19 Sawyer SM, Roberts KV. Sexual and reproductive health in young people with spina bifida. *Dev Med Child Neurol* 1999; **41**:671–5.

20 Calman KC. Definitions and dimensions of quality of life. In: Aaronson NK, Beckman J (Eds.). *The Quality of Life of Cancer Patients*. New York: Raven Press, 1987:1–9.

CHAPTER 6

Psychological aspects in bladder and bowel dysfunction

Alexander von Gontard

Department of Child and Adolescent Psychiatry, Saarland University Hospital, Homburg, Germany

Introduction

All types of incontinence are associated with a wide variety of psychological symptoms and disturbances, which can have a negative impact on treatment outcome—if they are not adequately assessed and treated [1]. The aim of this chapter is to provide a short overview of representative, population-based studies that are not influenced by selection effects and biases. The focus will be on manifest psychological disorders in children with daytime urinary incontinence (DUI) and fecal incontinence (FI). As nocturnal enuresis (NE) often coexists, relevant aspects will be summarized.

Subclinical symptoms

Subclinical psychological symptoms can be extremely distressing for child and parents. By definition, they do not fulfill all criteria for a psychological disorder according to standardized classification systems such as the DSM-5 [2] and the ICD-10 [3]. They are less severe and less frequent and have a shorter duration and less incapacitation. These "subthreshold" symptoms range from sadness, social withdrawal, anxiety, and negative cognitions to oppositional and provocative behavior [1]. Self-esteem and quality of life can be impaired (Chapter 5). Counseling of child and parents is usually sufficient [1]. These symptoms often resolve upon attaining dryness. Studies on children with DUI or FI are lacking, but self-esteem was shown to improve in the treatment of NE [4].

Pediatric Incontinence: Evaluation and Clinical Management, First Edition. Edited by Israel Franco, Paul F. Austin, Stuart B. Bauer, Alexander von Gontard and Yves Homsy.
© 2015 John Wiley & Sons, Ltd. Published 2015 by John Wiley & Sons, Ltd.

Clinical comorbid disorders

Clinical psychological disorders are more severe and have a greater impact on the child. Following professional child psychological and psychiatric assessment, they are diagnosed according to the classification systems of DSM-5 [2] or ICD-10 [3]. Two broad groups can be differentiated: Internalizing emotional disorders are characterized by "internal" symptoms such as depression and anxiety; in externalizing disorders, observable "external" behavior is typical such as in attention-deficit/hyperactivity disorder (ADHD) and oppositional defiant disorder (ODD).

These four disorders are more common in children with incontinence. As they are of special relevance, they shall be outlined. For further information, readers are referred to textbooks of child psychiatry [5].

Internalizing disorders

Major depression has a prevalence of 2–5%. The etiology is multifactorial with a 40–50% contribution of genetic factors. Symptoms include sadness, unhappiness, loss of enjoyment, lack of energy and interest, negative thinking, and sleep and appetite problems. Treatment includes counseling, cognitive behavioral, interpersonal, and psychodynamic psychotherapy, which can be combined with antidepressant medication.

Anxiety disorders affect 5% of children. The etiology is multifactorial, including family, temperament, and 40% genetic factors. Four subtypes predominate: *separation anxiety disorder,* characterized by fears associated with separation; *generalized anxiety disorder* with the main symptom of worrying; in *social phobia* avoidance of social situations is typical and in *phobia* a fear of objects. Treatment consists of counseling, cognitive behavioral therapy, relaxation, exposure and skills-based techniques, psychodynamic psychotherapy, and medication in severe cases (antidepressants).

Externalizing disorders

ADHD has a prevalence of 6% and a predominantly genetic etiology (70–80%) (Chapter 27). The main symptoms are inattention, hyperactivity, and impulsivity. Treatment includes counseling, parent training, and cognitive behavioral therapy. Medication plays a major role (mainly stimulants).

ODD is characterized by persistent hostile, provocative, and noncompliant behavior and affects 2–5% of children. The etiology is best explained by a gene–environment interaction, including a genetic disposition and dysfunctional parenting practices. Treatment consists of counseling, parent training, cognitive behavioral therapy, school-based interventions, but usually not medication.

Differences in types of incontinence

Overall, the comorbidity rates of psychological disorders are increased by a factor of two to five times in children with incontinence. In summary, 20–30% of children with enuresis, 20–40% of those with urinary incontinence, and 30–50% with encopresis have clinically relevant disorders [1]. Not only the overall prevalence, but also the spectrum of disorders varies among different types of incontinence.

NE

Externalizing disorders predominate in NE, but internalizing disturbances are also common and should not be overlooked (Chapter 27). In a large population-based study of 8242 7½-year-olds, the rates in children with NE were separation anxiety (8.0%), social anxiety (7.0%), specific phobia (14.1%), generalized anxiety (10.5%), depression (14.2%), ODD (8.8%), conduct disorders (8.5%), and ADHD (17.6%) [6]. In another population-based study of 1379 6-year-old children, 9.4% had clinically relevant ADHD symptoms—compared to 3.4% of nonwetting children [7].

The rate of psychological disorders is not increased in primary, but markedly so in secondary enuresis [8]. Relapses are precipitated by stressful life events [9]. Children with monosymptomatic enuresis are more affected by psychological symptoms and disorders than those with nonmonosymptomatic forms [10].

DUI

In DUI, externalizing disorders clearly predominate. In a population-based study of 8242 7½-year-olds, children with DUI had significantly increased rates of ADHD (24.8%), ODD (10.9%), and conduct disorders (11.8%) [11]. In another population-based study, 36.7% of children with urinary incontinence had ADHD—in comparison to 3.4% of dry children [7]. Children with voiding postponement are at special risk, especially for ODD [1].

FI and constipation

Children with FI are even more affected by psychological disorders than those with DUI and NE [1]. In a large population-based study of children aged 7½ years, children with FI had significantly increased rates of separation anxiety (4.3%), specific phobias (4.3%), generalized anxiety (3.4%), ADHD (9.2%), and ODD (11.9%) [12]. In other words, children with FI show a heterogeneous pattern of both internalizing and externalizing disorders. The comorbidity rates are comparable in children with constipation and nonretentive FI [13].

Conclusions and recommendations

Both subclinical symptoms and manifest psychological disorders are markedly increased in children with BBD. They cause emotional distress and children are incapacitated in their daily life. Although ADHD is very common, it is not the only comorbid disorder. ODD, but especially internalizing disorders such as depression and anxiety, can be overlooked. Therefore, screening with broadband question-naires such as the CBCL (Achenbach, 1991) or the SDQ (see appendix) in all patients with incontinence is recommended [1]. If marked symptoms are identi-fied, full child psychological or psychiatric assessment is recommended. Counseling and treatment should follow when indicated (see Chapters 23 and 27). Attending to both incontinence and behavioral/emotional needs will yield better outcomes and happier children and families.

Appendix   Short screening instrument for psychological problems in enuresis (SSIPPE)
Source: van Hoecke et al. [14]. Reproduced with permission from the American Urological Association/Elsevier.
- Parental questionnaire
- Validated, based on the Child Behavior Checklist (CBCL) [15]
- Seven items for emotional problems
- Three items for attention symptoms
- Three items for hyperactivity/impulsivity symptoms
- Yes/no format
- If more than two yes answers are given for any of the three problem areas (emotional, attention, hyperactivity/impulsivity), this should be followed by a more detailed questionnaire such as the CBCL. If the CBCL T-scores are in clinical range (or many problem items are answered with a "2"), then a detailed child psychiatric assessment should follow.

Short screening instrument for psychological problems in enuresis (SSIPPE)

Name ....   Date of birth.......

Emotional problems
If more than two positive items, full screening required

1. Does your child **sometimes** have the feeling that others are reacting negatively?	YES	NO
2. Does your child **sometimes** feel worthless and less confident?	YES	NO
3. Does your child **sometimes** have headaches?	YES	NO

4. Does your child **sometimes** feel sick?	YES	NO
5. Does your child **sometimes** have abdominal pain?	YES	NO
6. Is your child **sometimes** little active or lacking energy?	YES	NO
7. Does your child **sometimes** feel unhappy, sad, or depressive?	YES	NO

Inattention symptoms
If more than two positive items, full screening required

1. Does your child **frequently** pay insufficient attention to details or make careless defaults in schoolwork?	YES	NO
2. Does your child **frequently** have difficulties with organizing tasks and activities?	YES	NO
3. Does your child **frequently** forget in daily practice?	YES	NO

Hyperactivity/impulsivity symptoms
If more than two positive items, full screening required

4. Does your child **frequently** talk continuously?	YES	NO
5. Is your child **frequently** busy?	YES	NO
6. Does your child **frequently** run or climb in situations in which this is inappropriate?	YES	NO

Strengths and Difficulties Questionnaire (SDQ)

The Strengths and Difficulties Questionnaire (SDQ) is a brief behavioral screening questionnaire about 3–16-year-olds. It exists in several versions to meet the needs of researchers, clinicians, and educationalists. Official translations are available in 77 languages.

All versions of the SDQ ask about 25 attributes, some positive and others negative. These 25 items are divided between 5 scales.

1. Emotional symptoms (5 items)	1 to 4 added together to generate
2. Conduct problems (5 items)	a total difficulties score (based on
3. Hyperactivity/inattention (5 items)	20 items)
4. Peer relationship problems (5 items)	
5. Prosocial behavior (5 items)	

The Strengths and Difficulties Questionnaires, whether in English or in translation, are copyrighted documents that may not be modified in any way. Paper versions may be downloaded and subsequently photocopied without charge by individuals or nonprofit organizations provided they are not making any charge to families.

The questionnaires, scoring instructions, norms, and related articles can be downloaded free of charge at the following website: www.sdqinfo.org.

References

1 von Gontard A, Baeyens D, Van Hoecke E, et al.: Psychological and psychiatric issues in urinary and fecal incontinence. *J Urol* 2009;**185**:1432–1437.

2 American Psychiatric Association: *Diagnostic and Statistical Manual of Mental Disorders (DSM-5)*, 5th ed. Washington, DC: American Psychiatric Publishing, 2013.

3 World Health Organisation: *Multiaxial Classification of Child and Adolescent Psychiatric Disorders: The ICD-10 Classification of Mental and Behavioural Disorders in Children and Adolescents*. Cambridge: Cambridge University Press, 2008.

4 Longstaffe S, Moffat M, Whalen J: Behavioral and self-concept changes after six months of enuresis treatment: a randomized, controlled trial. *Pediatrics* 2000;**105**:935–940.

5 Rey J (ed.): *IACAPAP Textbook of Child and Adolescent Mental Health*. Geneva: International Association for Child and Adolescent Psychiatry and Allied Professions, 2012; http://iacapap.org/iacapap-textbook-of-child-and-adolescent-mental-health (accessed February 14, 2015).

6 Joinson C, Heron J, Emond A, et al.: Psychological problems in children with bedwetting and combined (day and night) wetting: a UK population-based study. *J Pediatr Psychol* 2007;**32**:605–616.

7 von Gontard A, Moritz AM, Thome-Granz S, et al.: Association of attention deficit and elimination disorders at school entry—a population-based study. *J Urol* 2011;**186**:2027–2032.

8 Feehan M, McGee R, Stanton W, et al: A 6 year follow-up of childhood enuresis: prevalence in adolescence and consequences for mental health. *J Paediatr Child Health* 1990;**26**:75–79.

9 Järvelin MR, Moilanen I, Vikeväinen-Tervonen L, et al.: Life changes and protective capacities in enuretic and non-enuretic children. *J Child Psychol Psychiatry* 1990;**31**:763–774.

10 Butler R, Heron J, Alspac Study Team: Exploring the differences between mono- and poly-symptomatic nocturnal enuresis. *Scand J Urol Nephrol* 2006;**40**:313–319.

11 Joinson C, Heron J, von Gontard A, ALSPAC Study Team: Psychological problems in children with daytime wetting. *Pediatrics* 2006;**118**:1985–1993.

12 Joinson C, Heron J, Butler U, et al.: Psychological differences between children with and without soiling problems. *Pediatrics* 2006;**117**:1575–1584.

13 Bennigna MA, Buller HA, Heymans HS, et al.: Is encopresis always the result of constipation? *Arch Dis Child* 1994;**71**:186–193.

14 Van Hoecke E, Baeyens D, Vanden Bossche H, et al.: Early detection of psychological problems in a population of children with enuresis: construction and validation of the short screening instrument for psychological problems in enuresis. *J Urol* 2007;**178**:2611.

15 Achenbach TM: *Manual for the Child Behavior Checklist/4-18 and 1991 profile*. Burlington: University of Vermont, 1991.

CHAPTER 7

Neuropsychiatric disorders and genetic aspects of bowel or bladder dysfunction

Israel Franco

Maria Fareri Children's Hospital, Valhalla, NY, USA

Introduction

Anyone who cares for the child with bowel and bladder dysfunction (BBD) will be able to confirm that there is a very close association between these issues and behavioral and psychiatric problems. Extensive epidemiologic studies have revealed that children with BBD have increased rates of psychological disorders [1–10]. (This topic is covered in Chapter 4 of this textbook.)

Up until recently, these were seen as just casual relationships and probably due to the stresses of BBD. Over the last decade or so with the advent of functional brain imaging, there came a greater level of understanding with the processes that are involved in voiding and also in neuropsychiatric disorders. Examination of the psychiatric literature has revealed some very interesting studies that may help explain our findings and further tie together the association between two seemingly disparate problems.

One of the first groups of patients who were recognized to have an increased incidence of BBD was that of patients who had ADHD, ADHD predominately inattentive subtype and patients with oppositional defiant disorder (ODD). For years, we have known that patients with ADHD were more difficult to treat than other children with incontinence or LUTS. These patients typically stand-out in the office and a causal relationship can easily be made in this group of patients. It was the patient who has milder forms of anxiety, depression, and OCD that was more difficult to pin down and identify, therefore making it less likely to associate these diagnoses with BBD. After careful observation of our patients over an extended period of time, we have begun to recognize that there is an increased association between other neuropsychiatric disorders and

Pediatric Incontinence: Evaluation and Clinical Management, First Edition. Edited by Israel Franco, Paul F. Austin, Stuart B. Bauer, Alexander von Gontard and Yves Homsy.
© 2015 John Wiley & Sons, Ltd. Published 2015 by John Wiley & Sons, Ltd.

LUTS, the literature tends to support these observation as well [11]. In our own series of patients we also found that it was clear that the patient did not have to carry a diagnosis of a neuropsychiatric disorder but as long as a family member had an issue, they could put that child at risk, the same as if the child had a diagnosis of a neuropsychiatric disorder. We have found that this phenomenon repeats in several studies that we have conducted in children, from patients with urgency/frequency syndrome to those who have autonomic dysfunction. Is there some connection between these neuropsychiatric disorders and LUTS in children?

The association of urinary incontinence and lower psychological well-being in the adult has also been noted by Botlero et al. [12]. Major depression can predict the onset of urinary incontinence in women in a population-based sample at risk [13]. One study found increased rates of enuresis in adult bipolar disorder (18%) [14]. There has also been an association with panic disorder and interstitial cystitis that has been described in the literature [15]. A publication in 1990 revealed that patients who were described as having psychoneuroticism were less likely to respond to treatment for detrusor instability than those who had no form of psychoneuroticism. Most good responders and one-third of non responders were free of psychiatric issues [16]. Of important note was that 25% of the patients in this study had IBS symptoms. These findings were no different than our data that indicates that patients with urge syndrome who are nonresponders have a 50% chance of having some form of neuropsychiatric problem. Enuresis was also found to be a premorbid developmental marker for schizophrenia (SCZ) [17]. The authors found that patients with SCZ had higher rates of childhood enuresis (21%) compared with siblings (11%) or controls (7%) and the relative risk for enuresis was increased in siblings.

There is increasing evidence that genetic factors play a major role in urinary incontinence in adults. Altman et al. [18] looked at the role of genetic influence on stress incontinence and pelvic organ prolapse. Hannestad et al. [19] looked at the familial risk of urinary incontinence in women using a population-based study. There are three twins' studies [20–22] that tend to confirm the existence of a correlation between UI and genetics. One study provides solid epidemiological evidence that among premenopausal female twins, depressive mood disorders (depressive symptoms and major depression) and neuroticism are positively associated with UI. However, the positive association between major depression and urge and mixed UI was explained by neuroticism [22].

In this chapter, we will try to present information, which is readily available in the psychiatric and neurologic literature that supports the concept that the underlying neurologic defect that is present may contribute to the fundamental problem of BBD. The author has examined this in a prior publication [23], but we seek to expand on this topic in this chapter.

Cortical thinning and neuropsychiatric disorders

In the work by Hyde et al. [17] evaluating patients with schizophrenia psychosis, family members (probands), and controls, they found that when they looked at the brain of these groups, they found the following: The voxel-based mapping (VBM) analysis of probands revealed frontal gray matter decreases in those with a history of enuresis (16 probands with enuresis and 66 probands without enuresis), specifically reductions of gray matter volume in the right superior frontal gyrus (BA 9), right middle frontal gyrus (BA 10), bilateral inferior frontal gyrus (BA 45), and right superior parietal cortex (BA 7). The VBM analysis on the subset of healthy controls also revealed areas of significantly decreased gray matter volume in those with a history of enuresis (11 healthy controls with enuresis and 91 healthy controls without enuresis). More specifically, they found reductions of gray matter volume in the right medial frontal gyrus (BA 11), right middle temporal gyrus (BA 21), left middle temporal gyrus (BA 22), and left cuneus (see Figure 7.1a and b).

In a review article by Thermenos et al. [24] on neuroimaging of schizophrenia, the authors' conclusions based on multiple studies in the literature were that there is evidence of reduced PFC volume at baseline in healthy relatives and patients with schizophrenia. These changes become more pronounced as time goes on and symptoms worsen in the patients with schizophrenia. There is also evidence that there are white matter changes in the PFC. The groups finding was that the PFC was the brain region most commonly altered in a genetic healthy relative when compared to controls. In the same review, there was data that there was evidence of structural defects in the ACC.

In the work performed on families at risk for depression by Peterson et al. [25], they looked to cortical imaging to try to find a link between a high-risk group that comprised patients who had moderate to severe, recurrent, and functionally debilitating major depressive disorder (MDD) and a control group composed of a sample of matched adults, ascertained from the same community, who had no discernible lifetime history of depression. Maps of cortical thickness demonstrated broad expanses of statistically significant thinning in the lateral aspect of the right hemisphere in the high-risk group, including the inferior and middle frontal gyri, somatosensory and motor cortices, dorsal and inferior parietal regions, the inferior occipital gyrus, and posterior temporal cortex. Thinning was absent in the lateral aspect of the left hemisphere of the high-risk group. Areas of statistically significant cortical thickening in the high-risk group were detected in the subgenual cortex, *anterior and posterior cingulate gyrus*, and medial orbitofrontal cortex of the right hemisphere. Findings were similar in analyses of children and adults separately, and no interaction of age with risk group was detected. Analyses of cortical volumes revealed regional differences across groups that were similar to those detected using measures of cortical thickness. Although cortical thickness was not associated with a lifetime history of MDD or anxiety disorder, cortical thickness did correlate significantly with the severity of current depression and

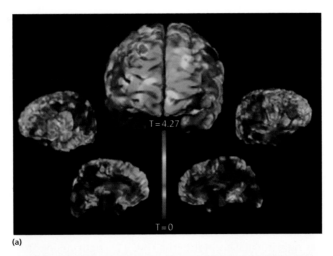

(a)

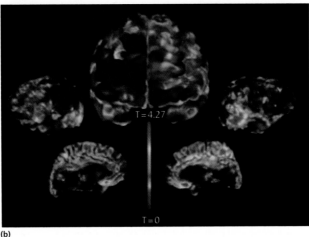

(b)

Figure 7.1 (a) Gray matter volume decreases in probands with enuresis compared with probands without enuresis. This figure depicts the statistical main effects of decreased regional gray matter volume comparing probands with a history of childhood enuresis to those without a history. The unthresholded VBM results are overlaid on an analysis of functional neuroimages (AFNI) of the pial surface and color coded for the statistical t-score. The central figure is the frontal view and the other figures, from the left to the right, are the left lateral, left medial, right medial, and right lateral hemispheric surface views. The most significant cluster of decreased gray matter volume in probands with enuresis is in the right superior frontal gyrus, BA 9. **(b) Gray matter volume decreases in controls with enuresis compared with controls without enuresis**. This figure depicts that the statistical main effects of regional gray matter volume decrease in healthy controls with a history of childhood enuresis versus those without a history. The unthresholded VBM results are overlaid on an analysis of functional neuroimages (AFNI) of the pial surface and color coded for the statistical t-score. The central figure is the frontal view and the other figures, from the left to the right, are the left lateral, left medial, right medial, and right lateral hemispheric surface views. The most significant cluster of reduced gray matter volume in healthy controls with enuresis is the left middle temporal gyrus, BA 22. There was also a cluster of decreased gray matter from the medial frontal gyrus, BA 11, extending into the subgenual cingulate. Source: Hyde et al. [17]. Reproduced with permission from Oxford University Press.

anxiety symptoms at the time of scan but primarily in the left rather than in the right hemisphere The impressive thinning of the cortical mantle in the right hemisphere of the high-risk compared with the low-risk group, and its independence both from a prior history of MDD or anxiety disorder and from current depressive or anxiety symptoms, naturally raises the questions of what the functional consequences of the cortical thinning may be and how those functional consequences may increase the risk for developing MDD or anxiety (see Figure 7.2).

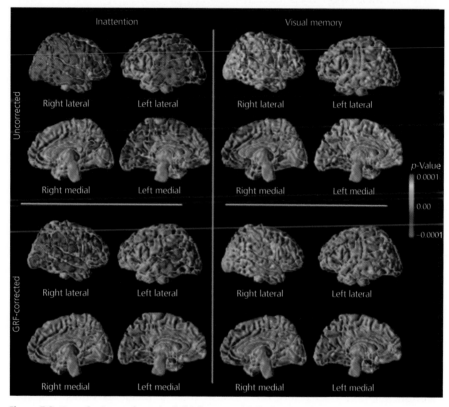

Figure 7.2 Correlations of cortical thickness with behavioral measures. Warm colors (yellow, orange, and red) represent significant positive correlations. Cooler colors (blue and purple) represent inverse correlations between cortical thickness and the behavioral measure. Statistical models for the correlations accounted for the degree of familial relatedness, age, and sex of the participants. Correlations are shown for high- and low-risk groups combined, although similar maps were found in both the high- and low-risk groups separately (data not shown). Findings did not change appreciably when covarying also for risk status, indicating that these correlations are not driven by differences in cortical thickness or memory scores across the two risk groups. Correlations are especially strong in the lateral surface of the right compared with the left hemisphere, and the general patterns of correlation are similar to those detected when comparing cortical thickness in the high- and low-risk groups. Maps that correct for multiple comparisons using the theory of Gaussian random fields (GRF) are shown in the lower half of each panel. (*Left*) Greater inattention accompanied proportionately thinner cortices (*n* ! 117). (*Right*) Worse visual memory performance accompanied proportionately thinner cortices (*n* ! 119). Source: Peterson et al. [25]. Reproduced with permission from PNAS. © National Academy of Sciences.

There are two distinct findings in depression regarding the PFC. There are increased activity (mainly in ventral and medial parts of PFC) and decreased (mainly in dorsal and lateral parts of PFC) activity of prefrontal regions. It is now widely accepted that dorsal and lateral parts of the PFC (DLPFC) are associated with more "cognitive" aspects of behavior, while ventral and medial (VMPFC) parts are mostly connected to "emotional" aspects of information processing [26]. It is also worth mentioning that medial and dorsal regions of the PFC are part of distinct, bigger brain circuits—namely, the frontoparietal or executive network (dorsal parts of the PFC) and the default mode network (medial parts of the PFC). Functional imaging studies convincingly indicate that depression is associated with opposite patterns of activity in ventromedial and dorsolateral parts of the PFC. Of particular importance is the fact that ventral parts of the PFC are usually hyperactive when measured in depressed populations and increase activity when symptoms remit [27]. This asymmetrical pattern of PFC activity with increased activity of "emotional" and decreased activity of "cognitive" regions is only one of many lines of evidence for abnormal PFC functioning in depression. A normally functioning PFC is critical for the control of the urge to urinate (see Chapter 3).

Results from brain stimulation studies employing transcranial magnetic stimulation (TMS) and electrical deep brain stimulation (DBS) targeting the dorsal and medial parts of the PFC confirm the aforementioned findings that these areas play distinct roles in pathophysiology and symptoms maintenance in depression [26].

Right frontal lobe and incontinence

Interestingly, right superior frontal damage has been associated with transient urinary incontinence in adulthood [28]. Other lesion studies have associated acquired frontal lobe lesions in adulthood with the development of urinary incontinence [29]. Conversely, there is also a higher incidence of depression in patients with right-sided brain injuries. In adult schizophrenic subjects, Hyde et al. [17] found that decreased volume of the right superior frontal gyrus was associated with persistent yet ultimately transient urinary incontinence in childhood. This finding suggests that at least in schizophrenic subjects, delayed or abnormal development of the right superior frontal gyrus (BA 9) may mediate childhood enuresis. The VBM analysis on adult probands revealed that a childhood history of enuresis was associated with decreased gray matter in several frontal regions (right BA 9, right BA 10, bilateral BA 45) and one parietal region (right BA 7). In controls, a somewhat different pattern emerged, with decreased gray matter in the frontal (right BA 11) and temporal (right BA 21, left BA 22) cortices and the left cuneus. The findings from subjects with SCZ and controls, along with worked sited throughout chapter 3 are in agreement with the proposition that the frontal lobes are intimately involved in the development and maintenance of volitional bladder control. The fact that these structural differences are present in adults with no current incontinence but a childhood history of enuresis suggests that they represent vestigial developmental pathology that is functionally compensated. The common finding among children that they wet without knowing can be accounted for by findings in the work by Peterson et al. [25]. They postulated that since the right cerebral hemisphere is thought to be dominant in mediating certain forms of attention and visuospatial memory [30, 31]. Thinner cortices in the right hemisphere were associated with greater degrees of inattention and with poorer performance on immediate and delayed visual memory tasks (Figure 7.3). Cortical thinning seen in the right hemisphere could produce social inattention and reduced visual memory. Social inattentiveness has been postulated to be a possible root cause of depression by Peterson. Their findings strongly suggest that the predisposition to familial depression derives from disturbances of cortical gray matter in the right cerebral hemisphere. The 28% average reduction in cortical thickness of the right hemisphere is remarkable for its magnitude and spatial extent, rivaling the magnitude and extent of cortical morphological abnormalities reported in the most severe neuropsychiatric disorders, including SCZ and Alzheimer's diseases [33, 34], and is perhaps all the more remarkable given that the thinning is present even in persons who have never suffered from MDD or anxiety disorder but who are biological descendants of a depressed relative. The presence of the findings in individuals with and without a prior lifetime history of depression who were at increased familial risk for MDD suggests that these abnormalities

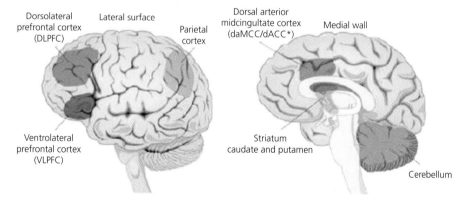

Figure 7.3 The cingulofrontal–parietal cognitive/attention network. The dorsal anterior midcingulate cortex (daMCC), dorsolateral prefrontal cortex (DLPFC), ventrolateral prefrontal cortex (VLPFC), and parietal cortex comprise the CFP network. These regions work in concert with each other and other regions such as the striatum and cerebellum to support normal cognition, attention, and motor control processes. All of these brain regions have been found to display functional and structural abnormalities in ADHD. Source: Bush [32]. Reproduced with permission from Elsevier.

are not simply a consequence of previously having been depressed or having been treated for depression. Rather, the findings suggest that thinning of the cortical mantle in the right hemisphere probably constitutes familial trait vulnerability for the development of MDD. The presence of the findings across a wide age range, the presence of the findings in children of the sample when analyzed separately, the absence of an interaction of age with risk group, and the increased rates of anxiety disorders and MDD in childhood and suggest that the determinants of the cortical thinning probably are operative early in development, either in utero or during early childhood.

ADHD

There has been an attempt to identify the pathophysiology of ADHD using imaging studies. This typically led to investigations centered on the dorsal anterior midcingulate cortex (daMCC), dorsolateral prefrontal cortex (DLPFC), ventrolateral prefrontal cortex (VLPFC), and, to a lesser extent, parietal cortex. Together, these regions comprise the main components of the cingulofrontal–parietal (CFP) cognitive/attention network (see Figure 7.3). These areas, along with the striatum, premotor areas, thalamus, and cerebellum, have been identified as nodes within parallel networks of attention and cognition [32]. The most consistent cross-study and cross-modality data identifying a region as dysfunctional in ADHD has been provided for the dorsal anterior midcingulate cortex (daMCC) [35, 36]. Structural studies have identified that the volumes of the cingulate cortices are reduced in adults and children with ADHD [32]. There is also evidence that volume decreases are present pretreatment and can persist posttreatment for ADHD [37]. Children with ADHD had significant global thinning of the cortex, most prominently in the cingulate and superior prefrontal regions [38]. These data in children were generally consistent with the findings by Makris et al. [39] that showed selective cortical thinning of the daMCC and CFP attention networks in adults with ADHD.

The daMCC integrates goal and feedback-related information from various sources and uses this information to modulate activity in executive brain regions that direct attention and produce motor responses. The daMCC thus acts within cognitive–reward–motor networks to increase the efficiency of decision-making and execution, and its proper function is, therefore, germane to ADHD [35]. Numerous functional, structural, connectionist, neurochemical, and pharmacological imaging studies have identified abnormalities of daMCC in ADHD. Specifically, many fMRI, PET, and event-related potential (ERP) studies have reported daMCC hypofunction in ADHD using a variety of tasks and techniques [35]. In a study looking at cerebral glucose metabolism in 25 treatment-naïve ADHD adults (compared to 50 adult controls), regional metabolism was specifically lower in ADHD in daMCC, premotor and somatosensory areas during

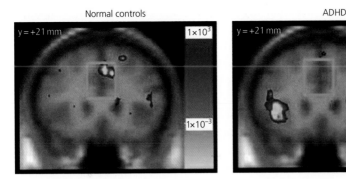

Figure 7.4 The daMCC shows hypofunction in ADHD during counting Stroop.
Dorsal anterior midcingulate cortex (daMCC) activated in healthy controls, but not in subjects
with ADHD, during the counting Stroop. Source: Bush [32]. Reproduced with permission
from Elsevier.

a continuous performance task [40]. Other fMRI studies to specifically inter-
rogate daMCC integrity in ADHD found that daMCC was hypoactive in
ADHD adults during cognitive/attention task performance (Figure 7.4).
Subsequent fMRI studies using a variety of tasks have similarly found relative daMCC hypofunction in ADHD compared to controls. These have
included an fMRI study of adolescent boys with ADHD using a Go/No Go task
[41] (see Figure 7.3). A meta-analysis of neuroimaging studies by Dickstein
et al. [42], shown in Figure 7.4, found daMCC to be among a limited number
of brain regions that were hypoactive in ADHD relative to healthy controls.
ADHD was additionally found to be associated with significant hypoactivity
of the DLPFC, VLPFC, superior parietal cortex, caudate, and thalamus.
Functional pharmacoimaging has been useful in identifying alteration in the
CFP neural circuitry that underlies ADHD. These pharmacoimaging studies
using fMRI and dopaminergic markers highlight the cingulate and frontal
effects of stimulant medications [32]. Variations in dopamine system dopamine transporter gene (SLC6A3) may be linked to alterations of daMCC
function [43].

The control of micturition in the patient with ADHD we can see that improper
function of the daMCC will be associated with unknowing incontinence and
even poor coordination of the sphincter.

Lateral prefrontal cortex

The dlPFC and vlPFC, as these regions are thought to support vigilance, selective
and divided attention, attention shifting, planning, executive control, and working memory functions. Also, the vlPFC in particular has been associated with

behavioral inhibition. Structural and functional data support the conclusion that lateral prefrontal cortex abnormalities contribute to ADHD. Structural imaging studies of ADHD have identified both 3–4% smaller global cerebral volumes in ADHD, as well as specifically smaller prefrontal volumes in ADHD [44, 45].

More recently, Monuteaux et al. [46, 47] found that among adults with ADHD, subjects with the 7-repeat allele of the dopamine D4 receptor (DRD4) gene had a significantly smaller mean volume of superior frontal cortex and cerebellum compared to subjects without this allele. Cortical thickness maturation delays have been found in ADHD, with delays most prominent in lateral prefrontal cortex, especially the superior and dlPFC regions [48]. In a separate study combining cortical thickness and genetics by the same group, cortical thinning of multiple regions, including the orbitofrontal cortex, inferior prefrontal cortex, and posterior parietal cortex, was associated with possession of the DRD4 7-repeat allele in both healthy children and those with ADHD [49]. These brain regions were generally thinner in ADHD than those in controls, though a complicating factor was that ADHD patients with the DRD4 7-repeat allele did better clinically. Cortical thickness results have not, however, always been consistent.

Diffusion tensor imaging and fMRI have been combined to help identify prefrontal cortical abnormalities in ADHD. This work has found that disruption of the frontostriatal connections may play a role in ADHD [50].

Additional work by Silk and colleagues [51] further helps confirm the frontostriatal and frontoparietal circuitry abnormalities in children with ADHD.

A number of functional imaging studies have reported prefrontal cortical abnormalities in ADHD. In particular, dysfunction of the dlPFC and vlPFC has been identified [32]. Also, beyond the global and daMCC hypometabolism discussed previously, the PET study by Zametkin and colleagues [40] also showed regional hypoactivity of superior prefrontal cortex and premotor cortex. The meta-analysis by Dickstein and colleagues [42] provided confirmatory evidence of wider CFP neurocircuitry dysfunction in ADHD. Also, they identified a more limited set of regions including the vlPFC, daMCC, parietal cortex, and caudate and precentral gyrus. Notably, the dlPFC was not included on this list. These data helped clarify that dlPFC and vlPFC abnormalities may contribute to ADHD in different ways. Pharmacoimaging studies have further supported the conclusion that CFP hypofunction occurs in ADHD. Bush and colleagues [52] have noted that aside from an increase in activity in the daMCC, 6 weeks of methylphenidate also increased activation of the dlPFC and vlPFC (and also the parietal cortex, caudate, thalamus, and temporal lobe). Nonstimulant medications used for ADHD have also been studied in healthy male adults with fMRI. Atomoxetine, a selective noradrenaline reuptake inhibitor, was found to increase both inhibitory control on a stop-signal task and right vlPFC activation [53].

Clearly, the accumulated data from these fMRI, PET, and ERP studies, along with the biochemical, genetic, cortical thickness, and volumetric data reviewed earlier, provide compelling evidence that daMCC and dlPFC and vlPFC dysfunction likely contributes to the pathophysiology of ADHD.

The dlPFC is more responsible for overall planning and goal setting, the vlPFC and daMCC are responsible for inhibiting excessive or inappropriate motor behavior, the heteromodal parietal cortex assists with target detection and attention shifts, and the daMCC integrates information from these inputs and helps to execute such plans by modifying behavior on a trial-by-trial basis. Dysfunction within components of the CFP network in ADHD could, therefore, lead to inattention by failing to detect targets or inadequately filtering noise within the system. Such an inability to filter noise may be the reason that children with ADHD will wet without even knowing that they wet.

White matter abnormalities

White matter (WM) structural abnormalities or white matter hyperintensities (WMH) are common in older people. These WMH have been associated with impairments in mobility, cognition, affect, and continence [54]. Kuchel et al. [54] studied 100 elderly adults with MRI studies and looked at WMH in the brain of these patients. Presence of WMH in right inferior frontal regions and selected WM tracts predicts incontinence, incontinence severity, and degree of bother. Our observations support the findings of recent functional MRI studies indicating a critical role for the cingulum in bladder control, while also suggesting potential involvement of other nearby WM tracts such as anterior corona radiata and superior fronto-occipital fasciculus. In a similar study involving WMH in the elderly, Haruta et al. [55] were able to show that performance on an inhibitory control task is decreased in patients with cerebral WM changes with detrusor overactivity (DO). These findings are in concordance with brain imaging findings that the prefrontal cortex accounts for overactive bladder and incontinence. The DO was independent of general cognitive status. This is in direct contrast to Alzheimer's where dementia is the predominant symptoms and early incontinence is extremely rare.

How does this correlate to children?

We now understand that there is a link between adult neuropsychiatric disorders that affect the right frontal cortex and voiding dysfunction. There is growing evidence that children as young as 2 years of age can have depression [56], which we have seen is associated with right frontal lobe dysfunction and cortical abnormalities. The present day feeling is that chronic mental illness is a disease of the young, or at least its seeds are present in childhood, and given certain epigenetic factors, it can become unmasked. If depression can be present at such a young age, can other neuropsychiatric problems be present as well and even at a younger age? There is compelling evidence from the work of J. Kagan and S. Rauch [57] from long-term longitudinal follow-up of patients with what was initially described as inhibited and uninhibited temperament. Children with an inhibited temperament tend to avoid people and objects that are novel or unfamiliar. Uninhibited children approach novel persons or objects readily. It has been shown that an inhibited temperament is a risk factor for the development of anxiety in both childhood and adolescence and in particular social phobia. The amygdala has been implicated as a major player in these patients with inhibited temperament and these patients are high reactors; it becomes activated even to novel nonthreatening faces in experimental studies. This occurs because the amygdala participates in states of vigilance, as well as fear [58]. The authors suggest that "the amygdala is specialized for the detection, processing and integration of stimuli that have potential biological import, of which threat is only one possible example." Since it is known that situations that are stressful for individuals will lead to the development of bypass mechanisms that lead straight to the amygdala and do not lead to the areas involved in executive decision-making (PFC and ACG), one can see where some childhood situations can lead to abnormal or elevated responses by the amygdala and the ensuing cascade of problems that can derive from these abnormal pathways.

These temperament changes can be seen as early as 4 months and many of these patients will outgrow their fearfulness. Children have been classified as inhibited (high reactive) or uninhibited (low reactive) and the inhibited ones are the ones that are more likely to go on and develop social anxiety disorders. It was found that by age 15, two-thirds of those who had been high reactors in infancy behaved pretty much like everybody else. There has been work done that shows that the PFC in high-reactive individuals increases in size. It is unclear if this is a mechanism for compensating for the overactivity of the amygdala in these patients and it allows them to suppress their fears. Taking things one step further, they separated the high reactors from those that did and did not have social anxiety, and they found that the ones that had social anxiety had significant cortical thinning. This confirms other findings of cortical thinning in the PFC in patients with anxiety, depression, ADHD, and SCZ.

The aforementioned findings have potential implications in the children that we see with incontinence. It gives us the ability to postulate why children seem to outgrow their urge incontinence and urgency problems. In these high-reactive patients, our treatments have allowed us to temporize and buy time so that eventually the brain has a chance to change and fix the problem. In some cases, the PFC does not compensate, and we are left with those patients who become adults with urgency and frequency. These findings parallel the findings of Stone et al. [59] where up to one-third of their patients did not get better by 18 years of age. If the amygdalar responses are left unchecked by a thinned PFC, these amygdalar responses due to their multiple innervation pathways to other areas of the brain, especially the hypothalamus, can lead to unwanted effects downstream in the spine and bladder.

A stressful situation in a bathroom, fear of going to the bathroom in a strange place, and fear of having a painful bowel movement because the last one was painful can all lead to exaggerated amygdalar responses, which in turn can lead to elevated norepinephrine levels that can be associated with problems in opening of the bladder neck and possibly straining to void and the development of inappropriate pelvic floor activation. Prolonged exposure or repetitions of these scenarios can lead to permanent changes due to abnormal behavior, elevated NE levels, or increased secretion of CRF. These effects can lead to further physiologic changes in receptors and even in the muscle and blood vessels of the bladder. These changes can lead to alterations in the expression of neurotransmitters and other proinflammatory agents, which could potentially lead to diseases as such as OAB and interstitial cystitis, and CP/CPPS.

Conclusion

The literature is full of articles that preach the bladder as the center of all evils when it comes to voiding problems [47]. There is a preponderance of data in the neuropsychiatric literature that point to the ACG, dlPFC, and vmPFC as centers of dysfunction in some of the most common neuropsychiatric disorders. These same sites are the areas that are intimately affected in the control of urge and vigilance of the need to urinate. We have very little data from functional imaging in children who have enuresis. We can only extrapolate at this time that some of the structural and functional changes that we see in adults can be present in children as well. What triggers changes in the brain areas that may be morphologically different to cause incontinence in some and not in others are questions that are yet to be discovered. Clearly more work needs to be done with functional imaging in the future in children.

References

1 Gontard A, Nevéus T. *Management of disorders of bladder and bowel control in childhood*. London: Mac Keith Press; 2006. xi, 355 p.
2 Tekgul S, Nijman RJM, Hoebeke P, Canning D, Bower W, von Gontard A. Diagnosis and management of urinary incontinence in childhood. In: Abrams P, Cardozo L, Khoury S, Wein A, editors. *Incontinence*. 4th ed. Paris: Health Publications Ltd; 2009. p. 701–92.
3 Bael A, Winkler P, Lax H, Hirche H, Gabel E, Vijverberg M, et al. Behavior profiles in children with functional urinary incontinence before and after incontinence treatment. *Pediatrics*. 2008;**121**(5):e1196–200.
4 Baeyens D. The relationship between attention-deficit/hyperactivity disorder (ADHD) and enuresis in children. Gent, Belgium; 2005.

5 Baeyens D, Roeyers H, Hoebeke P, Verte S, Van Hoecke E, Walle JV. Attention deficit/ hyperactivity disorder in children with nocturnal enuresis. *J Urol.* 2004;**171**(6 Pt 2):2576–9.

6 Joinson C, Heron J, Butler U, von Gontard A. Psychological differences between children with and without soiling problems. *Pediatrics.* 2006;**117**(5):1575–84.

7 Joinson C, Heron J, von Gontard A, Butler U, Golding J, Emond A. Early childhood risk factors associated with daytime wetting and soiling in school-age children. *J Pediatr Psychol.* 2008;**33**(7):739–50.

8 Robson WL, Jackson HP, Blackhurst D, Leung AK. Enuresis in children with attention-deficit hyperactivity disorder. *South Med J.* 1997;**90**(5):503–5.

9 Sureshkumar P, Jones M, Cumming R, Craig J. A population based study of 2,856 school-age children with urinary incontinence. *J Urol.* 2009;**181**(2):808–15; discussion 15–6.

10 Baeyens D, Roeyers H, Van Erdeghem S, Hoebeke P, Vande Walle J. The prevalence of attention deficit-hyperactivity disorder in children with nonmonosymptomatic nocturnal enuresis: a 4-year follow-up study. *J Urol.* 2007;**178**(6):2616–20.

11 Vrijens D, Drossaerts J, van Koeveringe G, Van Kerrebroeck P, van Os J, Leue C. Affective symptoms and overactive bladder—systematic review. *J Psychosomatic Res* 2015; **78**(2): 95–108.

12 Botlero R, Bell RJ, Urquhart DM, Davis SR. Urinary incontinence is associated with lower psychological general well-being in community-dwelling women. *Menopause.* 2010;**17**(2):332–7.

13 Melville JL, Fan MY, Rau H, Nygaard IE, Katon WJ. Major depression and urinary incontinence in women: temporal associations in an epidemiologic sample. *Am J Obstet Gynecol.* 2009;**201**(5):490.e1–7.

14 Henin A, Biederman J, Mick E, Hirshfeld-Becker DR, Sachs GS, Wu Y, et al. Childhood antecedent disorders to bipolar disorder in adults: a controlled study. *J Affect Disord.* 2007;**99**(1–3):51–7.

15 Weissman MM, Gross R, Fyer A, Heiman GA, Gameroff MJ, Hodge SE, et al. Interstitial cystitis and panic disorder: a potential genetic syndrome. *Arch Gen Psychiatry.* 2004;**61**(3):273–9.

16 Moore KH, Sutherst JR. Response to treatment of detrusor instability in relation to psycho-neurotic status. *Br J Urol.* 1990;**66**(5):486–90.

17 Hyde TM, Deep-Soboslay A, Iglesias B, Callicott JH, Gold JM, Meyer-Lindenberg A, et al. Enuresis as a premorbid developmental marker of schizophrenia. *Brain.* 2008;**131** (Pt 9):2489–98.

18 Altman D, Forsman M, Falconer C, Lichtenstein P. Genetic influence on stress urinary incontinence and pelvic organ prolapse. *Eur Urol.* 2008;**54**(4):918–22.

19 Hannestad YS, Lie RT, Rortveit G, Hunskaar S. Familial risk of urinary incontinence in women: population based cross sectional study. *BMJ.* 2004;**329**(7471):889–91.

20 Rohr G, Kragstrup J, Gaist D, Christensen K. Genetic and environmental influences on urinary incontinence: a Danish population-based twin study of middle-aged and elderly women. *Acta Obstet Gynecol Scand.* 2004;**83**(10):978–82.

21 Wennberg AL, Altman D, Lundholm C, Klint A, Iliadou A, Peeker R, et al. Genetic influences are important for most but not all lower urinary tract symptoms: a population-based survey in a cohort of adult Swedish twins. *Eur Urol.* 2011;**59**(6):1032–8.

22 Tettamanti G, Altman D, Iliadou AN, Bellocco R, Pedersen NL. Depression, neuroticism, and urinary incontinence in premenopausal women: a nationwide twin study. *Twin Res Hum Genet.* 2013;**16**(5):977–84.

23 Franco I. Neuropsychiatric disorders and voiding problems in children. *Curr Urol Rep.* 2011;**12**(2):158–65.

24 Thermenos HW, Keshavan MS, Juelich RJ, Molokotos E, Whitfield-Gabrieli S, Brent BK, et al. A review of neuroimaging studies of young relatives of individuals with schizophrenia: a developmental perspective from schizotaxia to schizophrenia. *Am J Med Genet B Neuropsychiatr Genet.* 2013;**162B**(7):604–35.

25 Peterson BS, Warner V, Bansal R, Zhu H, Hao X, Liu J, et al. Cortical thinning in persons at increased familial risk for major depression. *Proc Natl Acad Sci U S A*. 2009;**106**(15):6273–8.

26 Koenigs M, Grafman J. The functional neuroanatomy of depression: distinct roles for ventromedial and dorsolateral prefrontal cortex. *Behav Brain Res*. 2009;**201**(2):239–43.

27 Brzezicka A. Integrative deficits in depression and in negative mood states as a result of fronto-parietal network dysfunctions. *Acta Neurobiol Exp*. 2013;**73**(3):313–25.

28 Mochizuki H, Saito H. Mesial frontal lobe syndromes: correlations between neurological deficits and radiological localizations. *Tohoku J Exp Med*. 1990;**161** Suppl:231–9.

29 Sakakibara R, Fowler CJ, Hattori T. Voiding and MRI analysis of the brain. *Int Urogynecol J Pelvic Floor Dysfunct*. 1999;**10**(3):192–9.

30 Moratti S, Rubio G, Campo P, Keil A, Ortiz T. Hypofunction of right temporoparietal cortex during emotional arousal in depression. *Arch Gen Psychiatry*. 2008;**65**(5):532–41.

31 Posner MI, Petersen SE. The attention system of the human brain. *Annu Rev Neurosci*. 1990;**13**:25–42.

32 Bush G.. Cingulate, frontal, and parietal cortical dysfunction in attention-deficit/hyperactivity disorder. *Biol Psychiatry*. 2011;**69**(12):1160–7.

33 Narr KL, Bilder RM, Toga AW, Woods RP, Rex DE, Szeszko PR, et al. Mapping cortical thickness and gray matter concentration in first episode schizophrenia. *Cereb Cortex*. 2005;**15**(6):708–19.

34 Im K, Lee JM, Seo SW, Hyung Kim S, Kim SI, Na DL. Sulcal morphology changes and their relationship with cortical thickness and gyral white matter volume in mild cognitive impairment and Alzheimer's disease. *Neuroimage*. 2008;**43**(1):103–13.

35 Bush E. Dorsal and anterior midcingulate cortex: roles in normal cognition and attention-deficit/hyperactivity disorder. In: Vogt B, editor. *Cingulate neurobiology and disease*. Oxford: Oxford University Press; 2009. p. 245–74.

36 Vogt B, editor. *Dorsal anterior midcingulate cortex: roles in normal cognition and disruption in attention deficit/hyperactivity disorder*. Oxford: Oxford University Press; 2009.

37 Makris N, Seidman LJ, Valera EM, Biederman J, Monuteaux MC, Kennedy DN, et al. Anterior cingulate volumetric alterations in treatment-naive adults with ADHD: a pilot study. *J Atten Disord*. 2010;**13**(4):407–13.

38 Shaw P, Lerch J, Greenstein D, Sharp W, Clasen L, Evans A, et al. Longitudinal mapping of cortical thickness and clinical outcome in children and adolescents with attention-deficit/hyperactivity disorder. *Arch Gen Psychiatry*. 2006;**63**(5):540–9.

39 Makris N, Biederman J, Valera EM, Bush G, Kaiser J, Kennedy DN, et al. Cortical thinning of the attention and executive function networks in adults with attention-deficit/hyperactivity disorder. *Cereb Cortex*. 2007;**17**(6):1364–75.

40 Zametkin AJ, Nordahl TE, Gross M, King AC, Semple WE, Rumsey J, et al. Cerebral glucose metabolism in adults with hyperactivity of childhood onset. *N Engl J Med*. 1990;**323**(20):1361–6.

41 Tamm L, Menon V, Ringel J, Reiss AL. Event-related FMRI evidence of frontotemporal involvement in aberrant response inhibition and task switching in attention-deficit/hyperactivity disorder. *J Am Acad Child Adolesc Psychiatry*. 2004;**43**(11):1430–40.

42 Dickstein SG, Bannon K, Castellanos FX, Milham MP. The neural correlates of attention deficit hyperactivity disorder: an ALE meta-analysis. *J Child Psychol Psychiatry*. 2006;**47**(10):1051–62.

43 Brown AB, Biederman J, Valera EM, Doyle AE, Bush G, Spencer T, et al. Effect of dopamine transporter gene (SLC6A3) variation on dorsal anterior cingulate function in attention-deficit/hyperactivity disorder. *Am J Med Genet B Neuropsychiatr Genet*. 2010;**153B**(2):365–75.

44 Seidman LJ, Valera EM, Bush G. Brain function and structure in adults with attention-deficit/hyperactivity disorder. *Psychiatr Clin North Am*. 2004;**27**(2):323–47.

45 Valera EM, Faraone SV, Murray KE, Seidman LJ. Meta-analysis of structural imaging findings in attention-deficit/hyperactivity disorder. *Biol Psychiatry*. 2007;**61**(12):1361–9.

46 Monuteaux MC, Seidman LJ, Faraone SV, Makris N, Spencer T, Valera E, et al. A preliminary study of dopamine D4 receptor genotype and structural brain alterations in adults with ADHD. *Am J Med Genet B Neuropsychiatr Genet*. 2008;**147B**(8):1436–41.

47 Roosen A, Chapple CR, Dmochowski RR, Fowler CJ, Gratzke C, Roehrborn CG, et al. The prevalence of attention deficit-hyperactivity disorder in children with nonmonosymptomatic nocturnal enuresis. *Eur Urol*. 2009.

48 Shaw P, Eckstrand K, Sharp W, Blumenthal J, Lerch JP, Greenstein D, et al. Attention-deficit/hyperactivity disorder is characterized by a delay in cortical maturation. *Proc Natl Acad Sci U S A*. 2007;**104**(49):19649–54.

49 Shaw P, Gornick M, Lerch J, Addington A, Seal J, Greenstein D, et al. Polymorphisms of the dopamine D4 receptor, clinical outcome, and cortical structure in attention-deficit/hyperactivity disorder. *Arch Gen Psychiatry*. 2007;**64**(8):921–31.

50 Casey BJ, Epstein JN, Buhle J, Liston C, Davidson MC, Tonev ST, et al. Frontostriatal connectivity and its role in cognitive control in parent-child dyads with ADHD. *Am J Psychiatry*. 2007;**164**(11):1729–36.

51 Silk TJ, Vance A, Rinehart N, Bradshaw JL, Cunnington R. White-matter abnormalities in attention deficit hyperactivity disorder: a diffusion tensor imaging study. *Hum Brain Mapp*. 2009;**30**(9):2757–65.

52 Bush G, Spencer TJ, Holmes J, Shin LM, Valera EM, Seidman LJ, et al. Functional magnetic resonance imaging of methylphenidate and placebo in attention-deficit/hyperactivity disorder during the multi-source interference task. *Arch Gen Psychiatry*. 2008;**65**(1):102–14.

53 Chamberlain SR, Hampshire A, Muller U, Rubia K, Del Campo N, Craig K, et al. Atomoxetine modulates right inferior frontal activation during inhibitory control: a pharmacological functional magnetic resonance imaging study. *Biol Psychiatry*. 2009;**65**(7):550–5.

54 Kuchel GA, Moscufo N, Guttmann CR, Zeevi N, Wakefield D, Schmidt J, et al. Localization of brain white matter hyperintensities and urinary incontinence in community-dwelling older adults. *J Gerontol A Biol Sci Med Sci*. 2009;**64**(8):902–9.

55 Haruta H, Sakakibara R, Ogata T, Panicker J, Fowler CJ, Tateno F, et al. Inhibitory control task is decreased in vascular incontinence patients. *Clin Auton Res*. 2013;**23**(2):85–9.

56 Klein DN, Dougherty LR, Olino TM. Toward guidelines for evidence-based assessment of depression in children and adolescents. *J Clin Child Adolesc Psychol*. 2005;**34**(3):412–32.

57 Schwartz CE, Wright CI, Shin LM, Kagan J, Rauch SL. Inhibited and uninhibited infants "grown up": adult amygdalar response to novelty. *Science*. 2003;**300**(5627):1952–3.

58 Schwartz CE, Wright CI, Shin LM, Kagan J, Whalen PJ, McMullin KG, et al. Differential amygdalar response to novel versus newly familiar neutral faces: a functional MRI probe developed for studying inhibited temperament. *Biol Psychiatry*. 2003;**53**(10):854–62.

59 Stone JJ, Rozzelle CJ, Greenfield SP. Intractable voiding dysfunction in children with normal spinal imaging: predictors of failed conservative management. *Urology*. 2010;**75**(1):161–5.

SECTION 3

Evaluation of bowel and bladder dysfunction

Yves Homsy

Introduction

The lower bowel and the bladder are organs located in the pelvis. They have a similar and mostly shared blood and nerve supply. It should come as no surprise that dysfunction in one organ may affect the function of the other. The issue of bowel interference with bladder function has become prominent in the overall management of wetting problems. The terms "Voiding Dysfunction" and "Dysfunctional Elimination Syndrome" have been renamed "Bowel/Bladder Dysfunction" by the ICCS Nomenclature Committee, hence the importance of having a working knowledge of this condition, the pathophysiology of which resides within and encompasses elements from two pediatric subspecialties.

The tools used for the evaluation of Bowel/Bladder Dysfunction are initially based on a careful subjective history followed by non- or minimally invasive methods of investigation, reserving more invasive methods to "hard core" cases.

Chapter 8 is a step-by-step outline that elegantly demonstrates how to perform and interpret urodynamic studies in children. It is divided into noninvasive and invasive sections and emphasizes that sensate patients with nonneurogenic dysfunction must be carefully selected to undergo this type of testing and must be adequately and gently prepared for results to be reliable.

Chapter 9 explains in detail the components of uroflowmetry in different age groups. It is of the least invasive of all urodynamic tests. Parameters are described to properly perform and interpret uroflowmetry and thus save the patient from needing more invasive testing. Because of its noninvasiveness, the test may be readily repeated to ensure that the bladder was sufficiently full and that voiding was complete, as determined by immediate postvoid bladder ultrasonography.

Pediatric Incontinence: Evaluation and Clinical Management, First Edition. Edited by Israel Franco, Paul F. Austin, Stuart B. Bauer, Alexander von Gontard and Yves Homsy.
© 2015 John Wiley & Sons, Ltd. Published 2015 by John Wiley & Sons, Ltd.

Chapters 10 and 11 address the validity of questionnaires in assessing bladder and bowel dysfunction. A classification of nonneurogenic voiding disorders is provided in Chapter 10 to guide the reader in categorizing voiding disorders according to severity. The diagnosis and management of bowel issues in the voiding dysfunction context are discussed in depth in both Chapters 10 and 11. The eight tests that are currently in use for the evaluation of constipation/fecal incontinence are reviewed and placed in perspective. As it is mentioned in Chapter 18, because long-term recovery rates of constipation are low, ranging roughly from 50 to 70%, it is not a problem that all children will outgrow and long-term management will remain necessary.

CHAPTER 8

Urodynamics in the pediatric patient

Beth A. Drzewiecki[1] and Stuart B. Bauer[2]

[1] *Department of Urology, Children's Hospital at Montefiore, Bronx, NY, USA*
[2] *Department of Urology, Boston Children's Hospital, Harvard University, Boston, MA, USA*

Introduction

Urodynamic studies (UDS) have become common practice in the evaluation of infants and children with either neurogenic (NBD) or nonneurogenic bladder (NNBD) dysfunction or other associated conditions that might affect lower urinary tract function. Application of UDS in the infant, child, or adolescent requires adaptations to achieve meaningful results and accurate assessment of lower urinary tract (LUT) function leading to evidence-based programs for therapy. Standardization of techniques will permit reproducibility of results and comparison between centers.

This chapter is designed as a concise guide for pediatric urologists, nurse practitioners, or nurses involved with urodynamic testing on the technical aspects of performing UDS as well as the adaptations for children to optimize obtainment of meaningful results. A subsequent chapter will focus primarily on the noninvasive components of UDS such as uroflowmetry.

Evaluation of children prior to UDS

Initial assessment of a child with suspected or overt neuropathic bladder dysfunction, or functional LUT symptoms is multifaceted. Any method used to measure the function of the lower urinary tract function comprises urodynamics [1]. Therefore, the most important initial aspects of a UDS are a thorough history and a complete physical examination, voiding and defecation diaries that establish current bladder and bowel elimination patterns, information regarding UTIs and often a baseline ultrasonography, to identify

Pediatric Incontinence: Evaluation and Clinical Management, First Edition. Edited by Israel Franco, Paul F. Austin, Stuart B. Bauer, Alexander von Gontard and Yves Homsy.
© 2015 John Wiley & Sons, Ltd. Published 2015 by John Wiley & Sons, Ltd.

Table 8.1 Evaluation prior to UDS.

	Information to be obtained
History	Prenatal history Perinatal complications Family history
Physical examination	Spinal abnormalities Lower extremity reflexes, muscle mass, strength, gait, sensation Handedness, fine/gross motor coordination
Voiding diary	Characterization of incontinence; continuous, intermittent, day and/or night Fluid intake Frequency of catheterizations with/without incontinence between catheterization Frequency of voids Voided volumes
Defecation diary	Number of bowel movements per day Character of stool; hard, soft, diarrhea Presence of painful defecation Incontinence of stool episodes
Laboratory	Urinalysis and urine culture
Radiology	Spinal sonogram if indicated <3 months of age Renal bladder sonogram: bladder wall thickness, hydronephrosis, PVR, dilation of rectum VCUG: bladder contour, bladder neck appearance, urethral anatomy, VUR

any anatomic abnormalities of the upper or lower urinary tract. Components that make up this extensive investigation are listed in Table 8.1. If video imaging is not available, a voiding cystourethrogram should be obtained prior to the study, if warranted, to evaluate the bladder neck and proximal urethra, bladder contour, congenital abnormalities, or presence of vesicoureteral reflux.

Preparation of the child for UDS

One of the most important keys to success of UDS is having a dedicated and knowledgeable staff. Many children who present for UDS have already had prior invasive studies and thus may be traumatized and quite anxious. Involving both parents and the child throughout the study can increase the likelihood of a more comprehensive study with minimal artifact. Age appropriate distractions such as a pacifier, feeding with a bottle, watching television, or playing a video game can also be helpful to keep the child calm and quiet. Child life specialists, when available, can be extremely useful to ease the child's anxiety and keep them focused and calm throughout the procedure.

When age appropriate, a full explanation that involves what the test is about and why it needs to be done using visual aids, such as photos or a catheterizable doll, may decrease anxiety as the study progresses [1].

There is no standardization regarding timing of medications prior to UDS. It is these authors' opinion that bladder modulating medications should be given so their peak activity occurs around the time of the UDS. For most anticholinergic medications, this would be 2–3 h prior to the investigation. A rectal suppository or enema should be given the night before the UDS in children with severe constipation so as to minimize difficulty with rectal channel monitoring of abdominal pressure. This clean out may also eliminate changes in bladder function secondary to a distended rectum.

Invasive urodynamics

Invasive UDS include a cystometrogram to determine bladder capacity, contractility, compliance, emptying ability, and degree of continence [2]. In toilet-trained children, a uroflowmetry is also performed to obtain information on the voiding phase of the micturition cycle. Real-time viewing of UDS results can provide insight into the diagnosis, as well as accurate interpretation of findings. Urethral and rectal catheters are used to obtain intravesical and intra-abdominal pressure recordings, respectively, to denote any straining, especially when voiding. Detrusor pressure is calculated by continuous subtraction of the intra-abdominal from the intravesical pressure transducers to correct for changes that might occur during laughing, coughing, movement, or talking during the study.

Catheter and electrode placement

A latex-free environment should be maintained [3]. Prior to catheterization, intraurethral placement of topical 2% lidocaine jelly for several minutes improves placement of the catheter while reducing distress and crying, with minimal effect on UDS tracings [3]. A 6-Fr double lumen catheter is placed under aseptic technique and secured in place. In children with NGB, catheter placement allows for accurate assessment of the PVR as well as intravesical pressure at that volume that has taken place during natural filling.

This measurement has been labeled "pressure at residual volume."

Children with prior urethral surgery or high anxiety preventing easy catheter placement may require sedation, with or without cystoscopy, before the study [3].

A suprapubic catheter can also be inserted for natural fill cystometry. If this latter maneuver is required, a 6-Fr double lumen catheter is generally placed under sedation 6–24 h prior to the study [4].

A 7- or 10-Fr rectal balloon catheter is placed and is generally well tolerated by the child. If there has been an inadequate bowel clean out and stool is still palpable in the rectal vault, manual disimpaction should be performed to prevent defecation during the study or loss of the balloon catheter by extrusion.

Children can be positioned either supine or semirecumbent on the table or in the sitting position on a commode without a significant difference in the results [5]. In children who can sit, it is the preferred position for ease of voiding into the uroflowmeter and to reduce risk of losing catheters during repositioning. The feet should comfortably rest on either the floor or be supported by a foot stool.

Electromyography (EMG) of the striated component of the external sphincter and pelvic floor musculature is also an important component of UDS, and most centers utilize a patch EMG electrode with a capacity of at least 1000 Hz. Patch electromyography electrodes are placed on the perineum in the 3 and 9 o'clock positions or a 24-gauge needle electrode is positioned perineally in boys or paraurethral in girls. EMG needle electrodes can be employed during cystometry to provide the most accurate information on individual motor units at rest, in response to sacral reflexes, and during bladder filling and emptying in patients with suspected or known neurologic conditions and in whom sensation in the area is diminished or absent.

Cystometry

Filling the bladder should be performed at a rate of 5–10% of the age expected bladder capacity per minute with saline at a temperature of 21–37°C. The rate of filling may have an adverse effect on capacity, intravesical pressure, and compliance [1]. The expected bladder capacity can be calculated from the Hjalmas equation (expected capacity (mL) = 30 + (age in years × 30)). For children with myelodysplasia, it can be calculated using the formula 24.5 × age (years) + 62 [6]. Expected capacity in children who perform CIC can also be estimated by the largest recorded volume drained from the bladder during CIC, throughout the day, over a 3–4-day period.

A minimum of two filling cycles should be performed during the UDS once the child is as relaxed as possible. The first filling cycle is often artificial and inaccurate. If the child has NBD and no sensation, then the single cycle of filling may suffice. Filling should continue until one of the following conditions is met; the child has a strong urge to void, is uncomfortable, micturition occurs, detrusor pressure reaches a level that is >40 cm H_2O with an overactive contraction, volume of infused fluid exceeds at least 150% of expected capacity or the rate of leakage is greater than the rate of infusion. Some children with a much larger bladder may need additional filling to determine if they can initiate voiding only at these large volumes.

Alternatively, cystometry can be performed using the body's natural diuresis to fill the bladder, called natural fill cystometry or ambulatory urodynamics. In this setting, the child is permitted to be mobile and thus more compatible with his/her own environment, providing less overall psychological stress. The results of natural fill cystometry have identified several differences when compared to conventional filling. Natural fill studies elucidate lower voided volumes, higher voiding pressures, a dampened increase in the pressure rise during filling and increased sensitivity for detecting detrusor overactivity [4].

Combining fluoroscopic video imaging during the UDS can significantly improve the latter's diagnostic accuracy and lead to a more advanced level of interpretation. Information regarding the shape and contour of the bladder, detrusor pressure at leakage or VUR and evaluation of the bladder neck during filling and voiding as well as presence of simultaneous intrinsic sphincter deficiency can be obtained.

Sometimes, radionuclide cystography is performed simultaneously with cystometry to determine under what circumstances (children with) known reflux may occur, that is, an overactive contraction and/or a rise in detrusor pressure above a certain level.

Bladder storage function

Interpretation of the UDS should be performed by a trained pediatric urologist, UDS nurse practitioner or other urodynamicist. It is best accomplished in real time, while visualizing the study and observing the patient's behavior and response. In children who are too young to describe what they are feeling, curling of the toes and tightening of the abdomen may be signs that the bladder is becoming uncomfortably full and voiding is imminent.

Bladder storage function should be described in terms of the following [2]:
- Bladder sensation: first sensation, first desire, strong desire, unable to hold, correlation with contractions, markedly diminished, or absent
- Detrusor activity: normal, overactive, underactive [7]
- Bladder compliance: high or low
- Bladder capacity: less than expected ($\leq 70\%$), expected, or greater ($\geq 150\%$) than expected

Bladder sensation can only be ascertained in children who are old enough to understand and articulate their various bladder sensations. Diminished or absent bladder sensation may be identified on UDS when greater than expected bladder capacity has been reached without a change in sensation.

Bladder capacity and compliance

Bladder capacity in children does not change in a linear fashion with age, even though a linear formula is almost universally used to calculate capacity. Accepted values of normal compliance are either $10\,cm\,H_2O$ at capacity or 5% of the child's normal capacity per cm H_2O [1].

Uroflowmetry

The study should not be considered complete until there is a spontaneous void in children capable of performing it. Children who are toilet trained should void into a urimeter. They should be either well, but not overly, hydrated or have withheld urination for a period of time so they have a reasonable desire to void.

Information to be recorded from uroflow includes the following:
- Q_{max}—maximum voiding pressure that is sustained for $>2\,s$
- Q_{ave}—mean voiding pressure over the course of the void
- Flow time
- Volume voided
- Flow curve pattern: bell, tower shaped, staccato, plateau, interrupted

High voiding pressures with poor flow rates are indicative of either anatomic or functional bladder outlet or urethral obstruction. Functional obstruction is often the result of pelvic floor muscle contractions (registered and recorded on patch EMG) during voiding that may produce a staccato voiding pattern.

A persistently low flow rate during voiding is more suggestive of an anatomical obstruction, presuming the EMG activity of the sphincter is quiet. It is also important to evaluate whether or not the voiding pressure has been sustained throughout the entire contraction resulting in complete emptying of the bladder.

In children who are not toilet trained, observation of the void is important. Information such as sustained, strong stream, intermittent voiding associated with Valsalva, slow leakage, or dribbling should be noted with correlation of the bladder contraction and EMG.

Voiding pressures in infants trend higher than older children. Similarly, boys have higher median voiding pressures than girls, about $5–15\,cm\,H_2O$.

A PVR should be obtained within 5 min or less of completion of the voiding phase by emptying via the catheter or bladder echography if the catheter was removed. A range of 5–20 mL may be associated with incomplete emptying and that suggests repeating the study [2, 8].

Timing of UDS

In children born with a myelomeningocele, a tethered spinal cord, sacral agenesis, or an anorectal malformation, a baseline UDS should be obtained between 3 and 6 months of age and routinely yearly thereafter if the child is at risk for a changing neurological lesion. Changes in management, physical examination findings such as lower extremity weakness or pain, new onset or an increase in hydronephrosis, recurrent UTI and/or new onset of or worsening urinary incontinence, should prompt earlier UDS.

Other congenital obstructive abnormalities such as posterior urethral valves or obstructive ureteroceles may cause bladder outlet obstruction and UDS may identify the need for medications that modulate lower urinary tract function or surgery [1]. Changes in management, surgical interventions, or worsening renal function should also prompt repeat UDS.

Some children with nonneurogenic bladder dysfunction may also require UDS. Typically, all other conservative measures should have been attempted in these children before invasive UDS is performed to direct further management [9].

Conclusion

UDS in the pediatric population requires a dedicated staff and facility with extensive knowledge of proper techniques to achieve maximal results. When used appropriately, UDS can provide accurate clinical information for diagnosis and guide efficacious treatment decisions in the pediatric population.

References

1 de Jong TPVM, Klijn AJ. Urodynamics in pediatric urology. *Nat Rev Urol*. 2009; **6**: 585–94.

2 Nevéus T, von Gontard A, Hoebeke P, et al. The standardization of terminology of lower urinary tract function in children and adolescents: report from the Standardisation Committee of the International Children's Continence Society. *J Urol*. 2006; **176**: 314–24.

3 Gray M. Traces: making sense of urodynamic testing—part 13: pediatric urodynamics. *Urol Nurs*. 2012; **32**: 251–6.

4 Jorgenson B, Olsen LH, Jorgenson TM. Natural fill urodynamics and conventional cystometrogram in infants with neurogenic bladder. *J Urol*. 2009; **181**: 1862–9.

5 Lorenzo AJ, Wallis MC, Cook A, et al. What is the variability in urodynamic parameters with position change in children? Analysis of a prospectively enrolled cohort. *J Urol*. 2007; **178**: 2567–70.

6 Palmer LS, Richards I, Kaplan WE. Age related bladder capacity and bladder capacity growth in children with myelomeningocele. *J Urol*. 1997; **158**: 1261–4.

7 Austin PF, Bauer SB, Bower W, et al. The standardization of terminology of lower urinary tract function in children and adolescents: update report from the standardization committee of the International Children's Continence Society. *J Urol*. 2014; **191**: 1863–5.

8 Chang SJ, Chiang IN, Hseih CH, Lin CD, Yang SSD. Age and gender specific nomograms for single and dual post void residual urine in healthy children. *Neurorol Urodyn*. 2013; **32**: 1014–8.

9 Kaufman MR, DeMarco RT, Pope JC 4th, et al. High yield of urodynamics performed for refractory nonneurogenic dysfunctional voiding in the pediatric population. *J Urol*. 2006; **176**: 1835–7.

CHAPTER 9

Uroflowmetry and postvoid residual urine tests in incontinent children

Stephen Shei-Dei Yang and Shang-Jen Chang

Division of Urology, Taipei Tzu Chi Hospital, The Buddhist Medical Foundation, Tzu Chi University, New Taipei, and Buddhist Tzu Chi University, Hualien, Taiwan

Introduction

Uroflowmetry test is simple and noninvasive. Therefore, it is widely accepted as an initial diagnostic tool to evaluate the lower urinary tract function in children [1, 2]. It reflects the general performance of detrusor contractility and bladder outlet resistance. It helps pediatric urologists decide whether the child should undergo further invasive studies and receive treatments. Additionally, it can help us monitor the objective response to medical and surgical treatment [1, 2].

Indication for uroflowmetry and PVR tests

Uroflowmetry tests are indicated in toilet-trained children with lower urinary tract symptoms and urinary tract infections [1, 2]. With noninvasive characteristics, there existed no specific contraindication for the tests. However, we usually do not perform these tests when the child is in acute illness or active urinary tract infections.

Preparation

Before tests, the uroflowmeter should be calibrated and the scale of interpretation sheet should be adjusted to a $1:1$ ratio for flow rate (mL/s) versus time (s). The uroflowmeter should be placed in a quiet and private place that make the children feel comfortable and relaxed. Before tests, the child should be well hydrated. The suggested amount of fluids that the child need to intake 1 h before test is equal to the expected bladder capacity, that is, (age in years + 1) × 30 mL [1]. The child micturates at normal urge to void. The voiding posture for boy can be either standing or squatting. As for girls, both squatting and sitting are acceptable but good foot supported is a prerequisite.

Pediatric Incontinence: Evaluation and Clinical Management, First Edition. Edited by Israel Franco, Paul F. Austin, Stuart B. Bauer, Alexander von Gontard and Yves Homsy.
© 2015 John Wiley & Sons, Ltd. Published 2015 by John Wiley & Sons, Ltd.

Interpretation

The parameters generated from uroflowmetry tests included voided volume (mL), peak flow rate (maximal flow rate or Qmax, mL/s), time to peak flow rate (s), average flow rate (mL/s), voiding time (s), flow time (s), and uroflow patterns (Figure 9.1). Care should be taken to see if there is artifact (sharp peak in flow curve with duration less than 2 s) owing to accidental movement of the uroflowmeter when child is voiding. Among these parameters, the most relevant parameters for interpretation are voided volume (mL), Qmax (mL/s), and uroflow patterns. As these parameters generated from uroflowmetry were dependent on bladder capacity (voided volume + PVR), the optimal bladder

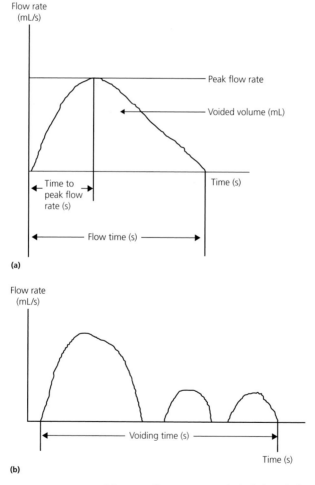

Figure 9.1 The parameters generated from uroflowmetry tests included voided volume (mL), peak flow rate (maximal flow rate or Qmax, mL/s), time to peak flow rate (s), average flow rate (mL/s), flow time (s), and voiding time (s).

capacity for interpretation of uroflowmetry tests is between 50 and 115% of expected bladder capacity [3, 4]. Uroflowmetry with voided volume of less 50 mL [5] is regarded as irrelevant for interpretation and the tests should be repeated. PVR should be checked in these children to rule out the possibility of overflow incontinence. Additionally, children with their urinary bladder overdistended (defined as bladder capacity >115% EBC or voided volume >100% EBC) tended to have more abnormal uroflow patterns and elevated PVRs [3, 6]. Therefore, care should be taken in interpreting the uroflowmetry if the child overdistended their bladder.

Peak flow rate (Qmax)

Peak flow rate is defined as the maximal flow rate during voiding with duration more than 2 s. Qmax is regarded by ICCS as the most relevant variable when assessing status of bladder outflow resistance [1]. Of the several existed nomograms for Qmax [7–10], Yang et al. chose the higher value of two consecutive uroflowmetry to construct the dual-Qmax nomogram with ranking method (Figure 9.2) [7]. Minimally acceptable Qmax, that is, around 5th to 10th percentile of nomogram, is defined as 11.5 mL/s in children below the age of 6 years and 15.0 mL/s in children with age 7 years old or above [7]. ICCS suggested that Qmax with value larger than square root of the VV is regarded as normal, which is around 10th–25th percentile of dual-Qmax nomograms.

Uroflow patterns

Under some conditions, detrusor contractility in children is so good that can overcome bladder outlet resistance, which makes the Qmax not be so reliable in the evaluation of bladder outlet resistance. Therefore, some pediatric urologists consider the uroflow pattern to be a more important parameter than the Qmax. The uroflow pattern could give us the clue to the possible underlying etiology of the lower urinary tract dysfunction of the children. ICCS suggested that uroflow patterns can be classified as bell-shaped, interrupted, staccato, tower, and plateau types [1]. Only bell-shaped curve is regarded as normal. Interrupted flow (Figure 9.3a) is defined as flow rate that reached zero during voiding, which may imply detrusor underactivity or pelvic flow overactivity during voiding. Plateau-shaped curve (Figure 9.3b) is defined as continuous, low amplitude, and flattened flow. Peak flow rate less than the age-specific minimally acceptable Qmax, and lasting for 4 s could be two useful parameters to define plateau curve, which implies bladder outlet mechanical obstruction or tonic sphincter contraction. Staccato flow pattern (Figure 9.3c) is defined as irregular and fluctuated flow curve, and the fluctuations between peak and trough should be larger than square root of Qmax. The etiology of staccato flow curve is assumed to be sphincter overactivity. Tower shaped (Figure 9.3d) is defined as sudden and high-amplitude flow, which is suggestive of overactive bladder. Peak flow rate more than age-specific 95th

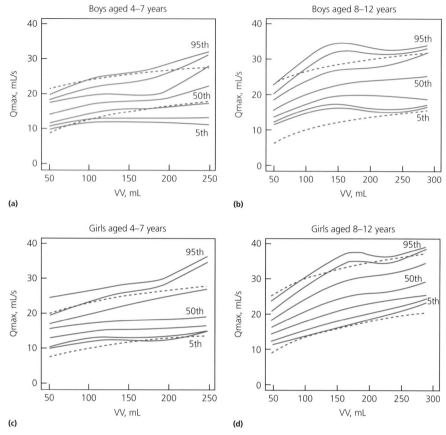

Figure 9.2 Dual-Qmax nomograms (the lines of percentiles were 5th, 10th, 25th, 50th, 75th, 90th, and 95th percentiles, respectively, from the bottom up) in boys and girls aged 4–7 and 8–12 years. The 5th and 95th percentile line of the Miskolc nomogram (dash lines) were plotted on the figures for comparison. Source: Yang et al. [7]. Reproduced with permission from Yang et al. and BJU International.

percentile of Qmax nomogram (ranking nomogram) may be regarded as high amplitude. In healthy children, the proportion of nonbell-shaped curves ranges widely from 2.8 to 37% [3, 11, 12], while only 3.8% of healthy children had repetitive nonbell-shaped curves, which can be defined as abnormal. In children with a diagnosis of dysfunctional voiding, nearly a third had an interrupted or mixed flow patterns and 14% had bell-shaped or depressed curves [13]. All types of abnormal flow pattern had been reported in healthy children. In addition, subjective uroflowmetry patterning is liable to personal bias [14] and there existed substantial interobserver disagreement in classifying the uroflow pattern into specific abnormal patterns [15]. Arguing specific type of abnormal flow pattern may not be clinically relevant. However, uroflowmetry serves as a good screening diagnostic tool in pediatric LUTD because interobserver's

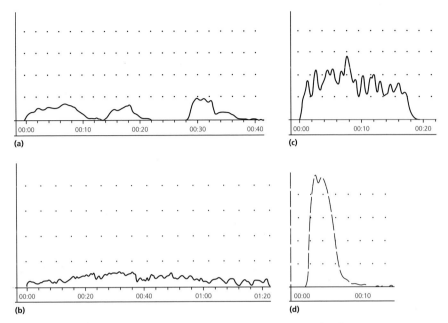

Figure 9.3 Patterns of uroflowmetry curves. (**a**) Interrupted curve. (**b**) Plateau curve.
(**c**) Staccato curve. (**d**) Tower curve.

agreement in normalcy of flow pattern is good [15]. One can determine whether further invasive urodynamic study is warranted if the child had repeated abnormal flow patterns.

EMG test during uroflowmetry test

The use of EMG during pediatric uroflowmetry is controversial. EMG may help us diagnose detrusor and sphincter/pelvic floor dyssynergy when the uroflow pattern showed staccato or interrupted flow patterns [13]. However, the perianal surface EMG may be compromised by artifact and may not reflect urinary sphincter activity.

Postvoid residual urine (PVR) tests

PVR should be checked with transabdominal ultrasound within 5 min after voiding. Though urethral catheterization may be more accurate, the major drawbacks, including invasiveness, possible complications of urinary tract infection, and associated discomfort, prevent its wide acceptability as screening tests. According to the nomograms generated from 1028 children (Figure 9.4), in children ≤6 years old, a single PVR >30 mL or >21% BC, or repetitive PVR >20 mL or >10% BC can be regarded as elevated. For children 7 years old, a single PVR >20 mL or 15% BC, or repetitive PVR >10 mL or 6% BC can be defined as elevated [16]. Due to high variability of PVR tests, repetitive test for PVR is warranted when the first PVR is high [17].

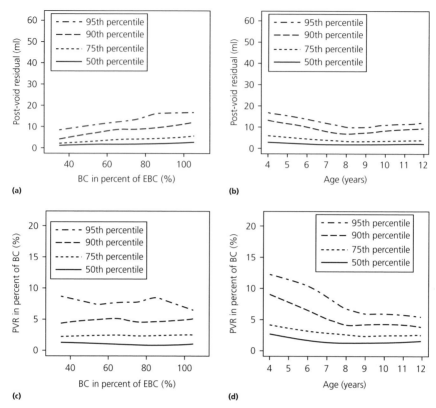

Figure 9.4 (need reprint permission) Dual-PVR nomogram for PVR in milliliter **(a** and **b)** and PVR in percent of bladder capacity, BC, **(c** and **d)** over varied age and BC/EBC. The lines of 50th, 75th, 90th, and 95th percentiles were plotted separately in the nomograms. Source: Chang et al. [16]. Reproduced with permission from Wiley Periodicals, Inc.

Bladder wall thickness can be measured with ultrasound when the urinary bladder is full and empty [18]. Increased bladder wall thickness may be associated with detrusor overactivity or neurogenic bladder, while decreased thickness may be associated with detrusor underactivity. However, a number of confounding variables and a lack of standardized methodology have resulted in discrepancies among studies. Therefore, reproducible diagnostic ranges or cutoff values have not been established.

Conclusion

Uroflowmetry is a good screening tool for toilet-trained children with lower urinary tract symptoms and dysfunction. To improve interobserver reliability and decrease discrepancy, we recommend a step-by-step approach in interpretation of uroflowmetry and PVR tests as shown in Table 9.1.

Table 9.1 Interpretation sheet for uroflowmetry and PVR.

Gender: ☐ boy   ☐ girl   Age: years

Expected bladder capacity (EBC):   mL, (age in years + 1) × 30 mL

PVR: mL. ☐ normal   ☐ elevated

Voided volume: mL   ☐ <50 mL   ☐ <50% (EBC)   ☐ >100% (EBC)

Bladder capacity: mL   ☐ <50 mL   ☐ <50% (EBC)   ☐ >115% (EBC)

Qmax: mL/s,   ☐ presence of artifact

Uroflow patterns:

Grade of normalcy: ☐ Normal, ☐ Probably normal, ☐ Equivocal, ☐ Probably abnormal, ☐ Abnormal

Specific abnormal pattern: ☐ interrupted, ☐ staccato, ☐ tower, ☐plateau

Recommendations:

☐ normal, no need of further tests

☐ repeat uroflowmetry tests

☐ further (video) urodynamic studies

References

1 Neveus T, von GA, Hoebeke P, Hjalmas K, Bauer S, Bower W, et al. The standardization of terminology of lower urinary tract function in children and adolescents: report from the Standardisation Committee of the International Children's Continence Society. *J Urol* 2006 Jul;**176**(1):314–24.

2 Chang SJ, Yang SS. Non-invasive assessments of pediatric voiding dysfunction. *LUTS* 2009;**1**(1):63–9.

3 Yang SS, Chang SJ. The effects of bladder over distention on voiding function in kindergarteners. *J Urol* 2008 Nov;**180**(5):2177–82.

4 Yang SS, Wang CC, Chen YT. Home uroflowmetry for the evaluation of boys with urinary incontinence. *J Urol* 2003 Apr;**169**(4):1505–7.

5 Norgaard JP, van Gool JD, Hjalmas K, Djurhuus JC, Hellstrom AL. Standardization and definitions in lower urinary tract dysfunction in children. International Children's Continence Society. *Br J Urol* 1998 May;**81**(Suppl 3):1–16.

6 Chang SJ, Yang SS, Chiang IN. Large voided volume suggestive of abnormal uroflow pattern and elevated post-void residual urine. *Neurourol Urodyn* 2011 Jan;**30**(1):58–61.

7 Yang SS, Chiang IN, Hsieh CH, Chang SJ. The Tzu Chi nomograms for peak flow rate in children: comparison with Miskolc nomogram. *BJU Int* 2014;**113**(3):492–7.

8 Kajbafzadeh AM, Yazdi CA, Rouhi O, Tajik P, Mohseni P. Uroflowmetry nomogram in Iranian children aged 7 to 14 years. *BMC Urol* 2005;**5**:3.

9 Szabo L, Fegyverneki S. Maximum and average urine flow rates in normal children—the Miskolc nomograms. *Br J Urol* 1995 Jul;**76**(1):16–20.

10 Gupta DK, Sankhwar SN, Goel A. Uroflowmetry nomograms for healthy children 5 to 15 years old. *J Urol* 2013 Sep;**190**(3):1008–13.

11 Bower WF, Kwok B, Yeung CK. Variability in normative urine flow rates. *J Urol* 2004 Jun;**171**(6 Pt 2):2657–9.

12 Mattsson S, Spangberg A. Urinary flow in healthy schoolchildren. *Neurourol Urodyn* 1994;**13**(3):281–96.

13 Wenske S, Van Batavia JP, Combs AJ, Glassberg KI. Analysis of uroflow patterns in children with dysfunctional voiding. *J Pediatr Urol* 2013 Nov;**10**(2):250–4.

14 Kanematsu A, Johnin K, Yoshimura K, Okubo K, Aoki K, Watanabe M, et al. Objective patterning of uroflowmetry curves in children with daytime and nighttime wetting. *J Urol* 2010 Oct;**184**(4 Suppl):1674–9.

15 Chang SJ, Yang SS. Inter-observer and intra-observer agreement on interpretation of uroflowmetry curves of kindergarten children. *J Pediatr Urol* 2008 Dec;**4**(6):422–7.

16 Chang SJ, Chiang IN, Hsieh CH, Lin CD, Yang SS. Age- and gender-specific nomograms for single and dual post-void residual urine in healthy children. *Neurourol Urodyn* 2013 Sep;**32**(7):1014–8.

17 Chang SJ, Yang SS. Variability, related factors and normal reference value of post-void residual urine in healthy kindergarteners. *J Urol* 2009 Oct;**182**(4 Suppl):1933–8.

18 Bright E, Oelke M, Tubaro A, Abrams P. Ultrasound estimated bladder weight and measurement of bladder wall thickness—useful noninvasive methods for assessing the lower urinary tract? *J Urol* 2010 Nov;**184**(5):1847–54.

CHAPTER 10

Evaluation of the child with voiding dysfunction

Yves Homsy

All Children's Hospital/Johns Hopkins Medicine, Saint Joseph's Children's Hospital, Tampa/St. Petersburg, FL, USA

Introduction

Voiding dysfunction disorders are reported to occur in about 20% of school-aged children [1]. Peak prevalence occurs at 5 to 6 years of age (10%), and it tapers down to 5% between 6 and 12 years and down further to 4% between 12 and 18 years [2]. These disorders are exhibited in approximately 40% of patients presenting to the pediatric urologist [3].

It is helpful to be prepared with the questions to ask in the course of the evaluation of the child with voiding dysfunction.

History and physical examination

The history and physical examination constitute an important part in the evaluation of the child with voiding dysfunction. History should be age appropriate and it should mirror the age, sex, and stage of development of the individual child. It should include questions addressing day and/or night wetting, urgency, frequency, posturing, history of febrile and afebrile urinary tract infection (UTI), dietary history, and stool habits (frequency, straining, consistency, and shape). Questions addressing the posture adopted on the toilet seat should be asked. Are the child's feet resting on the floor or on a footstool for urination and defecation (girls) and for defecation (boys)?

Pediatric Incontinence: Evaluation and Clinical Management, First Edition. Edited by Israel Franco,
Paul F. Austin, Stuart B. Bauer, Alexander von Gontard and Yves Homsy.
© 2015 John Wiley & Sons, Ltd. Published 2015 by John Wiley & Sons, Ltd.

Questionnaires and their validity

Since 2000, several validated questionnaires were developed to ensure uniform history taking in children with bladder dysfunction [4–6]. Despite the validity of these questionnaires, an extensive survey among a large number of Turkish pediatric urologists and nephrologists revealed that their utilization of validated questionnaires was scant and almost one half admitted that they were not appropriately evaluating their patients. In addition, only one quarter of children with lower urinary tract dysfunction were submitted to standard urotherapy, which is now considered to be one of the first steps in the management of this condition, before submitting patients to pharmacotherapy. Eighty-six percent of the physicians surveyed reported that the management of these children was being inadequately approached [7].

Most available questionnaires are similar and each uses its particular scoring system. The Vancouver is the most recent questionnaire and claims superiority on account of taking into consideration both validity and reliability [6] (Figure 10.1). While it is true that the care of children with bladder dysfunction can be quite time-consuming within the context of a busy practice, requiring much of a physician's time, some practices have trained specially designated nurses to help with this task and have achieved rewarding results.

It is important to remember that in addition to the voiding symptoms that usually constitute the main complaint, many patients are also enuretic and parents should be made to understand that daytime symptoms must be addressed before the enuresis component can be appropriately managed. This is because although some enuretics share etiological factors with daytime wetters, there are other factors that come into play in the etiology and management of enuresis (see chapters 22, 23 and 24).

Classification and major features of voiding dysfunction disorders

An overview of the different types of voiding dysfunction can be useful in the evaluation and in the charting of an appropriate treatment plan that could be tailored to the needs of each individual patient. The following classification of voiding dysfunction disorders may serve as a useful guide to help the reader navigate the different types of dysfunction and their possible repercussions on the upper urinary tract and renal function. Brief management guidelines are also provided.

Voiding dysfunction disorders may be classified into minor, moderate, and major according to their level of impact on the upper urinary tract [8]. Minor disorders have no impact on the upper urinary tract whereas moderate disorders may have some impact and major disorders have overt upper tract manifestations.

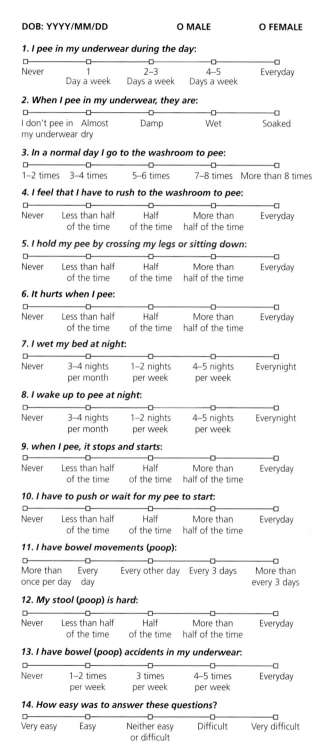

Figure 10.1 Vancouver Voiding Dysfunction Questionnaire. Source: Afshar et al. [6]. Reproduced with permission from the American Urological Association.

It thus becomes important to distinguish between these disorders, which all have wetting as their common denominator.

Minor voiding dysfunction disorders
Daytime urinary frequency syndrome
Giggle incontinence
Stress incontinence
Postvoid dribbling
Enuresis

Moderate voiding dysfunction disorders
Bladder/bowel dysfunction
Overactive bladder
Underactive bladder

Major voiding dysfunction disorders
Transient urodynamic dysfunction of infancy
Dysfunctional voiding
Hinman syndrome
Ochoa syndrome
Myogenic detrusor failure

Minor voiding dysfunction disorders
Daytime urinary frequency syndrome [9]
- Characterized by sudden onset of daytime-only frequency and urgency every 10–20 min.
- Nocturia or enuresis is rare.
- Very small amounts voided at a time.
- No associated UTIs.
- Seen in 3–8-year-olds.
- Very alarming to parents.
- No extensive investigation other than urinalysis/culture is needed as upper tracts are usually normal.
- Etiology is unknown although behavioral component is sometimes present.
- Recurrence is about 3%.

Management
- Condition is self-limiting but may take a few months to resolve.
- Reassurance is mainstay of therapy.
- Anticholinergics are of little help.

Giggle incontinence
- Massive unexpected detrusor contraction associated with complete bladder emptying.
- Starts around puberty.

- Episodes occur with giggling and laughter, sometimes with exertion.
- Although it was initially felt that the condition was limited to adolescence, it can persist into adulthood.
- No UTIs are found and the upper tracts are normal.
- Urodynamics may show mild uninhibited contractions.

Management
- Anticholinergics and sympathomimetics may help.
- Responds favorably to methylphenidate (Ritalin™) [10].
- Biofeedback alone or in combination with pharmacotherapy has met with success [11].
- Botulinum toxin injection in the detrusor has been reported in resistant cases [12].

Stress incontinence
- Not seen in childhood.
- Encountered in teenage girls.
- Prevalence in female college athletes is 28%.
- Increased incidence with high-impact sports.
- Found to be related to decreased foot flexibility possibly involving transmission of impact forces to pelvic floor.
- The upper tracts and urodynamics are normal but a high prevalence of urethral sphincteric incompetence is present.

Management
- Incontinence is minimal and is readily managed by timely bladder emptying.
- Sympathomimetics may be useful.

Post-void dribbling in girls (vaginal voiding)
- Careful history reveals that wetting typically occurs after micturition.
- Girls present with labiovulvar erythema and/or leucorrhea, burning, itching, and skin excoriation.
- Condition is due to trapping of urine in the vagina.
- Seen in small girls when the feet are unsupported during urination.
- In obese girls, the thighs are usually insufficiently separated during voiding.
- As the force of the urinary stream decreases toward the end of micturition, urine gets trapped in the lower vagina and then dribbles out.

Management
- Postural correction with either appropriate foot support, complete disrobing of pants and underwear that may interfere with appropriate thigh abduction.
- Sitting on the toilet bowl facing the wall usually corrects the problem.
- Steroid creams and antifungals to perineum as necessary.

Enuresis

- Primary monosymptomatic enuresis has no impact on the upper tracts unless it is associated with a condition that causes daytime wetting. (See chapters 22, 23 and 24).

Moderate disorders
Bladder/bowel dysfunction

- Frequently associated with fecal retention and/or retentive encopresis.
- Several studies have shown that there were more children with reflux found to have bladder and bowel disturbances often associated with UTIs. Ureteral reimplantation was required four times more frequently than in a cohort that did not have bowel disturbances. Even after successful reimplantation and reflux resolution in patients with bowel disturbances, the rate of recurrent UTIs remained four times higher [13].
- Unsuccessful surgical outcome of ureteral reimplantation is more likely in the presence of bladder/bowel dysfunction and should be avoided until this condition is resolved first [14].

Overactive bladder

- The most common voiding disorder encountered in children with peak incidence between 5 and 7 years.
- Commonly associated with fecal retention constituting bowel/bladder dysfunction.
- May be a cause of vesicoureteral reflux.
- Found in about 60% of incontinent children between 3 and 14 years.
- Gender prevalence is 60% girls : 40% boys.
- It is believed to be due to delay in acquisition of cortical inhibition over uninhibited detrusor contractions.
- Cortical control is usually acquired between 3 and 5 years of age.
- Symptoms include urgency, urge incontinence, and enuresis.
- Recurrent UTIs are common.
- Holding maneuvers such as leg crossing and squatting are common.
- Small functional bladder capacity for age is a constant finding due to bladder hypertonicity.
- Acquired vesicoureteral reflux is seen in 33–50%.
- Addressing the overactive bladder will triple the resolution rate of reflux compared to controls.
- Constipation contributes significantly to the etiology and symptoms of the overactive bladder and must be appropriately assessed and managed.
- Often associated with enuresis characterized by multiple wetting episodes during the night.

Management

The management of this condition is elaborated in detail in several other chapters in this book.

Underactive bladder

- Characterized by a desire to void only every 8–12 h with overflow incontinence between voids.
- May sometimes be considered as a progression to a decompensated stage of the untreated overactive bladder when a history of such is present.
- UTIs, straining to void, and constipation are common.
- The bladder is of large capacity, smooth walled, and hypotonic with elevated postvoid residuals in the absence of bladder outflow obstruction or neurological disease.

Management [15]

- Treat constipation first.
- Timed-voiding regimen.
- Alpha-blockers.
- Intermittent catheterization.

Major disorders

Transient urodynamic dysfunction of infancy

- High-grade reflux with thick-walled bladders noted prenatally.
- Absence of infravesical obstruction.
- Spontaneous resolution noted to reach 27% even with grade V reflux.
- May be associated with delay in maturation of the external urinary sphincter causing transient functional obstruction in some infants [16].

Management

- Vesicostomy is advised in the presence of elevated detrusor pressures and UTI.

Dysfunctional voiding

- Dysfunctional voiding must not be confused with "voiding dysfunction" from which it differs in occurring only during the act of voiding. The dysfunction is due to involuntary failure of relaxation or actual contraction of the urethral sphincter and pelvic floor muscles during voiding. This causes a rise of intravesical pressure that leads to incoordinated voiding although there is no identifiable neurologic lesion. When the condition is present in children with neurogenic bladder, it is called detrusor sphincter dyssynergia.
- The symptoms vary widely from mild frequency, postvoid dribbling, enuresis, urgency and urge incontinence, and UTIs so that it is difficult to distinguish it clinically from other voiding dysfunction disorders.
- Repeated testing with flowmetry/EMG will usually reveal pelvic floor muscle activity during voiding with an abnormal flow curve.
- Postvoid residuals are usually elevated and constipation is often present.
- The more severe forms share features with the Hinman syndrome (see the following text).

Hinman syndrome

- A severe voiding dysfunction encountered between childhood and puberty. It is associated with both bladder and urinary sphincter disturbances and is often accompanied by upper tract damage from vesicoureteral reflux or ureterovesical junction obstruction secondary to detrusor hypertrophy.
- There are no neurological stigmata nor is there anatomical infravesical obstruction. The disorder is acquired and psychopathological features are present in one half of the patients.
- Symptoms include daytime incontinence and enuresis, recurrent UTIs, constipation, and encopresis.
- Urodynamic findings vary with the stage of the disorder. Initially there is detrusor/sphincter dyssynergia which progresses to detrusor atony with decompensation and myogenic failure. Thus varying degrees of activity may be found in the bladder and urethral sphincter throughout the course of the disease.
- Progression to renal insufficiency is not uncommon.
- Surgical reconstructive procedures are usually unsuccessful so that urinary diversion may be necessary.
- Reeducation and suggestion therapy are helpful.
- Bowel regimens are important.
- Anticholinergics and alpha-blockers are helpful as well as Botox injections to the detrusor and urethral sphincter.
- Treatment is difficult and must be multimodal [17].

Ochoa (urofacial) syndrome

- A syndrome that has essentially the same features as the Hinman syndrome except that it is genetically transmitted and therefore runs in families.
- Characterized by an inversion in the muscles of facial expression that becomes more evident when smiling. The facial expression becomes a grimace that gives the appearance of sobbing or crying, making it possible to diagnose affected patients early in life.
- Some 200 cases have been described.
- The disorder is inherited in autosomal recessive manner. Mutations in the heparanase 2 (HPSE2) gene on chromosome 10q23q24 have been observed to cause the Ochoa syndrome [18].

Management

- Similar to Hinman syndrome.

Myogenic detrusor failure

- This disorder represents an end stage of bladder decompensation.
- It is easily recognizable in neuropathic bladders.
- May be encountered in older patients previously treated for posterior urethral valves [19, 20].

- Adequate voiding is usually accomplished although patients may carry a moderate amount of residual urine. They are more susceptible to episodes of lower UTI provided that they do not have reflux.
- Upper tract dilatation is a consequence of the initial lesion and tends to remain stable.

Management
- Alpha-blockers have been found to be of help in decreasing the amount of postvoid residual urine.

The bowel issue

It has become increasingly clear to researchers and clinicians alike that there is a tight relationship between the functions of the lower urinary tract and the lower gastrointestinal tract.

After having defined the voiding problem, it becomes quintessential to address bowel function issues. This can be a touchy subject because most parents do not understand the relationship between the lower gastrointestinal tract and the lower urinary tract until it is patiently explained to them. The task can be quite delicate because at the age of presentation, most parents are no longer as conscious of their child's bowel habits beyond the toddler years. It often comes as a surprise to them that detailed questions are asked about their child's bowel function. After all, that was not the reason why they consulted a urinary tract specialist in the first place.

At a time where there are many subspecialties in medicine, it would seem a simple matter to defer to a pediatric gastroenterologist for the evaluation of bowel function. It must be understood that this is not necessarily the best approach in most cases as it is likely to cause some dispersion of focus and may lead to poor compliance. A basic knowledge of the physiology of constipation thus becomes necessary for all medical and paramedical personnel involved in the management of voiding dysfunction. In cases where the constipation element is predominant and persistent, gastroenterology consultation should definitely be sought early. Bladder dysfunction is rarely if ever, the cause of bowel dysfunction although the two are frequently associated. On the other hand, fecal retention may affect bladder function to different degrees depending on the size and consistency of the retained fecal bolus in the rectosigmoid. Compression of the posterior bladder wall and the sensitivity of stretch receptors in the bladder wall may determine the threshold at which a detrusor contraction would be triggered. A rectum that is distended with stool would thus exert pressure on the bladder and lead to an overactive bladder.

The distended rectum may alternatively exert pressure on the pelvic nerve supply to the bladder and prevent the detrusor from contracting efficiently leading to an underactive bladder.

There is a spectrum in the severity and degree of fecal retention that may cause voiding dysfunction in some patients and not in others. Burgers et al. showed that in almost 70% of children with lower urinary tract symptoms, rectal distention significantly but unpredictably affected bladder capacity, sensation, and overactivity regardless of whether the children had constipation and independent of clinical features and baseline urodynamic findings. Urodynamics and management protocols for lower urinary tract symptoms that fail to recognize the effects of rectal distention may lead to unpredictable outcomes [21].

Although the exact mechanism of this relationship has not as yet been totally elucidated, it is a fact that when fecal retention is addressed and appropriately managed, the urinary symptoms will abate or completely disappear. Pharmacological agents should only be prescribed after constipation has come under control.

The relationship between constipation and voiding problems was analyzed in an elegant study of 234 constipated children by Loening-Baucke [22]. Twenty-nine percent of the patients had daytime urinary incontinence, 34% had nighttime incontinence, and 11% had UTIs. After 1 year when constipation was completely relieved in 52% of the patients, all ceased to have UTIs and 80% had daytime urinary incontinence corrected. Nighttime incontinence was also corrected in 63% of cases. It is interesting to note that children who have had problems with chronic constipation can accommodate a rectal balloon with up to 120 mL before they feel the sensation to defecate. Normal children only accommodate a balloon with a volume of 20 mL before they have a sudden urge to defecate. This indicates that many of these children have retention of stool in the rectal vault. Thus, confirmation by parents that the children have bowel movements every day is usually not an adequate reason to assume that their child is not constipated.

One way of explaining fecal retention to parents is to illustrate what Siggaard called the "iceberg phenomenon" where it is known that only a small portion of the iceberg is visible floating above the surface with the majority being submerged (Figure 10.2).

Constipation can be readily diagnosed and monitored in a uniform and objective manner, and patient progress can be followed using the Bristol Stool Form Scale (Figure 10.3), which has been validated in adults and is readily and reliably applicable to children who are often more aware of the appearance of their bowel movements than are their parents [23]. When the Bristol Stool Form Scale is coupled with a transabdominal sonogram of the rectum, this adds an additional objective validated parameter that helps in monitoring progress. A rectal diameter exceeding 30 mm is indicative of fecal retention [24].

A history of chronic abdominal discomfort, particularly periumbilical discomfort, is usually associated with issues of constipation in children who have overactive bladder [25]. The ICCS Standardization Committee has issued a multidisciplinary report on the management of functional constipation in children with lower urinary tract symptom [26].

The Iceberg Phenomenon
(Siggaard C, ICCS Ghent 2005)
Eliminated stool
Retained stool
can be several times
larger than eliminated
stool

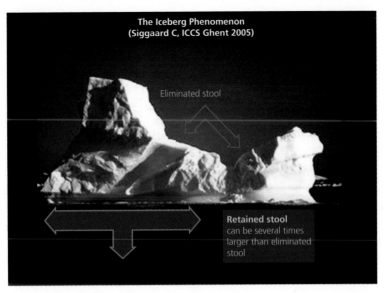

Figure 10.2 The "iceberg phenomenon." Source: Adapted from Siggaard C, (Personal Communication 2005).

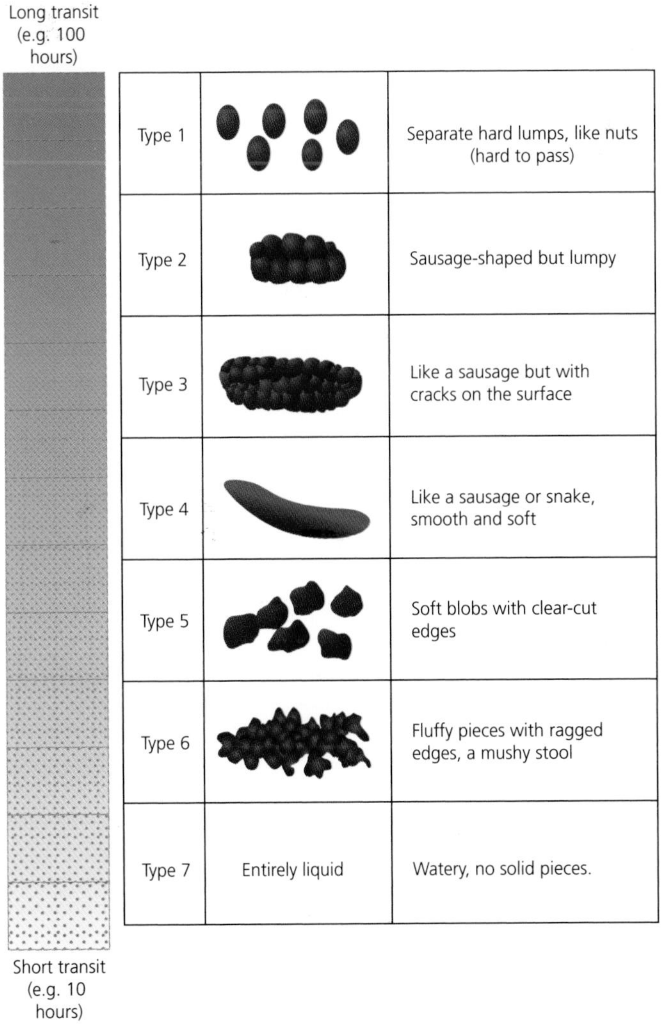

Long transit
(e.g. 100
hours)
Type 1
Separate hard lumps, like nuts
(hard to pass)
Type 2
Sausage-shaped but lumpy
Type 3
Like a sausage but with
cracks on the surface
Type 4
Like a sausage or snake,
smooth and soft
Type 5
Soft blobs with clear-cut
edges
Type 6
Fluffy pieces with ragged
edges, a mushy stool
Type 7
Entirely liquid
Watery, no solid pieces.
Short transit
(e.g. 10
hours)

Figure 10.3 Bristol Stool Form Scale. Source: Adapted from Lewis and Scand [27].

There is evidence of "cross-talk" between the lower gastrointestinal tract and the lower urinary tract. There is compelling evidence of bidirectional neural cross-talk between colon and lower urinary tract in a rat model [28, 29].

A convergence of multiple pelvic organ inputs (bladder, urethra, colon, and penis) was demonstrated in rat rostral medullary reticular formation neurons [30].

Animal data indicate that tegaserod has an effect in the spinal cord. It is possible that the better stool propulsion and the elimination of unwanted colonic contractions lead to the elimination of detrusor hyperactivity [31, 32].

References

1 Sureshkumar P, Jones M, Cumming R, Craig J. A population based study of 2856 school-age children with urinary incontinence. *J Urol.* 2009;**181**(2):808–15; discussion 815–6.

2 Bloom DA, Seeley WW, Ritchey ML, McGuire EJ. Toilet habits and continence in children: an opportunity sampling in search of normal parameters. *J Urol.* 1993 May;**149**(5):1087–90.

3 Snodgrass W. Relationship of voiding dysfunction to urinary tract infection and vesicoureteral reflux in children. *Urology.* 1991 Oct;**38**(4):341–4.

4 Farhat W, Bägli DJ, Capolicchio G, O'Reilly S, Merguerian PA, Khoury A, McLorie GA. The dysfunctional voiding scoring system: quantitative standardization of dysfunctional voiding symptoms in children. *J Urol.* 2000 Sep;**164**(3 Pt 2):1011–5.

5 Akbal C, Genc Y, Burgu B, Ozden E, Tekgul S. Dysfunctional voiding and incontinence scoring system: quantitative evaluation of incontinence symptoms in pediatric population. *J Urol.* 2005;**173**(3):969–73.

6 Afshar K, Mirbagheri A, Scott H, MacNeily AE. Development of a symptom score for dysfunctional elimination syndrome. *J Urol.* 2009;**182**(4 Suppl):1939–43.

7 Silay MS, Aslan AR, Erdem E, Tandogdu Z, Tekgul S. Evaluation of functional lower urinary tract dysfunction in children: are the physicians complying with the current guidelines? *Sci World J.* 2013:**341606**.

8 Homsy YL, Austin PF. Dysfunctional voiding disorders and enuresis. In Belman AB, King LR, Kramer SA (eds.) *Clinical Pediatric Urology.* Fourth edition. London: Martin Dunitz, 345 (2002).

9 Koff SA, Byard MA. The daytime urinary frequency syndrome of childhood. *J Urol.* 1988;**140**(5 Pt 2):1280–1.

10 Berry AK, Zderic S, Carr M. Methylphenidate for giggle incontinence. *J Urol.* 2009 Oct;**182**(4 Suppl):2028–32.

11 Richardson I, Palmer LS. Successful treatment for giggle incontinence with biofeedback. *J Urol.* 2009;**182**(4 Suppl):2062–6.

12 Wefer B, Seif C, van der Horst C, Jünemann KP, Braun PM. Botulinum toxin A injection for treatment-refractory giggle incontinence. *Urologe A.* 2007; **46**(7):773–5.

13 Koff SA, Murtagh DS. The uninhibited bladder in children: effect of treatment on recurrence of urinary infection and on vesicoureteral reflux resolution. *J Urol.* 1983; **130** (6): 1138–41.

14 Elder JS, Diaz M. Vesicoureteral reflux—the role of bladder and bowel dysfunction. *Nat Rev Urol.* 2013; **10**(11): 640–8.

15 Miyazato M, Yoshimura N, Chancellor MB. The other bladder syndrome: underactive bladder. *Rev Urol.* 2013;**15**(1):11–22.

16 Kokoua A, Homsy Y, Lavigne JF, Williot P, Corcos J, Laberge I, Michaud J. Maturation of the external urinary sphincter: a comparative histotopographic study in humans. *J Urol.* 1993; **150**(2 Pt 2):617–22.

17 Silay MS, Tanriverdi O, Karatag T, Ozcelik G, Horasanli K, Miroglu C. Twelve-year experience with Hinman-Allen syndrome at a single center. *Urology.* 2011;**78**(6):1397–401.

18 Pang J, Zhang S, Yang P, Hawkins-Lee B, Zhong J, Zhang Y, Ochoa B, Agundez JA, Voelckel MA, Fisher RB, Gu W, Xiong WC, Mei L, She JX, Wang CY. Loss-of-function mutations in HPSE2 cause the autosomal recessive urofacial syndrome. *Am J Hum Genet.* 2010;**86**(6):957–62.

19 Androulakakis PA, Karamanolakis DK, Tsahouridis G, Stefanidis AA, Palaeodimos I. Myogenic bladder decompensation in boys with a history of posterior urethral valves is caused by secondary bladder neck obstruction? *BJU Int.* 2005;**96**(1):140–3.

20 De Gennaro M, Capitanucci ML, Capozza N, Caione P, Mosiello G, Silveri M. Detrusor hypocontractility in children with posterior urethral valves arises before puberty. *Br J Urol.* 1998;**81**(3 Suppl):81–5.

21 Burgers R, Liem O, Canon S, Mousa H, Benninga MA, Di Lorenzo C, Koff SA. Effect of rectal distension on lower urinary tract function in children. *J Urol.* 2010:**184**(4 Suppl):1680–5.

22 Loening-Baucke V. Urinary incontinence and urinary tract infection and their resolution with treatment of chronic constipation of childhood. *Pediatrics.* 1997;**100**:228.

23 Heaton KW, Radvan J, Cripps H, Mountford RA, Braddon FE, Hughes AO. Defecation frequency and timing, and stool form in the general population: a prospective study. *Gut.* 1992;**33**:818.

24 Joensson IM, Siggaard C, Rittig S, Hagstroem S, Djurhuus JC. Transabdominal ultrasound of rectum as a diagnostic tool in childhood constipation. *J Urol.* 2008;**179**(5):1997–2002.

25 Chase JW, Homsy Y, Siggaard C, Sit F, Bower WF. Functional constipation in children. *J Urol.* 2004;**171**(6 Pt 2):2641–3.

26 Burgers RE, Mugie SM, Chase J, Cooper CS, von Gontard A, Rittig CS, Homsy Y, Bauer SB, Benninga MA. Management of functional constipation in children with lower urinary tract symptoms: report from the Standardization Committee of the International Children's Continence Society. *J Urol.* 2013;**190**(1):29–36.

27 Lewis SJ, Heaton KW. Stool form scale as a useful guide to intestinal transit time. *Scand J Gastroenterol.* 1997;**32**:920.

28 Pezzone MA , et al. A model of neural cross-talk and irritation in the pelvis: implications for the overlap of chronic pelvic pain disorders. *Gastroenterology.* 2005; **128**: 1953

29 Ustinova EE, Fraser MO, Pezzone MA. Cross-talk and sensitization of bladder afferent nerves. *Neurourol Urodyn.* 2010;**29**(1):77–81.

30 Kaddumi EG, Hubscher CH. Convergence of multiple pelvic organ inputs in the rat rostral medulla. *J Physiol.* 2006;**572**(Pt 2):393–405.

31 Franco I. Overactive bladder in children. Part 1: Pathophysiology. *J Urol.* 2007;**178**(3 Pt 1): 761–8; discussion 768.

32 Franco I. Overactive bladder in children. Part 2: Management. *J Urol.* 2007;**178** (3 Pt 1): 769–74.

CHAPTER 11

Evaluation of constipation and fecal incontinence

Marc A. Benninga

Department of Pediatric Gastroenterology and Nutrition, Emma Children's Hospital/Academic Medical Center, Amsterdam, The Netherlands

Definitions

There is a clear need for consensus regarding the definitions of constipation and fecal incontinence (FI) in order to make a diagnosis and to allow different researchers to study the same disorder. Since 2006, clinicians and researchers use the Rome III criteria to define functional gastrointestinal disorders in children, including constipation and FI [1] (Tables 11.1 and 11.2).

Four main groups of children present with FI: (i) children who have functional fecal retention with overflow incontinence, (ii) children with functional nonretentive fecal incontinence (FNRFI), (iii) children with anorectal malformations, and (iv) children with spinal problems [2]. More than 80% of the children with FI have retentive FI [3]. Functional FI in children can also be subclassified as either primary, in those children who have never been toilet trained, or secondary, in those in which the incontinence returns after successful toilet training [4]. According to the Rome III criteria, FI is defined as the involuntary loss of stool into the underwear in a child over the age of 4 years.

Normal defecation pattern

The stool frequency gradually declines from more than four stools per day during the first week of life to one to two stools per day by the age of 4 years [5–7]. During the first 3 months of life, the defecation frequency is significantly higher, and the stools are softer in healthy breastfed infants compared to formula-fed infants [6]. The type of feeding does, however, not influence the stooling

Pediatric Incontinence: Evaluation and Clinical Management, First Edition. Edited by Israel Franco, Paul F. Austin, Stuart B. Bauer, Alexander von Gontard and Yves Homsy.
© 2015 John Wiley & Sons, Ltd. Published 2015 by John Wiley & Sons, Ltd.

Table 11.1 Rome III criteria for pediatric functional constipation.

Diagnostic criteria must include the following:
- Two or more criteria for at least 1 month in infants up to 4 years
- Two or more symptoms for at least once per week for at least 2 months in children of at least 4 years, without fulfilling irritable bowel syndrome criteria
  - Two or fewer defecations per week
  - At least one episode of fecal incontinence per week
  - History of retentive posturing or excessive stool retention
  - History of painful or hard bowel movements
  - History of large-diameter stool that may obstruct the toilet
  - Presence of a large fecal mass in the rectum

Table 11.2 Rome III criteria for pediatric functional nonretentive fecal incontinence.

Diagnostic criteria must include all of the following in children of at least 4 years of age, for at least 2 months prior to diagnosis:
- Defecation into places inappropriate to the social context at least once per month
- No evidence of an inflammatory, anatomic, metabolic, or neoplastic process that explains the subject's symptoms
- No evidence of fecal retention

quantity [8]. From 5 years of age, the majority of children pass stools daily or every other day without straining or withholding [8].

Epidemiology

The worldwide prevalence of functional constipation in children varies from 0.7 to 29.6%, with this condition occurring in all pediatric age groups, from newborns to young adults [9]. Like constipation, FI is also a widespread problem with prevalence rates ranging from 0.8 to 4.1% in the West and 2 to 7.8% in Asia [10]. FI is more common in younger children with a prevalence of 4.1% in children ranging from 5 to 6 years of age and 1.6% in 11- to 12-year-olds [10]. A study from Sri Lanka showed that the majority of children (80%) with FI had constipation-associated (retentive) FI and only 20% had FNRFI [11]. FI is more common among males and children from low socioeconomic strata [11]. Furthermore, bullying, psychological stress, behavioral and upbringing problems, and poor social and school performances are more often reported in children with FI [12].

Clinical evaluation and diagnosis
The clinical presentation of constipation and/or FI in children is obvious in the majority but may be subtle and nonspecific in a subset of children. There are, however, no well-designed studies that determine which aspects of a history are

Table 11.3 Alarm signs and symptoms in constipation and fecal incontinence.

Constipation starting very early in life (<1 month)
Passage of meconium >48 h
Family history of Hirschsprung's disease
Blood in the stools in the absence of anal fissures
Failure to thrive/respiratory problems
Growth delay, developmental delay
Fever
Bilious vomiting
Abnormal thyroid gland
Severe abdominal distension
Explosive stool and air from the rectum upon withdrawal of examining finger
Perianal fistula
Anal stenosis
Abnormal position of anus
Absent anal or cremasteric reflex
Decreased lower extremity strength/tone/reflex
Tuft of hair on spine
Sacral dimple
Gluteal cleft deviation
Urinary bladder distension
Extreme fear during anal inspection
Smearing with feces
Anal scars

pertinent. The physician should be aware of symptoms and signs of organic causes or red flag symptoms, as presented in Tables 11.3, 11.4, and 11.5 [3]. It is important to emphasize that constipation and FI are clinical diagnoses that are primarily based on symptoms in the absence of red flag symptoms, and therefore in the majority of patients no further testing is needed.

Medical history

The medical history of children with constipation and FI should include questions about the time of the first bowel movement after birth, the age of onset, the time of toilet training, the defecation frequency, the stool characteristics (consistency, caliber, and size), whether the child experiences pain during defecation, the presence of episodes and timing of FI, and the stool withholding behavior. Children suffering from extreme fecal impaction may have FI episodes even during the night. The Amsterdam infant stool scale and the modified Bristol Stool Form Scale are simple instruments assessing consistency, amount and color of stools in infants and older children [13, 14]. The accuracy of the defecation history in children as provided by the child and/or parents can be

Table 11.4 Causes of constipation in children.

Intestinal causes	Hirschsprung's disease
	Anorectal malformation
	Neuronal intestinal dysplasia
Neuropathic conditions	Spinal cord abnormalities
	Spinal cord trauma
	Neurofibromatosis
	Static encephalopathy
	Tethered cord
Metabolic, endocrine causes	Hypothyroidism
	Diabetes mellitus
	Hypercalcemia
	Hypokalemia
	Vitamin D intoxication
Drugs	Opioids
	Anticholinergics
	Antidepressants
Other causes	Anorexia nervosa
	Sexual abuse
	Scleroderma
	Cystic fibrosis
	Dietary protein allergy

Table 11.5 Causes of fecal incontinence in children.

Functional causes	Functional constipation-associated FI
	Functional nonretentive fecal incontinence (FNRFI)
Organic causes	Repaired anorectal malformation
	Postsurgical Hirschsprung's disease
	Spinal dysraphism
	Spinal cord trauma
	Spinal cord tumor
	Cerebral palsy
	Myopathies affecting the pelvic floor and external anal sphincter

improved with use of a bowel diary [3]. Accompanying symptoms including abdominal pain, loss of appetite, nausea, vomiting, weight loss or poor weight gain, neuromuscular development, and psychological or behavioral problems should be assessed as well. Dietary history and a history of previous treatment strategies for constipation should be investigated. Finally, it is important to ask for life-altering events, such as death in the family, birth of a sibling, school problems, and sexual abuse, which might contribute to the development of retentive behavior.

Children with FNRFI typically visit the outpatient clinic at an older age (age of 9.2 years vs. 6.5 years) compared to children with constipation [10]. It has been postulated that parents postpone a visit to a health-care professional because of the shame they feel not being capable of properly toilet training their child. The majority of children with FNRFI have, in contrast to constipated children, episodes of FI happening after school during the late afternoon and before bedtime [10]. Besides FI, they have a (normal) defecation frequency of at least three times per week with stools normal in size and consistency.

An association between constipation and urinary tract dysfunction (i.e., urine incontinence and recurrent urinary tract infections) is well established [15]. A higher frequency of daytime and nighttime urinary incontinence is reported in children without constipation (around 45%), while daytime and nighttime enuresis is found in 25–29% of those with constipation [15]. A high prevalence of urine incontinence in children with FNRFI, suggests an overall delay in the achievement of toilet training or the neglect of normal physiological stimuli to go to the toilet.

Between 25 and 75% of the children with anorectal anomalies and myelomeningocele, respectively, continue to have FI despite long-lasting and invasive treatment, such as colonic irrigation [4, 16], whereas 50% of the children continue to have FI after corrected surgery.

Physical examination

A comprehensive physical examination including rectal- and detailed neurological examination can often help to discriminate functional from organic defecation disorders [3]. Physical examination should start with measurement of weight and height. Obesity is a predisposing factor for developing chronic constipation and metabolic or endocrine disorders may lead to short statue and growth restriction. Abdominal examination may reveal the accumulation of gas or feces, particularly in the left quadrant. Evaluation of the perianal region provides valuable information about the anal position, evidence of FI, skin irritation, eczema, fissures, hemorrhoids, and signs of possible sexual abuse. The anorectal digital examination assesses the perianal sensation, anal tone, size of the rectum, and contraction and relaxation of the anal sphincter. A patulous anal sphincter may suggest a neurological disorder as the cause of impaired sphincter function. The lumbosacral area should be inspected for the presence of a sacral dimple, a tuft of hair, gluteal cleft deviation, or flat buttocks, which may indicate sacral dysraphism. It has been recommended to perform at least one rectal examination in children with defecation disorders. In children fulfilling more than one criterion of functional constipation, however, a rectal examination is not necessary. Extreme fear during anal inspection or rectal examination should alert the health-care professional of possible sexual abuse.

Laboratory investigations

In the far majority of cases, routine laboratory testing rarely uncovers an underlying disorder such as hypothyroidism, hypercalcemia, or celiac disease in children with functional defecation disorders [3]. A recent study showed that only 1.7% was diagnosed with celiac disease, only 0.6% with hypothyroidism and none with hypercalcemia [17]. The likelihood of finding patients with an organic cause decreases even further in children who present with constipation as their only symptom [17]. The ESPGHAN/NASPGHAN constipation guideline does not recommend routine allergy testing to diagnose cow's-milk allergy in children with functional constipation, since current evidence is clearly conflicting [3]. Still, a 2–4-week trial of avoidance of cow's milk protein may be indicated in a child with intractable constipation [3].

Abdominal radiograph

Abdominal X-rays are far too frequently requested by health-care professionals to evaluate and objectify fecal loading in children with both organic and functional defecation disorders. Despite the existence of several scoring systems to evaluate fecal loading in children with constipation, it is well known, however, that evaluating an abdominal X-ray is prone to a low inter- and intraobserver variability for assessing fecal loading [18]. The current guidelines strongly recommend not to use an abdominal X-ray to diagnose functional constipation [3, 19]. Based on expert opinion, however, a plain abdominal X-ray may be used in a child in whom fecal impaction is suspected but in whom physical examination is unreliable/impossible because of obesity, refusal, or psychological factors (sexual abuse) [3].

Colonic transit time measurement

In children with functional constipation and in children with spinal abnormalities, a low defecation frequency and a high number of FI episodes in combination with a palpable rectal mass correlate well with prolonged total colonic transit time with particular delay in the rectosigmoid [18, 20]. Moreover, a prospective, observational case–control study showed that stool form, as measured by the Bristol Stool Form Scale, rather than stool frequency, also correlates with total colonic transit time in both constipated and nonconstipated children [21]. In children with FNRFI, a normal colonic transit time is found in more than 90% of the children, and therefore, colonic transit time measurement is valuable in discriminating children with FI secondary to constipation and children with FNRFI [3]. Furthermore, colonic transit measurement may be helpful in children in which the medical history is unreliable. Colonic scintigraphy and wireless pressure/ pH capsules are more sophisticated and more costly methods to assess colonic transit, whose clinical usefulness in children is only now beginning to be explored [22, 23].

Transabdominal rectal ultrasonography

Transabdominal rectal ultrasonography is considered a simple, noninvasive, and reliable technique to demonstrate fecal loading in children with constipation. Several studies have shown that a rectal diameter larger than 30 mm is considered as enlarged [18]. Not surprisingly the rectal diameter is significantly larger among constipated children compared to healthy children. Despite these data, transabdominal is not recommended to diagnose functional constipation but might only be used to replace digital rectal examination in the evaluation of fearful children with constipation [3, 24].

Contrast enema

A contrast enema is useful in identifying anatomic abnormalities, such as a distended rectum or colon, primary or secondary to a more distal holdup. A transition zone between aganglionic and ganglionic bowel is suggestive for Hirschsprung's disease. On the other hand, a contrast enema has the lowest sensitivity compared with rectal suction biopsy and anorectal manometry (70% vs. 93% and 91%, respectively), leading to false-negative results [25]. Pediatric surgeons often use this test to assess the extent of the aganglionic segment before surgery.

Rectal suction biopsy with cholinesterase staining is the most accurate test in the diagnostic workup of patients suspected of having Hirschsprung's disease. Recently, calretinin, a calcium binding protein, has been reported to be a new marker in Hirschsprung's disease and may be superior to ACE activity with respect to the diagnosis of total aganglionosis, superficial biopsies, and prematurity [26].

Both contrast enema and rectal suction biopsy are not recommended as initial diagnostic tools for the evaluation of children with functional constipation [3].

Defecography

Defecography is used to visualize the anal canal and rectum at rest and during defecation and provides useful information about anatomical and functional anorectal changes [27]. A normal test excludes a perineal descent syndrome or anatomic obstruction as a cause of constipation (e.g., internal rectal prolapse, rectocele). In patients with outlet obstruction, the anorectal angle may not widen and the contrast will be partially expelled. This may be due to failure of the puborectalis muscle to relax. Currently, defecography is not recommended in the diagnostic workup of childhood constipation but should be regarded as an adjunct to clinical and manometric assessment of anorectal function [3]. Though there are some advantages, its drawbacks include radiation exposure, embarrassment, interobserver bias, and inconsistent methodology.

Magnetic resonance imaging

In rare cases, neurological abnormalities of the lower spinal cord are the cause for constipation and FI. Spinal cord abnormalities (such as an intradural lipoma or tethered cord) were only found in 3% of children with constipation, constipation-associated FI, and FNRFI [28]. The majority of these patients with neurological abnormalities on magnetic resonance imaging (MRI) had deviation of the gluteal cleft on physical examination [28]. Despite these neurological abnormalities, all patients responded to intense medical and behavioral therapy, and none needed neurosurgical intervention [28]. Currently, evidence does not support the use of MRI of the spine in patients with intractable constipation without neurological abnormalities [3]. Imaging of the spinal cord is only recommended when physical examination reveals abnormalities such as lipoma or hemangioma on the lower back, asymmetry of the buttocks, or sensory or motor abnormalities of the lower limb and perineum [3].

Anorectal manometry

Anorectal manometry assesses anorectal function. Its main indication is to demonstrate the presence of the rectoanal inhibitory reflex (RAIR). The RAIR is absent in children with Hirschsprung's disease or in children with anal achalasia or ultrashort segment Hirschsprung's disease [29]. Other features that can be evaluated with this test are anal resting pressures and defecation dynamics. The presence of anal spasms on anorectal manometry may indicate an underlying tethered or retethered cord and then MRI is indicated [30].

Colonic manometry

Colonic manometry is a diagnostic test performed in specialized motility centers to differentiate between normal colonic motor function and colonic neuromuscular disorders in the evaluation of children with intractable constipation [31].

Other indications are clarifying the pathophysiology of persisting lower GI symptoms after surgery for Hirschsprung's disease, evaluating colonic involvement in a child carrying a diagnosis of intestinal pseudo-obstruction, assessing function of a diverted colon prior to possible reanastomosis, and assessing colonic motor activity prior to intestinal transplantation in order to find out whether or not the colon should be kept at the time of transplant [31]. Furthermore, colonic manometry testing resulted in recommendation to change therapy (mostly surgical) in 93% of patients with refractory defecation disorders [31]. Moreover, manometry may help in predicting whether antegrade enema treatment through a Malone stoma or cecostomy will be successful [31]. Again, colonic manometry is not recommended in the initial diagnostic work up of children with functional or organic defecation disorders.

Conclusion

A comprehensive history and a thorough physical examination are essential steps in the evaluation of all children presenting with either a functional or an organic defecation disorder. A variety of radiographic and motility tests are currently available and provide useful information in selected circumstances, but additional diagnostic testing is rarely necessary. Only in cases presenting with alarming features, the diagnostic workup should be expanded.

References

1 Rasquin A, Di Lorenzo C, Forbes D, et al. Childhood functional gastrointestinal disorders: child/adolescent. *Gastroenterology*. 2006;**130**:1527–37.

2 Di Lorenzo C, Benninga MA. Pathophysiology of pediatric fecal incontinence. *Gastroenterology*. 2004;**126**(Suppl 1):S33–40.

3 Tabbers MM, Dilorenzo C, Berger MY, et al. Evaluation and treatment of functional constipation in infants and children: evidence-based recommendations from ESPGHAN and NASPGHAN. *J Pediatr Gastroenterol Nutr*. 2014;**58**:265–81.

4 Ambartsumyan L, Nurko S. Review of organic causes of fecal incontinence in children: evaluation and treatment. *Expert Rev Gastroenterol Hepatol*. 2013;**7**:657–67.

5 Corazziari E, Staiano A, Miele E, Greco L. Bowel frequency and defecatory patterns in children: a prospective nationwide survey. *Clin Gastroenterol Hepatol* 2005;**3**:1101–6.

6 Steer CD, Emond AM, Golding J, Sandhu B. The variation in stool patterns from 1 to 42 months: a population-based observational study. *Arch Dis Child*. 2009;**94**:231–3.

7 Benjasuwantep B, Ruangdaraganon N. Bowel movements of normal Thai infants. *Southeast Asian J Trop Med Public Health*. 2009;**40**:530–7.

8 Weaver LT. Bowel habit from birth to old age. *J Pediatr Gastroenterol Nutr*. 1988;**7**:637–40.

9 Mugie SM, Benninga MA, Di Lorenzo C. Epidemiology of constipation in children and adults: a systematic review. *Best Pract Res Clin Gastroenterol*. 2011;**25**:3–18.

10 Rajindrajith S, Devanarayana NM, Benninga MA. Review article: faecal incontinence in children: epidemiology, pathophysiology, clinical evaluation and management. *Aliment Pharmacol Ther*. 2013;**37**:37–48.

11 Rajindrajith S, Devanarayana NM, Benninga MA. Constipation-associated and nonretentive fecal incontinence in children and adolescents: an epidemiological survey in Sri Lanka. *JPediatr Gastroenterol Nutr.* 2010;**51**:472–6.

12 Joinson C, Heron J, Butler U, et al. Psychological differences between children with and without soiling problems. *Pediatrics.* 2006;**117**:1575–84.

13 Bekkali N, Hamers SL, Reitsma JB, Van Toledo L, Benninga MA. Infant stool form scale: development and results. *J Pediatr.* 2009;**154**:521–6.

14 Lane MM, Czyzewski DI, Chumpitazi BP, Shulman RJ. Reliability and validity of a modified Bristol stool form scale for children. *J Pediatr.* 2011;**159**:437–41.

15 Burgers RE, Mugie SM, Chase J, et al. Management of functional constipation in children with lower urinary tract symptoms: report from the standardization committee of the international Children's continence society. *J Urol.* 2013;**190**:29–36.

16 Bischoff A, Levitt MA, Peña A.Bowel management for the treatment of pediatric fecal incontinence. *Pediatr Surg Int.* 2009;**25**:1027–42.

17 Chogle A, Saps M. Yield and cost of performing screening tests for constipation in children. *Can J Gastroenterol.* 2013;**27**:e35–8.

18 Berger MY, Tabbers MM, Kurver MJ, et al. Value of abdominal radiography, colonic transit time, and rectal ultrasound scanning in the diagnosis of idiopathic constipation in children: a systematic review. *J Pediatr.* 2012;**161**:44–50.

19 Bardisa-Ezcurra L, Ullman R, Gordon J, Guideline Development Group. Diagnosis and management of idiopathic childhood constipation: summary of NICE guidance. *BMJ.* 2010;**1**:340.

20 Velde SV, Pratte L, Verhelst H, et al. Colon transit time and anorectal manometry in children and young adults with spina bifida. *Int J Colorectal Dis.* 2013;**28**:1547–53.

21 Russo M, Martinelli M, Sciorio E, et al. Stool consistency, but not frequency, correlates with total gastrointestinal transit time in children. *J Pediatr.* 2013;**162**:1188–92.

22 Yik YI, Cain TM, Tudball CF, et al. Nuclear transit studies of patients with intractable chronic constipation reveal a subgroup with rapid proximal colonic transit. *J Pediatr Surg.* 2011;**46**:1406–11.

23 Green AD, Belkind-Gerson J, Surjanhata BC, et al. Wireless motility capsule test in children with upper gastrointestinal symptoms. *J Pediatr.* 2013;**162**:1181–7.

24 Burgers R, de Jong TP, Benninga MA. Rectal examination in children: digital versus transabdominal ultrasound. *J Urol.* 2013;**190**:667–72.

25 de Lorijn F, Kremer LC, Reitsma JB, Benninga MA. Diagnostic tests in hirschsprung disease: a systematic review. *J Pediatr Gastroenterol Nutr.* 2006;**42**:496–505.

26 Volpe A, Alaggio R, Midrio P, et al. Calretinin, β-tubulin immunohistochemistry, and submucosal nerve trunks morphology in Hirschsprung disease: possible applications in clinical practice. *J Pediatr Gastroenterol Nutr.* 2013;**57**:780–7.

27 Zhang SC, Wang WL, Liu X. Defecography used as screening entry for identifying evacuatory pelvic floor disorders in childhood constipation. *Clin Imaging.* 2014;**38**:115–21.

28 Bekkali NL, Hagebeuk EE, Bongers ME, et al. Magnetic resonance imaging of the lumbosacral spine in children with chronic constipation or non-retentive fecal incontinence: a prospective study. *J Pediatr.* 2010;**156**:461–5.

29 Chumpitazi BP, Fishman SJ, Nurko S. Long-term clinical outcome after botulinum toxin injection in children with nonrelaxing internal anal sphincter. *Am J Gastroenterol.* 2009;**104**:976–83.

30 Siddiqui A, Rosen R, Nurko S. Anorectal manometry may identify children with spinal cord lesions. *J Pediatr Gastroenterol Nutr.* 2011;**53**:507–11.

31 Dinning PG, Di Lorenzo C. Colonic dysmotility in constipation. *Best Pract Res Clin Gastroenterol.* 2011;**25**:89–101.

SECTION 4

Treatments of functional bowel and bladder dysfunction

Paul F. Austin

Introduction

The complexity of the multiple regulatory mechanisms of bladder and bowel function requires a thorough understanding of the pathophysiologic aspects of bladder and bowel dysfunction (BBD) followed by a careful, detailed evaluation to delineate the heterogeneous influences responsible for BBD. It is this characterization of the pathophysiology of BBD that guides the practitioner toward a treatment plan that is tailored to the child and their family. Because of the heterogeneity of BBD, there are numerous efficacious therapeutic approaches that mandate the capability of a multidisciplinary approach. In this section, all treatment modalities are presented in the care of children with BBD. These include urotherapy, pharmacotherapy, bowel therapy, neuromodulation, and psychotherapy.

Wendy F. Bower and Janet W. Chase discuss in detail in Chapter 12 the role of standard urotherapy for all patients with BBD and the use of specific targeted therapies that is further outlined in the conceptual focused case presentations in Chapter 13. Ann Raes and Catherine Renson provide a detailed, pragmatic description in Chapter 14 of using specific targeted urotherapy in the form of biofeedback. Israel Franco and I then explore the multiple medical therapeutics that are available for the treatment and modulation of BBD in Chapter 15. Pharmacotherapy targeting the bladder body and bladder outlet (internal and external sphincter complexes) as was as emerging extravesical targets (brain, spinal cord, and peripheral nerves) is comprehensively covered. It is fitting that Chapter 16 addresses the comorbidity of constipation and/or fecal incontinence that commonly occurs with bladder dysfunction (hence the term "BBD"). Vera

Pediatric Incontinence: Evaluation and Clinical Management, First Edition. Edited by Israel Franco, Paul F. Austin, Stuart B. Bauer, Alexander von Gontard and Yves Homsy.
© 2015 John Wiley & Sons, Ltd. Published 2015 by John Wiley & Sons, Ltd.

Loening-Baucke and Alexander Swidsinski methodically describe the management of functional bowel dysfunction in all ages beginning with infants and toddlers and ending with children and adolescents.

The next three chapters tackle neuromodulation and illustrate the different available options of instituting neuromodulation with pediatric BBD. Mario De Gennaro and Maria L. Capitanucci present one of the more new neuromodulation therapeutics with posterior tibial nerve stimulation in Chapter 17. Yuri E. Reinberg and coauthors present their impressive and expanding experience in Chapter 18 using implantable sacral nerve stimulation therapy for the treatment of bladder dysfunction in a selected cohort of patients. Finally, Ubirajara Barroso Jr. presents his exciting work using sacral transcutaneous electrical nerve stimulation in Chapter 19 and is one of a handful of investigators that has validated neuromodulation for pediatric OAB by performing one of the few randomized placebo-controlled trials.

Piet Hoebeke is the first person to publish using botulinum toxin for refractory OAB in neurologically intact children and presents an excellent historical perspective of the therapeutic merits of botulinum toxin as well as the applicability in today's treatment choices for pediatric BBD in Chapter 20. Monika Equit and Alexander von Gontard complete this section on therapeutics with their thoughtful psychological approach in Chapter 21. The hallmark of standard urotherapy (demystification, education, diaries, etc.) reflects the psychological importance of managing the child with BBD. The association of neuropsychiatric comorbidities with BBD is gaining proper recognition, and cognitive-based therapy is a valuable asset in these patients.

In summary, treatment of pediatric BBD requires multiple modalities that encompass multiple disciplines. This is most evident in cases involving complex pathophysiologic mechanisms or in cases that are refractory to treatment. The treatment of BBD does not warrant a broad, shotgun approach but rather a thoughtful, tailored approach with specific therapies available as warranted.

CHAPTER 12

Implementation of urotherapy

Wendy F. Bower[1] and Janet W. Chase[2]

[1] Department of Epidemiology and Preventive Medicine, School of Public Health and Preventive Medicine, Health Services Unit, Monash University, Melbourne, Australia

[2] Victorian Children's Continence Clinic, Cabrini Hospital, Melbourne, Australia

Implementation of urotherapy

Treatment of bladder and bowel dysfunction (BBD) involves multidisciplinary input to promote routine bladder filling and unopposed emptying. Initial intervention is referred to as urotherapy, but also includes attention to bowel function.

The goals of urotherapy relate to signs and symptoms identified on initial assessment of each child (Table 12.1). The components of a therapy program (Box 12.1) are targeted to address the underlying dysfunctions, and involve a combination of therapies. Efficacy of urotherapy is evaluated by reduction in the number of wet episodes, improvement in bladder emptying, and resolution of associated symptoms such as episodes of urinary tract infection, constipation, and grade of vesicoureteric reflux.

Urotherapy is delivered in packages of care, with standard therapy being augmented by specific targeted interventions. The distinction between approaches is mentioned only to clarify the terms as they appear in relevant publications. Box 12.1 summarizes the hierarchy of implementing urotherapy.

Standard therapy begins with education of the child and family, exploring each person's understanding of the lower urinary tract and explaining the child's specific dysfunction. Visual aids that are age appropriate, backed up by written information for parents, are vital as health literacy has been shown to predict treatment adherence. Motivation is an integral part of intervention success; a child who cannot conceive of any upside to resolution of his or her dysfunction may not be ready to commence therapy [1].

Pediatric Incontinence: Evaluation and Clinical Management, First Edition. Edited by Israel Franco, Paul F. Austin, Stuart B. Bauer, Alexander von Gontard and Yves Homsy.
© 2015 John Wiley & Sons, Ltd. Published 2015 by John Wiley & Sons, Ltd.

Table 12.1 Goals of urotherapy.

Sign/symptom	Goal
Incontinence	Long-term dryness
Urinary urgency	Void when convenient; normal bladder wall thickness on ultrasound
Fecal incontinence	Regular bowel emptying; no fecal soiling
Urinary tract infection	No further episodes of UTI
Abnormal voiding dynamics	Continuous uroflow curve Routine postvoid residual volume of urine < 10 mL
Pelvic girdle activity during voiding	PFM relaxation during void; silent perineal EMG
Vesicoureteric reflux	Reduction in grade of VUR
Reduced or enlarged age-expected bladder capacity	Normalized bladder capacity

Box 12.1 Components of a urotherapy program; items in italics constitute *standard therapy* with the remaining interventions considered *specific targeted therapies*.

- *Explain normal bladder behavior and specific changes underlying the child's symptoms (demystification and education)*
- *Screen for coexisting bowel disorder; facilitate routine bowel emptying*
- *Implement voiding routine to ensure child passes urine at regular intervals*
- *Cognitive behavioral therapy*
- *Registration of symptoms and voiding behavior*
- Teach pelvic floor muscle (PFM) awareness and coordination
  - To achieve PFM recruitment and relaxation with minimal accessory muscle activity
- Train optimal voiding mechanics and posture
- Teach specific PFM relaxation at initiation of void
- Adjunctive neuromodulation
  - Clean intermittent catheterization if large postvoid residual volumes of urine persist
- Bowel retraining

One of the aims of standard urotherapy is to achieve routine bladder filling. Drinking acceptable volumes of fluid regularly will reverse voluntary dehydration and assist in reestablishing a cycle of routine filling and emptying. Normal urine concentration associated with adequate hydration will relieve some symptoms of irritative urgency and facilitate LUT rehabilitation. There is no evidence to support a curative association between high fluid intake and resolution of bladder symptoms; normalized gut transit or defecation dynamics and subsequently moderate, regular fluid intake are the goals.

Standardizing a child's voiding interval follows adequate hydration. Voiding every 2–3 h minimizes pelvic floor holding maneuvers and prevents routine bladder overdistension. Regular voiding may also reestablish sensory awareness for age-appropriate volumes of urine. The crucial factor is that voiding should be unopposed by pelvic girdle or urethral muscular activity.

Two elements of traditional cognitive therapy, namely monitoring and organizing oneself, are fundamental to the success of standard urotherapy [2]. Children are taught how to fill out bladder diaries, frequency volume charts, and bowel diaries and to self-monitor voiding frequency. In some cases, a timed voiding schedule may be augmented with a vibrating wrist watch or preset alarm.

Specific interventions

Children with urgency, dysfunctional voiding, or abnormal defecation dynamics may have an altered pattern of pelvic girdle and sphincter muscle relaxation during elimination. Successful retraining begins with teaching pelvic floor muscle awareness, then effective contraction and relaxation, followed by task specificity.

Pelvic floor muscle awareness can be taught via a whole body approach, using techniques such as progressive relaxation, seated ball work, and known synergistic patterning. Once the child achieves some proprioception of pelvic girdle muscles, activity of the abdominal and corset muscles can be explained. A full-length mirror is helpful to demonstrate rectus and oblique activity and to teach active relaxation (often perceived as a lengthening) of the lower abdominal muscles.

It has been suggested that pelvic floor muscle contraction cannot occur during transversus abdominal relaxation [3]. Thus, pelvic floor muscle relaxation may be trained using visual feedback or self-palpation of the relaxed lower abdominal muscles that share a common fascia with the PF. A handheld mirror may provide visual feedback to a child who has difficulty understanding the concept of pelvic floor/perineal elevation and descent associated with contraction and relaxation. Dysfunctional voiding is not an indication for pelvic floor muscle strength training.

Children who require additional support to identify pelvic floor structures may be offered a course of biofeedback therapy. Electrodes that detect activity within underlying muscles are placed on the perineum, around the anal sphincter, inside the anal canal, or on the abdominal wall. Children use the visual and auditory feedback, often via an interface with games, to rehearse appropriate contraction and relaxation of pelvic girdle muscles. Since it is possible to use accessory muscles or other maneuvers to generate the required pressures, a biofeedback training system should be used with supervision.

Motor training in urotherapy must be specific to voiding and defecation. First ensure that toilet posture facilitates maximal pelvic muscle relaxation. Ensure adequate leg support, either by feet on the ground, when the legs are long, or on a footstool. Legs should be abducted to shoulder width, hips flexed, lumbar extension, trunk neutral but inclined forward, and elbows resting on knees. Active abdominal relaxation without Valsalva should precede the voiding effort.

Therapy can include home training of optimal voiding using a portable uroflow unit or handheld EMG machine. Voiding technique should be reviewed frequently and the child offered more intense training if either voiding coordination or symptoms do not improve. Strategies may include half-day training, a longer series of biofeedback sessions, referral to a tertiary center, hospitalization for intensive training, or attendance at a live-in bladder rehabilitation camp.

When children with over or under active bladder presentations cannot self-manage their symptoms, pharmacotherapy is usually offered. Another option is neuromodulation. The underlying rationale is that current has a direct effect on the central nervous system by artificially activating neural structures, thereby facilitating both neural plasticity and normative afferent and efferent activity of the lower urinary tract [4]. The application of electric current is also known to change the availability of neurotransmitters and in the case of bladder overactivity to both reduce cholinergic and increase beta adrenergic activity [5].

In children with an overactive bladder, transcutaneous and percutaneous neuromodulation delivered over either the sacral outflow or peroneal region of the ankle at a frequency between 10 and 25 Hz has proven a useful adjunctive treatment [6, 7]. Less frequently, intravesical stimulation can target an underactive bladder. Treatment can be clinic based or delivered on a daily basis at home.

Clean intermittent catheterization is considered when a child has infrequent voiding or does not adequately empty their bladder following standard urotherapy advice. Usually taught by the team nurse, this technique prevents stasis of urine and allows the detrusor muscle to begin a voiding contraction at a more appropriate length–tension ratio. Even quite young children can be taught to empty their bladder with clean intermittent catheterization [8]. Over time, both sensation of bladder fullness and detrusor contractile ability may improve.

Bowel therapy

When a child with BBD presents for treatment, initial management concentrates on normalizing bowel function [9]. Improvement of lower urinary tract symptoms is less likely if constipation and fecal incontinence persist [10]. Active bowel management (Box 12.2) continues for a minimum of 6 months with

Box 12.2 Urotherapy cascade for bowel retraining.

- Education, remove blame/guilt, establish realistic expectations of treatment
- Bowel diary
- Abdominal palpation to identify fecal mass
- Evaluation of rectal diameter or identification of impacted rectum
- Bowel disimpaction using oral laxatives
- Maintenance of regular soft stools (stool softeners/laxatives for at least 4–6 months)
- Age-appropriate postprandial toileting regime and optimal defecation mechanics
- Hygiene, skin care, strategies to manage fecal incontinence
- Advocacy, liaising with school, ongoing review and support
- Addressing behavioral issues

progress monitored via a bowel diary, abdominal palpation, and ultrasound examination of rectal diameter. If 6 months of documented and consistent treatment with laxatives and a toileting program has not improved symptoms, a referral to a pediatric gastroenterologist is recommended.

References

1 Butler RJ, Redfern EJ, Holland P. Children's notions about enuresis and the implications for treatment. *Scand J Urol Nephrol Suppl* 1994;**163**:39–47.
2 Von gontard A and Neveus T. Eds of *Management of disorders of bladder and bowel control in childhood*. Cambridge University Press, London, 2006. Chapter 5.
3 Sapsford R. Rehabilitation of pelvic floor muscles utilizing trunk stabilization. *Man Ther* 2004;**9**(1): 3–12.
4 Bower WF, Yeung CK. A review of non-invasive electroneuromodulation as an intervention for non-neurogenic bladder dysfunction in children. *Neurourol Urodyn* 2004;**23**(1):63–67.
5 Bower WF, Diao M. Acupuncture as a treatment for nocturnal enuresis. *Auton Neurosci* 2010;**157**(1–2):63–67.
6 Hoebeke P, Renson C, Petillon L et al. Transcutaneous electrical nerve stimulation in children with therapy resistant nonneuropathic bladder sphincter dysfunction: a pilot study. *J Urol* 2002;**168**(6):2605–2607.
7 Bower WF, Moore KH, Adams RD. A pilot study of the home application of transcutaneous neuromodulation in children with urgency or urge incontinence. *J Urol* 2001;**166**(6): 2420–2422.
8 Pohl HG, Bauer SB, Borer JG, Diamond DA, Kelly MD, Grant R, et al. The outcome of voiding dysfunction managed with clean intermittent catheterization in neurologically and anatomically normal children. *BJU Int* 2002;**89**(9):923–927.
9 Borch L, Hagstrom S, Bower WF, Siggaard Rittig C, Rittig S, Djurhuus JC. Bladder and bowel dysfunction (BBD) and the resolution of urinary incontinence with successful management of bowel symptoms in children. *Acta Paediatr* 2013;**102**(5):e215–e220.
10 Loening-Baucke V. Urinary incontinence and urinary tract infection and their resolution with treatment of chronic constipation of childhood. *Pediatrics* 1997;**100**(2 Pt 1):228–232.

CHAPTER 13

The concept of physiotherapy for childhood BBD

Janet W. Chase[1] and Wendy F. Bower[2]

[1] Victorian Children's Continence Clinic, Cabrini Hospital, Melbourne, Australia
[2] Department of Epidemiology and Preventive Medicine, School of Public Health and Preventive Medicine, Health Services Unit, Monash University, Melbourne, Australia

The concept of physiotherapy for childhood bladder and bowel dysfunction

It is accepted that the best approach to the treatment of bladder and bowel dysfunction (BBD) in adults and children is multidisciplinary. This is reflected in the membership of Societies such as the ICS and ICCS and national continence organizations.

Continence team members have areas of common expertise and areas that are discipline specific. This chapter will not elaborate on things we can all do—for example, incontinence assessment, initial screening of behavioral comorbidities, education of child/family, voiding/bowel regimes, and use of bed-wetting alarms. Instead, it aims to elucidate the concept of physiotherapy and specific areas of expertise.

Bladder and bowel functions depend on the interplay between the somatic and autonomic nervous systems, coordinated sensorimotor functions, and smooth and striated muscle actions. Understanding this interplay is fundamental to delivering continence physiotherapy. For example, breathing patterns, posture, pain, anxiety, and spinal stability can all contribute to pelvic floor muscle (PFM) activity and disruption of bladder and bowel emptying mechanics [1–4]. Understanding the therapeutic use of electrical stimulation, the effect of differing electrical parameters, and currents on autonomic or somatic functions gives an ability to tailor treatment to neuromodulate these functions or dysfunctions.

Continence physiotherapy is a specialist area. "... experience in a very specific area of practice, arising from a detailed and particular knowledge base.

Pediatric Incontinence: Evaluation and Clinical Management, First Edition. Edited by Israel Franco,
Paul F. Austin, Stuart B. Bauer, Alexander von Gontard and Yves Homsy.
© 2015 John Wiley & Sons, Ltd. Published 2015 by John Wiley & Sons, Ltd.

Professional strength lies in the depth of understanding … underpinned by clinical reasoning and decision making" [5]. Continence/pelvic floor physiotherapists working with children have appropriate postgraduate qualifications, with previous training in neurodevelopment, both normal and abnormal, and motor learning. They are skilled at assessing muscle dysfunction and prescribing exercise such as PFM relaxation in the setting of lower urinary tract (LUT) and lower gastrointestinal tract (LGIT) dysfunction, training for strength or endurance in children with lung disease or obesity, or reestablishing balance in functional muscle groups. The physiotherapeutic approach is to train for specificity of action and then incorporate this into functional use.

In the realm of childhood incontinence intervention, physiotherapy contributes to musculoskeletal assessment, movement analysis, and understanding of the source of LUT and LGIT dysfunction. Physiotherapists use real-time transabdominal ultrasound (TAUS) for the noninvasive assessment of pelvic floor and abdominal muscle function and to deliver biofeedback, as well as the more common uses of measuring postvoid residual urine (PVR), rectal diameter, and bladder wall thickness. For comprehensive evidence-based pelvic floor physiotherapy, the reader is directed to Bo et al. [6].

Two case studies in the following demonstrate a discipline-specific stepwise approach to treatment.

Case 1

AB is an 11-year-old boy referred for retraining of defecation dynamics prior to reversal of his stoma. Weight gain and growth were satisfactory. He has a defunctioning ileostomy, having developed toxic colitis related to severe fecal retention 15 months earlier. He had a long-standing history of constipation and fecal incontinence, a normal colonic biopsy excluding Hirschsprung's disease, and normal gastric emptying studies. Previous enuresis and urinary urgency had resolved.

Prior to referral, he had (i) antegrade gas enema of his colon that showed normal size and (ii) a nuclear medicine marked stool placed through the distal limb of the stoma—showing severe anorectal retention with some reflux of contents. AB had support from a stomal therapy nurse and psychologist.

On assessment, AB was a slim, quiet boy, attentive and motivated. Prior to surgery, abdominal and anal pains were present, and his protective posture reflects that—fixed thoracic and lumbar flexion, little lumbopelvic movement, a rigid and retracted abdominal wall, and upper chest breathing. He had poor proprioceptive awareness of breathing, abdominal relaxation, or pelvic floor/sphincter activity. AB played no sport; his general fitness was assessed as being low–moderate. Table 13.1 lists the aims, management, and progression of treatment.

Table 13.1 Case 1.

Aim	Management	Progression
To establish trust, education, and expectations of treatment and provide ongoing support/problem solving	Educational DVD bowel function, age-appropriate charts regarding muscle functions, pelvic model, etc.	Reinforce and reinform and explain as necessary Regular contact
To retrain defecation dynamics	Retrain breathing, abdominal stretches, postural correction	Step-by-step at AB's pace/ability using principles of motor learning
	Train awareness of anal relaxation, PFM/transversus abdominis (TA) cocontraction/relaxation, gentle rectus abdominis release, and anal sphincter relaxation	Use transabdominal ultrasound for education and BFB
	Incorporate into toilet posture and function, that is, defecation	Abdominal EMG, no rectal/anal electrodes because of previous pain/anxiety
	Teach increasing IAP using external obliques without increasing anal closure pressure	Possible internal anal sphincter overactivity if progress limited—if so, medication or electrical neuromodulation?
To assist with pain management as needed	General relaxation	Physical agents—heat (prior), cold (postdefecation), TENS
To establish a postsurgery bowel regime	Postprandial toileting Bowel diary Aim for Bristol Stool 5	Consider electrical neuromodulation, for example, interferential therapy (IFT) to assist bowel motility:
	Increase soluble fiber intake	Allergy testing
	Laxatives	
To improve fitness level	Identify fitness activity that is appealing to AB and enhances socialization	Avoid activity that may be detrimental to his progress, for example, over development of global abdominal musculature

Case 2

CD is a 7-year-old otherwise well girl with a 3-year history of constipation, four symptomatic urinary tract infections over the last year, nonmonosymptomatic enuresis, and day wetting. Diagnoses of bladder overactivity and dysfunctional voiding established. No renal abnormality on ultrasound. Bowel and voiding regimes in place, hygiene issues addressed. Previous use

Table 13.2 Case 2.

Aim	Management	Progression
To reinforce previous education, support the child/family	Educational DVD bladder function, age-appropriate pictures, cartoons, charts regarding muscle functions, pelvic model	Use TAUS measurements, uroflowmetry to inform regarding progress and consolidate learning
To monitor bowel function	Bowel diary	Assess by abdominal palpation, TAUS rectal measurement, rectal perception, soiling. Ongoing monitoring of laxative use
To inhibit bladder overactivity	Neuromodulation—TENS 3rd sacral foramina	If limited response, consider other inhibitory pathways—pudendal afferents, S3, S4 dermatome, transcutaneous posterior tibial nerve, suprapubic [7]
To teach relaxed unopposed voiding	Relaxed lower chest breathing Correct toilet posture Awareness of muscle contraction versus relaxation Abdominal "release" Pubococcygeal (PC) awareness and relaxation—specificity of action Apply to voiding, especially in different environments and different toilets	Consider CD's ability to selectively attend, level of arousal and motivation to learn, memory, and sensoriperceptual awareness and teach accordingly. Set achievable yet specific goals. Ensure feedback of correct movement and prescribe a suitable practice regime Use TAUS to visualize effect of PC contraction/relaxation on the bladder neck EMG as indicated Monitor PVR urine on US Monitor flow curve
To treat urinary incontinence	Reinforce voiding/drinking schedules Monitor day wetting frequency and severity Identify any nocturnal polyuria or OAB Monitor enuresis episodes	If another UTI, consider prophylactic antibiotics Vibrating watch Dry days recording Repeat frequency volume chart Assessment of enuresis when LUTS resolved Treat enuresis

of anticholinergic medication with behavioral side effects, increased PVR, and constipation.

On assessment, CD is a busy and sociable child, with symptoms of bladder overactivity. She has no specific developmental or musculoskeletal deficits such as joint hypermobility or postural limitations. She does well at school and there are no concerns about her social development despite her continence difficulties. Her diet and activity levels are appropriate for age. Table 13.2 lists the aims, management, and progression of treatment.

Conclusion

Continence physiotherapists are part of the multidisciplinary pediatric continence team and bring specific skills of sensorimotor retraining, exercise prescription, therapeutic use of electrical current, and other physical modalities to treat BBD and promote, maintain, and restore physical, psychological, and social well-being.

References

1 Hodges PW, Sapsford R, Pengel LH. Postural and respiratory functions of the pelvic floor muscles. *Neurourology and Urodynamics* 2007;**26**(3):362–71.
2 Sapsford RR, Richardson CA, Maher CF, Hodges PW. Pelvic floor muscle activity in different sitting postures in continent and incontinent women. *Archives of Physical Medicine and Rehabilitation* 2008 Sep;**89**(9):1741–7.
3 Sapsford R, Hodges PW, Richardson CA, Cooper DH, Markwell SJ, Jull GA. Co-activation of the abdominal and pelvic floor muscles during voluntary exercises. *Neurourology and Urodynamics* 2001;**20**(1):31–42.
4 Sapsford RR, Clarke B, Hodges PW. The effect of abdominal and pelvic floor muscle activation patterns on urethral pressure. *World Journal of Urology* 2013 Jun;**31**(3):639–44.
5 Chartered Society of Physiotherapy. *Scope of Physiotherapy Practice 2008*. London: Chartered Society of Physiotherapy. 2008.
6 Bo K, Berghmans B, Morkved S, Van Kampen M, editors. *Evidence-Based Physical Therapy for the Pelvic Floor*. Second edition. London: Churchill Livingstone Elsevier; 2014.
7 Fall M, Lindstrom S. Functional electrical stimulation: physiological basis and clinical principles. *International Urogynecology Journal and Pelvic Floor Dysfunction* 1994;**5**:296–304.

CHAPTER 14

Biofeedback for the treatment of functional voiding problems

Ann Raes and Catherine Renson

Department of Pediatric Nephrology, Ghent University Hospital, Gent, Belgium

Introduction

Biofeedback was introduced in the 1970s and was relatively forgotten until the late 1990s. Since then the devices used to perform biofeedback have become more sophisticated [1]. The principle of biofeedback in children with dysfunctional voiding, without neurological disorder, is that they gain information about their disturbed voiding pattern and that they develop voluntary control techniques to relax the pelvic floor thereby decreasing their dysfunctional voiding pattern without the need for medications or invasive procedures. Before the biofeedback treatment is started, most children already received standard therapy, consisting of instructions about adequate toilet posture in order to reach an optimal relaxation of the pelvic floor and an individually adapted voiding and drinking schedule. Because compliance for these life-style modifications is often not optimal, it is certainly worthwhile to repeat these instructions.

The dietary log and voiding chart

The voiding and drinking chart is a diagnostic and therapeutic tool [2]. It is used to identify the habits that may contribute to their incontinence and to teach the child to deal consciously with the bladder and its function. The chart should be attainable and applicable to child and family. During the diagnostic phase, the parents are asked to record accurately for 2 weeks the voiding frequency, urine volume, fluid intake, number of wet and/or dirty pants, and number of wet/dry nights and stoolpattern. In the therapeutic phase, the voiding and drinking chart has to be completed by the child and evaluated at regular time to discuss

Pediatric Incontinence: Evaluation and Clinical Management, First Edition. Edited by Israel Franco,
Paul F. Austin, Stuart B. Bauer, Alexander von Gontard and Yves Homsy.

improvement. Some children need to adapt their quantity and/or the quality of liquid intake. A voiding frequency of five to seven times a day with a regular fluid intake spread during the day is advised. Some children need to avoid or significantly reduce their intake of soft drinks, for example, caffeine, carbonated beverages, ice-cool drinks, citrus juices or heavily sugared drinks, and milk. Some of these can induce detrusor instability or osmotic polyuria.

Toilet posture

The children are advised to void while sitting down with the thighs spread sufficiently (to relax the perineum), while leaning forward slightly with a straight back. For children who cannot reach the floor a small bench or support is placed under the feet. Small children may need a toilet reducer. It has been previously described that this posture results in optimal relaxation of the pelvic floor and in better emptying of the bladder. During voiding the children are asked to count or to sing to ensure quiet breathing in case of straining. After voiding they stay a few seconds. These simple adaptations can help and can avoid urine that trickles from the vagina in girls with vaginal micturition [3].

Relaxation biofeedback training

The process of biofeedback training is labor-intensive and time-consuming and requires a positive working relationship between an excellent skilled professional and a motivated child of appropriate developmental age (typically older than 5 years) [1, 4]. Biofeedback helps the child to coordinate the relaxation of the pelvic floor muscles during bladder contraction by means of a signal. This signal can be visual, audible, or tactile. It is of utmost importance to select the ideal candidate.

There are some conditions that a child must meet: The child has to be motivated, mature, and has to show good cooperation. Age has been mentioned by many authors as an important factor for success. It is important that the child has a well-developed body awareness that enables it to listen to the signals of his/her body. To raise the awareness of the pelvic floor and the pelvic floor muscles, the therapist first explains the location of the anus, urethra, and pelvic floor muscles with imagery (Figure 14.1). Secondly the contraction and relaxation of the pelvic floor muscles is practiced. For this, the therapist needs to evaluate when and to what extent the contraction and relaxation occurs. By manual testing of the pelvic floor, this proprioceptive examination is performed (Figure 14.2). The child is placed in the lateral recumbent position with the bottom leg stretched backward and the top leg bent forward. The therapist places one (for girls) or two fingers crosswise on the perineum and asks the child to do as though it wants to hold urine. The pelvic

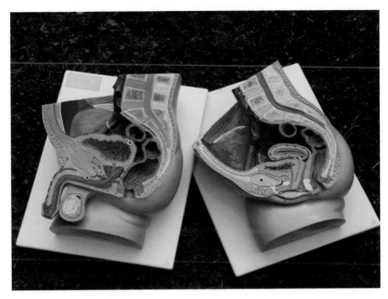

Figure 14.1 Imagery.

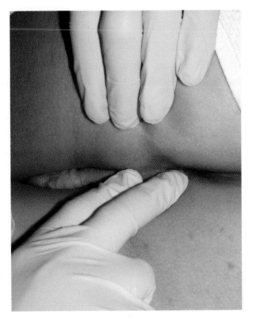

Figure 14.2 Manual exercises.

floor muscles have to be able to be contracted as selectively as possible, without involvement of the gluteus muscle. This technique stimulates the proprioception of the pelvic floor which enables the child to localize and gain control over the pelvic floor [5]. These exercises can be complemented by feedback.

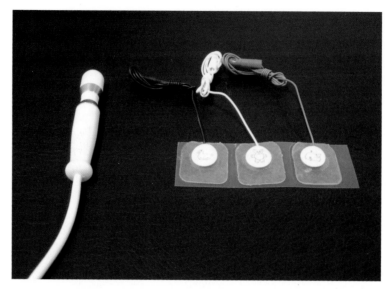

Figure 14.3 Anal plug and surface electrodes.

Myo-biofeedback: With this technique, the child gets direct insight in the activity of the pelvic floor muscle using electromyography (EMG) by means of a visual or audible signal, so it can be used as biofeedback. The muscle activity can be registered by use of a small anal plug or a surface electrode. The child lies down in lateral recumbent position in a relaxed position and the anal plug has to be introduced very carefully (Figure 14.3). The use of the anal plug is preferable because the signals are more reliable. The muscle activity is then reflected as a trace on a computer screen (or auditory feedback). The child becomes aware of the grade of relaxation and toning of the pelvic floor muscles as the curve goes up with contraction and falls down with relaxation. In this way, both relaxation and toning of the pelvic floor can be practiced. Through the direct feedback, the child is able to relax the pelvic floor muscles to attain the desired EMG tracing. One session consists of 20–30 cycles. One cycle consists of 3 s of strong contraction followed by prolonged relaxation (about 30 s). The aim of prolonged relaxation is to learn to empty the full bladder without interference of the pelvic floor muscles.

Uroflow-biofeedback: For those children where the introduction of the anal plug is experienced to be invasive, uroflow-biofeedback is an alternative (Figure 14.4). The child is asked to void while the flow curve is visualized on a screen. A normal shape is a bell curve, which is compatible with complete absence of pelvic floor activity during the urine flow. After micturition the child is immediately informed about the shape of the curve and indirect about the pelvic floor activity during micturition [6]. The child learns to recognize a disturbed pattern and can make corrections during micturition to gain an optimal uroflow curve. After each uroflow-biofeedback, an ultrasound is performed to identify residual urine. Some authors use EMG to get additive information about the use of the

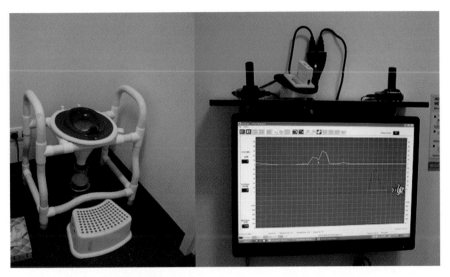

Figure 14.4 Uroflow biofeedback.

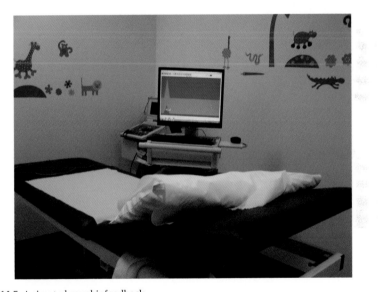

Figure 14.5 Animated myobiofeedback.

pelvic floor during voiding. A surface electrode is then placed at the perineal musculatures. This needs a skilled professional and there may be artifacts that occur when the child voids on the electrodes.

The nonanimated biofeedback techniques described above require the child to use auditory and visual signals in helping to identify the correct muscles. This can be challenging and frustrating for even the motivated child. Recently animated biofeedback became available (Figure 14.5) and several studies have documented similar results in less time [7].

The goal of each biofeedback program is improvement of the incontinence problem and cessation of urinary tract infections. Appropriate positive reinforcement and rewards should be part of the management approach. The therapy is considered successful with disappearance of lower urinary tract symptoms, normalization of the flow curve, and good pelvic floor relaxation at the start of the session. The treatment can be stopped when there are no symptoms or complaints anymore during a period of 6 months follow up.

Biofeedback efficacy

Many studies documented the success of biofeedback for managing childhood incontinence in large groups of children of different ages. Desantis carried out a systematic review and concluded that biofeedback, including electromyographic tracings, uroflows, or a combination of the two, is an effective, noninvasive method of treating functional voiding problems and that approximately 80% of children benefited from this treatment [1]. However, the observation that most reports were retrospective reviews and the possible biases in inclusion and classification of the treated groups may influence the findings.

Conclusion

Biofeedback has been shown to be very effective in children to correct continence problems secondary to dysfunctional voiding. It can be used as monotherapy or as a part of combination program. The outcome is directly related to the cooperation and motivation of the child and his environment, to practice the learned skills on a daily basis.

References

1 Desantis DJ, Leonard MP, Preston MA, Barrowman NJ, Guerra LA. Effectiveness of biofeedback for dysfunctional elimination syndrome in pediatrics: a systematic review. *Journal of Pediatric Urology.* 2011 Jun;**7**(3):342–8. PubMed PMID: 21527216.

2 Vande Walle J, Rittig S, Bauer S, Eggert P, Marschall-Kehrel D, Tekgul S, et al. Practical consensus guidelines for the management of enuresis. *European Journal of Pediatrics.* 2012 Jun;**171**(6):971–83. PubMed PMID: 22362256. Pubmed Central PMCID: 3357467. Epub 2012/03/01. eng.

3 Zeng F, Chen HQ, Qi L, Zhang XY, Li Y. Comparative study of pelvic floor biofeedback training and tolterodine for treatment of detrusor after-contraction in posturination dribbling in children. *The Journal of International Medical Research.* 2012;**40**(6):2305–10. PubMed PMID: 23321187.

4 Kjolseth D, Madsen B, Knudsen LM, Norgaard JP, Djurhuus JC. Biofeedback treatment of children and adults with idiopathic detrusor instability. *Scandinavian Journal of Urology and Nephrology.* 1994 Sep;**28**(3):243–7. PubMed PMID: 7817166.

5 Wennergren H, Oberg B. Pelvic floor exercises for children: a method of treating dysfunctional voiding. *British Journal of Urology.* 1995 Jul;**76**(1):9–15. PubMed PMID: 7648068.

6 van Gool JD, Vijverberg MA, Messer AP, Elzinga-Plomp A, de Jong TP. Functional daytime incontinence: non-pharmacological treatment. *Scandinavian Journal of Urology and Nephrology Supplementum* 1992;**141**:93–103; discussion 4–5. PubMed PMID: 1609257.

7 Kajbafzadeh AM, Sharifi-Rad L, Ghahestani SM, Ahmadi H, Kajbafzadeh M, Mahboubi AH. Animated biofeedback: an ideal treatment for children with dysfunctional elimination syndrome. *The Journal of Urology.* 2011 Dec;**186**(6):2379–84. PubMed PMID: 22019033.

CHAPTER 15

Pharmacotherapy of the child with functional incontinence and retention

Paul F. Austin[1] and Israel Franco[2]

[1] Division of Urologic Surgery, Washington University in St. Louis, School of Medicine, St. Louis Children's Hospital, St. Louis, MO, USA

[2] Maria Fareri Children's Hospital, Valhalla, NY, USA

Lower urinary tract symptom management

Every child with lower urinary tract (LUT) dysfunction should receive standard urotherapy as outlined in the ICCS standardization documents and as outlined in earlier chapters of this book [1–3]. The decision to implement pharmacotherapy is determined by the characteristics of the bladder function obtained from the clinical history, elimination diaries, and noninvasive urodynamics [4, 5]. It is advisable to use a tailored, selective approach in therapy decisions.

Overactive bladder

The clinical history of urinary urgency is the hallmark of overactive bladder (OAB) [1]. Urinary frequency is often associated with OAB as well as urge incontinence. In the past, an empirical approach with anticholinergics was undertaken but with increased understanding of LUT function in children, this blinded approach has been abandoned. We know that OAB can occur in children with a small functional bladder capacity but also in a large-sized bladder with incomplete emptying (Figure 15.1). It is the child with a small OAB and complete bladder emptying that will respond the best to pharmacotherapy. There are several choices for pharmacotherapy in the clinical management of these small OAB (Figure 15.2).

Pediatric Incontinence: Evaluation and Clinical Management, First Edition. Edited by Israel Franco, Paul F. Austin, Stuart B. Bauer, Alexander von Gontard and Yves Homsy.

© 2015 John Wiley & Sons, Ltd. Published 2015 by John Wiley & Sons, Ltd.

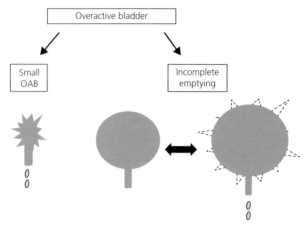

Figure 15.1 OAB subtypes.

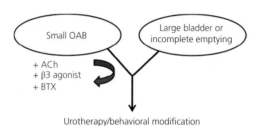

Figure 15.2 Pharmacotherapy choices for OAB.

Anticholinergics

Many classes of drugs have been studied or proposed for the treatment of symptoms of OAB in adults. Several pitfalls limit the quality of clinical studies in children, heterogeneity of the patients and their symptoms and the fact that many patients can have more than one confounding problem. The clinical trials performed in children have generally utilized patients with neurogenic voiding problems and have not concentrated on the nonneurogenic patients.

Oxybutynin is the prototype anticholinergic that targets detrusor overactivity. Furthermore, there is level 1 evidence of the efficacy of anticholinergics in treating OAB [6]. Oxybutynin has been extensively studied in the pediatric neurogenic bladder population and has both FDA and EMA labeling for this purpose. For OAB in neurologically intact children, the usage is considered off-label but nevertheless has an extensive track record in the published literature.

The mechanism of action for anticholinergics is their antimuscarinic effect. Anticholinergics competitively inhibit the binding of acetylcholine to muscarinic receptors at the neuromuscular junction. The bladder consists of primarily M2 and M3 muscarinic receptor subtypes that the anticholinergics will selectively target. Recent data suggests that antimuscarinics may be functioning more at the sensory limb of the reflex arc in neurologically intact patients than at the motor side [7].

Unfortunately, there are risks of potential side effects with the usage of anticholinergic therapy for OAB. The side effect profile is secondary to the metabolites that will target other muscarinic receptor subtypes located in other areas of the body. For example, oxybutynin is metabolized to desethyloxybutynin after passage through the hepatobiliary system, and desethyloxybutynin will target muscarinic receptor subtypes located in the salivary glands, skin, and brain. Although dry mouth is the most common side effect, constipation, gastroesophageal reflux, blurry vision, urinary retention, and cognitive side effects can all occur in children. The potential for adverse cognitive effects and delirium due to antimuscarinic drugs can occur in children but it is generally limited to overdosing situations.

Other delivery systems such as transdermal applications can be used to minimize the side effects or alternatively, different formulations of anticholinergics may be used as well. In one placebo-controlled trial, the patch caused local skin erythema in more than half the subjects (3% of cases were severe) and was associated with pruritus in up to 17%. The different anticholinergics that have been used in children can be referenced in Chapter 29.

α-Blockers

Aside from the role that α-blockers play in the management of bladder neck dysfunction and urinary retention, one of the authors (IF) has found them to be useful in ameliorating the symptoms of urgency and urge incontinence in some children [8]. In many cases, terazosin is the first-line drug for urgency and frequency due to its nonselective properties and the potential to cross the blood–brain barrier. It is well understood that there are α-1D receptors in the bladder and these receptors can modulate sensory signals from the bladder [9]. Also, the nonselective α-blockers can bind presynaptically [10, 11] and inhibit acetylcholine release, potentially reducing the instability. More selective α-blockers such as tamsulosin and alfuzosin are better suited for the management of bladder neck dysfunction, which can lead to detrusor hypertrophy and instability, but they have been documented to relieve symptoms of instability as well in adult studies [12]. Because nonselective α-blockers can cause postural hypotension, they require a gradual titration of the dose and must be used carefully. In patients where there is a family history of easily fainting or postural hypotension, dose titration is essential even with the selective α-blockers. For the most part, children tolerate α-blockade well, and we have used terazosin in children as young as 2 years old for bladder neck dysfunction associated with high-grade vesicoureteral reflux. Further research is needed to determine the optimal use of α-blockers.

β3-Agonists

An emerging treatment for OAB is β3-agonists. In a "quasi" meta-analysis and review, stimulation of the β3-adrenoceptors results in relaxation of the detrusor smooth muscle and decreased afferent signaling from the bladder [13]. Additionally, the β3-agonists improve bladder compliance and increase bladder capacity. Mirabegron is the β3-agonist with FDA, EMA, and Japanese labeling for adult indication and usage in the treatment of OAB [13]. Pediatric usage for OAB is off-label.

In randomized controlled trials in adult OAB, mirabegron decreases the number of micturitions and incontinence episodes in a 24 h period compared with placebo [13]. There is a potential for adverse drug interactions with other CYP2D6 substrates that may result in tachycardia.

Botulinum toxin

For refractory OAB, botulinum toxin (BTX) is an alternative treatment for OAB. The usage of BTX in the treatment of pediatric nonneuropathic bladder dysfunction is off-label and is discussed in detail in Chapter 22.

Urinary retention/incomplete bladder emptying

Internal urethral sphincter discoordination
α-Adrenergic antagonists (α-blockers)

α-Adrenergic receptors are located in large concentration at the bladder neck and throughout the urethra [14]. Stimulation of these α-adrenergic receptors results in smooth muscle contraction and increased outlet resistance, whereas α-adrenergic blockade results in smooth muscle relaxation and decreased bladder outlet resistance. α-Blocker therapy is routinely used to facilitate bladder emptying in adult patients but is "off-label" in pediatric patients. In selected children with LUT dysfunction characterized by incomplete bladder emptying, α-blockers have been demonstrated to be efficacious in several reports [15–21]. Other than postural hypotension in some patients, there are few complications associated with α-blocker treatment of LUT dysfunction in children [20–22], and the safety profile appears to be good.

α-Blocker treatment selection of children with LUT dysfunction is either done through a comprehensive treatment program that involves an escalating treatment paradigm [2, 4] or by identifying patients with characteristic uroflow abnormalities [23]. The uroflow finding of a prolonged "EMG lag time" is associated with bladder neck and internal urethral sphincter discoordination and may be used to select patients for α-blocker therapy [24, 25].

The EMG lag time is the time duration after the external sphincter relaxes and the flow of urine (Figure 15.3). A prolonged lag time of greater than 6 s is suggested as a reliable indicator of tailoring LUT dysfunction treatment with

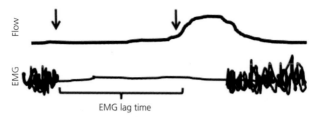

Figure 15.3 Schematic of EMG lag time assessment.

α-blocker therapy [24]. Further validation is needed to investigate the reliability and reproducibility of these uroflow findings.

Antidepressants

Tricyclics

We (IF) have found imipramine, a tricyclic antidepressant with both anticholinergic and α-adrenergic effects and, possibly, a central effect on voiding reflexes, to be effective in controlling urge incontinence in some children who were refractory to antimuscarinic therapy (Franco, unpublished data). We have used this medication in children who are refractory to conventional therapy and have achieved a 65% complete success rate, and another additional 10% had partial response to the medication. Dosing is initiated slowly with 10 mg as the initial dose and by increasing the dose to 75 mg total per day (2–3 mg/kg/day). We will typically not exceed the 75 mg dose since we have found that few need more than 50 mg/day and have seen no improvement with doses higher than 75 mg.

Imipramine is known to have a cocaine-like blocking effect on amine reuptake in nerve terminal in the rat brain, potentiating the effect of NE and 5-HT on postsynaptic membranes. It has also been shown that imipramine can modulate vesicourethral motility by elevating the threshold of the micturition reflex at Onuf's nucleus, most likely via the aforementioned blocking effect [26].

Imipramine has been shown to increase diastolic blood pressure [27] but in some cases can cause postural hypotension and cardiac conduction abnormalities and thus must be used carefully. A careful review of the literature reveals that the all cases of cardiac toxicity with the use of imipramine were all related to overdoses of the medication or in patients with conduction abnormalities. Caution should be used when the drug is used in conjunction with other drugs that have sympathomimetic effects since these are potentiated especially in the younger patients. On the other hand, desipramine has been associated with cardiac toxicity at normal dosing levels. Amitriptyline, another tricyclic, has been used more frequently for the management of interstitial cystitis and OAB in adults, and its use in children are limited.

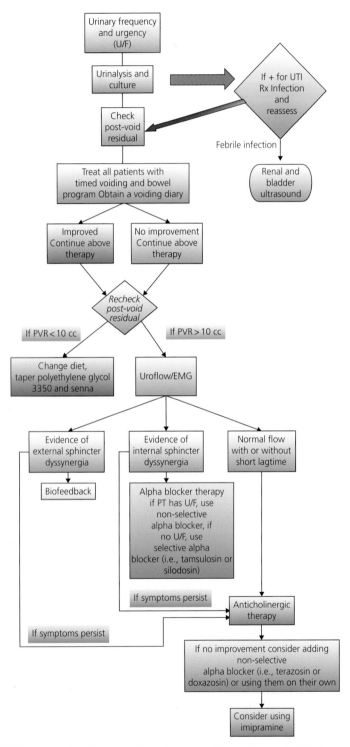

Figure 15.4 Treatment algorithm for urinary frequency. Source: Franco 2012 [5]. Reproduced with permission from Elsevier.

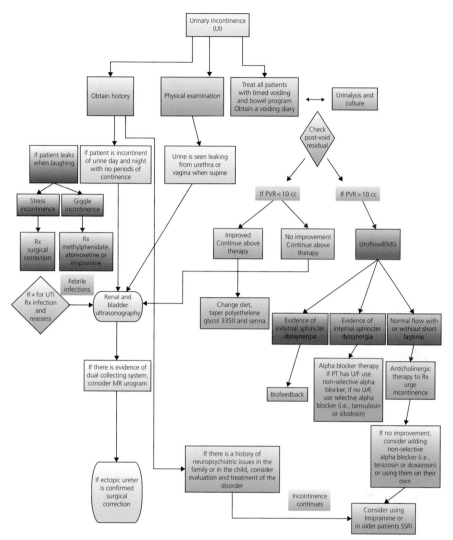

Figure 15.5 Treatment algorithm for urinary incontinence. Source: Franco 2012 [5]. Reproduced with permission from Elsevier.

SSRI/SNRI

The use of duloxetine, a known SSRI and SNRI, has been shown to be effective in animal studies in increasing the maximal bladder capacity to as much as five-fold in an acetic acid irritative study [28] and can increase the electromyographic activity of the sphincter up to eightfold [29]. These characteristics can increase bladder capacity and sphincter tone without interfering with the normal voiding cycle. SSRIs and SNRIs such as duloxetine have been useful in older patients with stress and mixed urinary incontinence [30]. We have found it to be useful in some patients who have unresponsive OAB especially when there is evidence of anxiety disorders of clinical significance.

Other drugs

The role of phosphodiesterase inhibitors in OAB is something that needs further exploration, and only time will tell if it may also play a useful role [31, 32].

External urethral sphincter discoordination
BTX

BTX is an emerging medical therapy for the treatment of children who are refractory to treatment for dysfunctional voiding [33–37]. The use of BTX in the treatment of patients with dysfunctional voiding is discussed in detail in Chapter 22.

Conclusion

In summary, there are several options of medical therapy for the treatment of the child with OAB, functional incontinence, and retention. A suggested treatment algorithm for OAB (Figure 15.4) and incontinence (Figure 15.5) is included in this chapter. The selection of pharmacotherapy is made after proper determination and identification of the underlying factor(s) of the LUT dysfunction and tailoring therapy accordingly.

References

1 Austin PF, Bauer SB, Bower W, Chase J, Franco I, Hoebeke P, et al. The standardization of terminology of lower urinary tract function in children and adolescents: update report from the standardization committee of the international Children's continence society. *The Journal of Urology*. 2014.

2 Chase J, Austin P, Hoebeke P, McKenna P. International Children's continence S. The management of dysfunctional voiding in children: a report from the standardisation committee of the international Children's continence society. *The Journal of Urology*. 2010; **183**(4):1296–302.

3 Hoebeke P, Bower W, Combs A, De Jong T, Yang S. Diagnostic evaluation of children with daytime incontinence. *The Journal of Urology*. 2010;**183**(2):699–703.

4 Thom M, Campigotto M, Vemulakonda V, Coplen D, Austin PF. Management of lower urinary tract dysfunction: a stepwise approach. *Journal of Pediatric Urology*. 2012;**8**(1):20–4.

5 Franco I. Functional bladder problems in children: pathophysiology, diagnosis, and treatment. *Pediatric Clinics of North America*. 2012;**59**(4):783–817.

6 Andersson KE, Chapple CR, Cardozo L, Cruz F, Hashim H, Michel MC, et al. Pharmacological treatment of overactive bladder: report from the international consultation on incontinence. *Current Opinion in Urology*. 2009;**19**(4):380–94.

7 Finney SM, Andersson KE, Gillespie JI, Stewart LH. Antimuscarinic drugs in detrusor over-activity and the overactive bladder syndrome: motor or sensory actions? *BJU International.* 2006;**98**(3):503–7.

8 Franco I CS, Collett T, Reda E. The use of alpha blockers to treat urgency/frequency syndrome in children.

9 Ishihama H, Momota Y, Yanase H, Wang X, de Groat WC, Kawatani M. Activation of alpha1D adrenergic receptors in the rat urothelium facilitates the micturition reflex. *The Journal of Urology.* 2006;**175**(1):358–64.

10 Somogyi GT, Tanowitz M, de Groat WC. Prejunctional facilitatory alpha 1-adrenoceptors in the rat urinary bladder. *British Journal of Pharmacology.* 1995;**114**(8):1710–6.

11 Szell EA, Yamamoto T, de Groat WC, Somogyi GT. Smooth muscle and parasympathetic nerve terminals in the rat urinary bladder have different subtypes of alpha(1) adrenoceptors. *British Journal of Pharmacology.* 2000;**130**(7):1685–91.

12 Athanasopoulos A, Gyftopoulos K, Giannitsas K, Fisfis J, Perimenis P, Barbalias G. Combination treatment with an alpha-blocker plus an anticholinergic for bladder outlet obstruction: a prospective, randomized, controlled study. *The Journal of Urology.* 2003;**169**(6):2253–6.

13 Andersson KE, Martin N, Nitti V. Selective beta(3)-adrenoceptor agonists for the treatment of overactive bladder. *The Journal of Urology.* 2013;**190**(4):1173–80.

14 Ek A. Adrenergic innervation and adrenergic mechanisms. A study of the human urethra. *Acta Pharmacol Toxicology.* 1978;**43** Suppl 2:35–40.

15 Austin P. The role of alpha blockers in children with dysfunctional voiding. *The Scientific World Journal.* 2009;**9**:880–3.

16 Yucel S, Akkaya E, Guntekin E, Kukul E, Akman S, Melikoglu M, et al. Can alpha-blocker therapy be an alternative to biofeedback for dysfunctional voiding and urinary retention? a prospective study. *The Journal of Urology.* 2005;**174**(4 Pt 2):1612–5; discussion 5.

17 Donohoe JM, Combs AJ, Glassberg KI. Primary bladder neck dysfunction in children and adolescents II: results of treatment with alpha-adrenergic antagonists. *The Journal of Urology.* 2005;**173**(1):212–6.

18 Bogaert G, Beckers G, Lombaerts R. The use and rationale of selective alpha blockade in children with non-neurogenic neurogenic bladder dysfunction. *Official Journal of the Brazilian Society of Urology.* 2004;**30**(2):128–34.

19 Yang SS, Wang CC, Chen YT. Effectiveness of alpha1-adrenergic blockers in boys with low urinary flow rate and urinary incontinence. *Journal of the Formosan Medical Association = Taiwan yi zhi.* 2003;**102**(8):551–5.

20 Cain MP, Wu SD, Austin PF, Herndon CD, Rink RC. Alpha blocker therapy for children with dysfunctional voiding and urinary retention. *The Journal of Urology.* 2003;**170**(4 Pt 2):1514–5; discussion 6–7.

21 Austin PF, Homsy YL, Masel JL, Cain MP, Casale AJ, Rink RC. Alpha-adrenergic blockade in children with neuropathic and nonneuropathic voiding dysfunction. *The Journal of Urology.* 1999;**162**(3 Pt 2):1064–7.

22 Vanderbrink BA, Gitlin J, Toro S, Palmer LS. Effect of tamsulosin on systemic blood pressure and nonneurogenic dysfunctional voiding in children. *The Journal of Urology.* 2009;**181**(2):817–22; discussion 22.

23 Van Batavia JP, Combs AJ, Horowitz M, Glassberg KI. Primary bladder neck dysfunction in children and adolescents III: results of long-term alpha-blocker therapy. *The Journal of Urology.* 2010;**183**(2):724–30.

24 Van Batavia JP, Combs AJ, Fast AM, Glassberg KI. Use of non-invasive uroflowmetry with simultaneous electromyography to monitor patient response to treatment for lower urinary tract conditions. *Journal of Pediatric Urology.* 2014;**10**(3):532–7.

25 Van Batavia JP, Combs AJ, Hyun G, Bayer A, Medina-Kreppein D, Schlussel RN, et al. Simplifying the diagnosis of 4 common voiding conditions using uroflow/electromyography, electromyography lag time and voiding history. *The Journal of Urology.* 2011;**186**(4 Suppl):1721–6.

26 Hunsballe JM, Djurhuus JC. Clinical options for imipramine in the management of urinary incontinence. *Urological Research.* 2001;**29**(2):118–25.

27 Rapoport JL, Mikkelsen EJ, Zavadil A, Nee L, Gruenau C, Mendelson W, et al. Childhood enuresis. II. Psychopathology, tricyclic concentration in plasma, and antienuretic effect. *Archives of General Psychiatry.* 1980;**37**(10):1146–52.

28 Thor KB. Serotonin and norepinephrine involvement in efferent pathways to the urethral rhabdosphincter: implications for treating stress urinary incontinence. *Urology.* 2003;**62**(4 Suppl 1):3–9.

29 Thor KB, Katofiasc MA. Effects of duloxetine, a combined serotonin and norepinephrine reuptake inhibitor, on central neural control of lower urinary tract function in the chloralose-anesthetized female cat. *The Journal of Pharmacology and Experimental Therapeutics.* 1995;**274**(2):1014–24.

30 Steers WD, Herschorn S, Kreder KJ, Moore K, Strohbehn K, Yalcin I, et al. Duloxetine compared with placebo for treating women with symptoms of overactive bladder. *BJU International.* 2007;**100**(2):337–45.

31 Oger S, Behr-Roussel D, Gorny D, Denys P, Lebret T, Alexandre L, et al. Relaxation of phasic contractile activity of human detrusor strips by cyclic nucleotide phosphodiesterase type 4 inhibition. *European Urology.* 2007;**51**(3):772–80; discussion 80–1.

32 Werkstrom V, Svensson A, Andersson KE, Hedlund P. Phosphodiesterase 5 in the female pig and human urethra: morphological and functional aspects. *BJU International.* 2006;**98**(2):414–23.

33 Vricella GJ, Campigotto M, Coplen DE, Traxel EJ, Austin PF. Long-term efficacy and durability of botulinum-A toxin for refractory dysfunctional voiding in children. *The Journal of Urology.* 2014;**191**(5 Suppl):1586–91.

34 Franco I, Landau-Dyer L, Isom-Batz G, Collett T, Reda EF. The use of botulinum toxin A injection for the management of external sphincter dyssynergia in neurologically normal children. *The Journal of Urology.* 2007;**178**(4 Pt 2):1775–9; discussion 9–80.

35 Radojicic ZI, Perovic SV, Milic NM. Is it reasonable to treat refractory voiding dysfunction in children with botulinum-A toxin? *The Journal of Urology.* 2006;**176**(1):332–6; discussion 6.

36 Mokhless I, Gaafar S, Fouda K, Shafik M, Assem A. Botulinum A toxin urethral sphincter injection in children with nonneurogenic neurogenic bladder. *The Journal of Urology.* 2006;**176**(4 Pt 2):1767–70; discussion 70.

37 Cruz F, Silva C. Botulinum toxin in the management of lower urinary tract dysfunction: contemporary update. *Current Opinion in Urology.* 2004;**14**(6):329–34.

CHAPTER 16

Treatment of functional constipation and fecal incontinence

Vera Loening-Baucke[1] and Alexander Swidsinski[2]

[1] Pediatrics Department, General Pediatric Division, University of Iowa, Iowa City, IA, USA
[2] Medizinische Klinik und Poliklinik, Gastroenterologie, Hepatologie and Endokrinologie, Charité, Universitaetsmedizin Berlin, Campus Charite Mitte, Berlin, Germany

In a primary care clinic in North America, 3% of infants suffered from functional constipation in the first and 10% in the second year of life [1]. In 4–7-year-olds, 18% had suffered from constipation and 4.4% from functional fecal incontinence (≥1/week) [2]. The functional fecal incontinence was associated with constipation in 95% and was not associated with constipation or underlying disease in 5% (functional nonretentive fecal incontinence).

The aims of this chapter are to discuss the treatment of these defecation disorders and to report on outcome.

Treatment of functional constipation in infants and toddlers

The diagnosis of constipation is based upon the history and physical examination. However, in the very young infant, an organic condition needs to be ruled out, if alarming symptoms, such as a history of delayed passage of meconium or passage of a meconium plug at birth is given or if the physical examination shows abdominal distention, or failure to thrive.

Fiber or diet: Acute, simple constipation in infants and toddlers is usually treated first with sorbitol containing juices, such as prune, pear, and apple juice; addition of pureed fruits and vegetables; formula changes; or medication with high sugar content, such as 1 tsp of barley malt extract or 1 tsp of corn syrup. The amount and frequencies of these can be increased until the desired stool consistency is reached. Dietary changes can include decreasing excessive milk intake. An allergy to milk has not been confirmed as a cause of constipation. In addition, no evidence supporting the use of prebiotic and probiotic was found [3].

Pediatric Incontinence: Evaluation and Clinical Management, First Edition. Edited by Israel Franco, Paul F. Austin, Stuart B. Bauer, Alexander von Gontard and Yves Homsy.
© 2015 John Wiley & Sons, Ltd. Published 2015 by John Wiley & Sons, Ltd.

Laxative: If despite dietary changes the stool is still hard and painful to evacuate, then osmotic laxatives are given, such as polyethylene glycol (dose, 0.7 g/kg body weight/day) or lactulose, sorbitol, or milk of magnesia (dose, 1–3 mL/kg body weight/day). The key to effective treatment is assuring painless defecation. Behavior modification using rewards for successes in toilet learning is helpful in older toddlers.

Outcome

Dietary changes resolved the constipation in infants and toddlers in 25% [1]. Ninety-two percent of constipated infants and toddlers responded to laxative treatment [1].

One study specifically targeted 90 younger constipated children (<4 years). After a mean follow-up of 7 years, 63% had recovered [4].

Infant dyschezia and **infrequent bowel movements in breastfed infants**, both accompanied by soft to loose stools, are often misinterpreted as constipation. Infant dyschezia is the term used for otherwise healthy infants in the first few months of life who appear to have significant discomfort and excessive straining associated with defecation and crying for over 10 min, followed by successful passage of a soft to liquid stool. These symptoms resolve over time. Breastfed infants may defecate after each feeding or have infrequent soft to loose bowel movements up to every 14 days [1]. This bowel pattern in breastfed infants is considered normal and no treatment is necessary. Still with very infrequent stooling, a physical examination, including abdominal and rectal examination, should be performed.

Treatment of functional constipation with and without fecal incontinence in children and adolescents

Most children with functional constipation with or without fecal incontinence and often urinary incontinence and/or abdominal pain benefit from a precise, well-organized plan. The treatment is comprehensive and has four phases including education, disimpaction, prevention of reaccumulation of stools, and withdrawal of treatment.

Education: Effective education is important in the treatment and includes developmentally appropriate explanation to parents and child of the anatomy and physiology of defecation, explanation of the prevalence of constipation and that fecal incontinence is most often involuntary, and discussion of the related shame, embarrassment, and social issues. We stress that the defecation problem is most often not caused by a disturbance in the psychological behavior of the child and is not the parents' fault. A caring relationship is established, because the treatment of functional constipation with or without fecal incontinence is a long-term process. Without the family's and the child's compliance, the recommended therapy will not be successful.

Disimpaction: The fecal impaction can be resolved comfortably with oral laxatives, such as polyethylene glycol, with or without electrolytes. A study by Youssef et al. [5] demonstrated that 1.5 g/kg body weight/day of electrolyte-free polyethylene glycol for 3 days was efficient in removing the rectal fecal impaction within 5 days. The fecal impaction can also be softened and liquefied with large quantities of oral mineral oil, lactulose, or mineral oil (2 mL/kg body weight twice daily) for several days, but the fecal incontinence increases till the fecal impaction is resolved.

The rapid removal of the fecal retention with hypertonic phosphate enema (6 mL/kg body weight, up to 135 mL twice) is now rarely used. The use of cleansing soapsuds enemas is not advised; it can cause bowel necrosis, bowel perforation, and death. The use of tap-water enemas is not advised, because it is most often not effective and multiple water enemas can lead to dilution of serum electrolytes and may result in seizures and death.

Prevention of reaccumulation of stools (maintenance therapy)

Behavior modification: The child needs to be reconditioned to normal bowel habits by regular toilet use. The child is encouraged to sit on the toilet for up to 5 min, three to four times a day following meals. The children and their parents need to be instructed to keep a daily record of bowel movements, fecal and urinary incontinence, and medication use. This helps to monitor compliance and helps to make appropriate adjustments in the treatment program by parents and physician. If necessary positive reinforcement and rewards for compliant behavior are given for effort and later for success, using star charts, little presents or television viewing or computer game time as rewards.

Fiber: Normalization of the fiber content of the diet is recommended. A recent review concluded that there was no evidence to support the use of fiber supplements [3].

Laxatives: In most constipated patients, daily defecation is maintained by the daily administration of laxatives beginning in the evening of the clinic visit. Suggested dosages of commonly used laxatives are given in the Table 16.1.

First-line laxatives: Polyethylene glycol (PEG) without added electrolytes (PEG 3350, MiraLax®, Braintree Laboratories, Inc., Braintree, MA, United States) is tasteless, odorless, and colorless and has no grit when stirred in juice, Kool-Aid, or water for several minutes. PEG is not degraded by bacteria, is not readily absorbed, and, thus, acts as an excellent osmotic agent and is safe. PEG 3350 with electrolytes (Movicol®, Norgine Pharmaceuticals Ltd., United Kingdom) and PEG 4000 with electrolytes (Forlax®, Ipsen, Paris, France) are not tasteless, but are only available in some countries.

Since PEG has become available, milk of magnesia, lactulose, sorbitol, and mineral oil have become *second-line laxatives*. Mineral oil should never be force-fed or given to patients with dysphagia, gastroesophageal reflux, or vomiting because of the danger of aspiration pneumonia.

Table 16.1 Suggested medications and dosages for maintenance therapy in constipation with or without fecal incontinence.

Medication	Age	Dose
First-line treatment		
Polyethylene glycol		
3350 (MiraLax®)	>1 month	0.4–0.7 g/kg body weight/day
3350 + electrolytes (Movicol®)	>6 months	13.8–40 g/day
4000 (Forlax®)	>6 months	0.5 g/kg body weight/day
Second-line treatment		
Lactulose, sorbitol, milk of magnesia, mineral oil	>1 months	1–3 mL/kg body weight/day
Stimulant laxatives		
Senna	>2–6 years	2.5–5 mg 1–2× daily
	>6 years	7.5–10 mg 1–2× daily
Sodium picosulfate	>1 month	2.5–10 mg once daily
	>4 years	2.5–20 mg once daily
Rectal treatment		
Bisacodyl suppository	>10 years	5–10 mg/day
Phosphate enema	>10 years	6 mL/kg body weight up to 135 mL/day
Glycerin enema	>10 years	20–30 mL/day (1/2 glycerin + 1/2 normal saline)

We use senna (5–10 mL or 1–2 tablets) when liquid stools produced by osmotic laxatives are retained. The North American Society for Pediatric Gastroenterology, Hepatology, and Nutrition recommended senna for short-term therapy. It has been suggested that senna could produce changes in the ganglion cells, but that has not been proven [6, 7].

A newer drug used as a stimulant is sodium picosulfate (2.5–20 mg once a day). Occasionally, I advise rectal treatment, such as a daily 10 mg bisacodyl suppository or a daily phosphate or glycerin enema, as initial treatment for several months in an older child who would like immediate control of the incontinence (see Table 16.1).

The choice of medication for functional constipation with or without fecal incontinence does not seem as important as the child's and parents' compliance with the treatment regimen. There is only a starting dosage for each child (Table 16.1) that must be adjusted to induce one to two bowel movements per day that are loose enough to ensure complete daily emptying of the lower bowel and to prevent fecal incontinence and abdominal pain.

No evidence exists to support the use of *fiber supplements* or *biofeedback treatment* alone in the treatment of constipation that is severe enough to require medical attention [3, 8].

Psychological treatment: Functional constipation and particularly fecal incontinence affect the lives of these children and families in several areas—physically, psychologically, educationally, and socially—and in terms of self-esteem. Most often, coexisting behavior problems improve with treatment but can persist and be associated with poor treatment outcome. Children who do not improve should be referred for further evaluation.

Follow-up visits and weaning from medication

Since the management of functional constipation with or without fecal incontinence requires considerable patience and effort on the part of the child and parents, it is important to provide necessary support and encouragement through regularly scheduled office visits. Progress should be initially assessed monthly by review of the stool records and repeat of the abdominal and often the rectal examination in order to assure that the problem is adequately managed. If necessary, dosage adjustment is made and the child and parents are encouraged to continue with the regimen. After regular bowel habits are established, the frequency of toilet sitting is reduced and the medication dosage is gradually decreased to a dosage that maintains one bowel movement daily and prevents the fecal incontinence. Once the child feels the urge to defecate and initiates toilet use on his/her own, then the scheduled toilet times are discontinued. After 6–12 months, reduction with discontinuation of the medication is attempted. Treatment (laxatives and/or toilet sitting) needs to resume if constipation, fecal incontinence, urinary incontinence, and/or abdominal pain recurs.

What can go wrong in the treatment?

Physician and the parents and children make frequent mistakes. Frequent mistakes by physicians are as follows: treating with stool softeners and laxatives but not removing the fecal impaction, removing the fecal impaction but failing to start maintenance therapy, giving too low a laxative dose, not controlling the adequacy and success of therapy with follow-up visits, stopping the laxative too soon, and not providing education, anticipatory guidance, continuing support, and regular follow-up. Rarely is the diagnosis of functional constipation not correct. Frequent mistakes by the parents and children are as follows: not insisting that the child uses the toilet at regular times for defecation trials; not giving the medication daily or, worse, discontinuing the laxatives as soon as the fecal incontinence has disappeared; or not restarting the laxative after the child had a relapse.

Outcome

Outcome in most publications of functional constipated children (>4 years of age) with or without fecal incontinence was assessed by rates of successful treatment and recovery (off laxatives).

Behavior modification: There is only one study that examined behavior modification as monotherapy—36% had recovered 1 year later with behavior modification alone, and 51% with behavior modification plus laxative treatment.

Laxatives and behavior modification

1-year outcome: Nine well-designed 1-year outcome studies have been reviewed previously [8]. Laxative treatment with behavior modification dramatically improved constipation, abdominal pain, and functional fecal incontinence. Four of these studies, evaluating children with constipation with or without functional fecal incontinence, showed recovery rates of 31–59%. Five studies evaluated children with functional constipation with fecal incontinence. The 1-year recovery rates with laxatives such as milk of magnesia, lactulose, or polyethylene glycol in children with constipation and fecal incontinence ranged from 33 to 51%.

Long-term outcome: Long-term outcome studies (4–10-year follow-up) report recovery rates between 48 and 69% [8]. The largest long-term follow-up study is by van Ginkel et al. [7]. They initially enrolled 418 children with functional constipation, 2/3 with and 1/3 without fecal incontinence. All were older than 5 years of age at initiation of therapy. The recovery rate of 193 children was 63% after 5 years and 68% of 48 children had recovered after 8 years [9]. However, 50% of recovered children had at least one relapse and approximately 30% of children, who had reached adolescence, were still having problems with constipation or fecal incontinence. These findings show that constipation with or without fecal incontinence is not a problem, which all children will eventually outgrow.

Treatment of nonretentive fecal incontinence

It has been recognized that 5–20% of children with fecal incontinence have no underlying constipation. They have functional nonretentive fecal incontinence. The diagnosis is made on the basis of a history of normal bowel movement frequency and no evidence of constipation by history and physical examination. The underlying mechanism is largely unknown.

The treatment approach consists of education, toilet sitting (3–4 times daily, 5 min after meals without any distractions), and filling out a bowel diary. Rewards, such as praise, small gifts, and TV or computer time, can enhance motivation. An appropriate diagnosis of functional nonretentive fecal incontinence is important, because these patients do not benefit from laxatives.

Outcome

Voskuijl et al. [10] studied 114 children with functional nonretentive fecal incontinence for approximately 10 years. Recovery was defined as having <1 episode of fecal incontinence in 2 weeks while not using medication, such as loperamide, for at least 1 month. After 2 years of intensive medical and behavioral treatment, only 29% had recovered. At the age of 12 years, 49% of patients still had not recovered, and at age 18 years, 15% had not recovered. No prognostic factors for success were found [10].

Because the etiology of functional nonretentive fecal incontinence is not known, further studies and evaluation of different treatments will be necessary to come up with better treatment recommendations.

References

1 Loening-Baucke V. Prevalence, symptoms and outcome of constipation in infants and toddlers. *J Pediatr* 2005;**146**:359–63.
2 Loening-Baucke V. Prevalence rates for constipation, faecal incontinence and urinary incontinence in children evaluated in primary care clinics. *Arch Dis Child* 2007;**92**:486–9.
3 Tabbers MM, Di Lorenzo C, Berger MY, et al. Evaluation and treatment of functional constipation in infants and children: evidence-based recommendations from ESPGHAN and NASPGHAN. *J Pediatr Gastr Nutr* 2014;**58**:258–74 .
4 Loening-Baucke V. Constipation in early childhood: patient characteristics, treatment, and long-term follow up. *Gut* 1993;**34**:1400–4.
5 Youssef NN, Peters JM, Henderson W, et al. Dose responses of PEG 3350 for the treatment of childhood fecal impaction. *J Pediatr* 2002;**141**:410–4.
6 Kiernan JA, Heinicke EA. Resistance of myenteric neurons in the colon of the rat or mouse. *Neuroscience* 1989;**30**:837–42.
7 Heinicke, EA, Kierman JA. Resistance of myenteric neurons in the rat's colon to depletion by 1,8-dihydroxyanthraquinone. *J Pharm Pharmacol* 1990;**42**:123–5.
8 Loening-Baucke V, Swidsinski A. Constipation. In: Faure C, Di Lorenzo C, Thapar N (eds), *Pediatric Neurogastroenterology: Gastrointestinal Motility and Functional Disorders in Children.* Springer Science+Business Media, New York. 2013:413–28.
9 van Ginkel R, Reitsma JB, Bueller HA, et al. Childhood constipation: longitudinal follow-up beyond puberty. *Gastroenterology* 2003;**125**;357–63.
10 Voskuijl WP, Reitsma JB, van Ginkel R, et al. Longitudinal follow-up of children with functional nonretentive fecal incontinence. *Clin Gastroenterol Hepatol* 2006;**4**:67–72.

CHAPTER 17

Peripheral tibial nerve stimulation therapy for the treatment of functional voiding problems

Mario De Gennaro and Maria Luisa Capitanucci

Urology Unit, Department of Nephrology and Urology, Children's Hospital Bambino Gesu', Rome, Italy

Introduction

Peripheral tibial nerve stimulation (PTNS) was initially tested in clinical trials more than 25 years ago [1]. Several studies and randomized controlled trials in adult patients upgraded PTNS to level 1 of evidence [1]. These landmark reports led to resurgent interest in PTNS as a potential treatment option also in children with refractory lower urinary tract dysfunction (LUTD).

Among different neuromodulation techniques, transcutaneous electrical nerve stimulation (TENS) and PTNS offer minimally invasive, nonsurgical, and reversible second-line means to treat LUTD in children [2]. Using surface suprapubic or sacral electrodes, TENS has been widely popularized to treat refractory OAB in children [3]. On the contrary, since needle insertion is required to perform PTNS, few experiences have been reported with this technique in children. However, published uncontrolled cohort studies seem to indicate good tolerability and efficacy of PTNS in children with OAB and dysfunctional voiding (DV) [4–6]. Comparing TENS versus PTNS, Barroso et al. [7] found that TENS is more effective in resolving OAB symptoms than PTNS, which matches parental perception. However, there were no statistically significant differences in the evaluation by dysfunctional voiding symptom score, or in complete resolution of urgency or diurnal incontinence between the two techniques.

Pediatric Incontinence: Evaluation and Clinical Management, First Edition. Edited by Israel Franco, Paul F. Austin, Stuart B. Bauer, Alexander von Gontard and Yves Homsy.
© 2015 John Wiley & Sons, Ltd. Published 2015 by John Wiley & Sons, Ltd.

Technique

Technique of PTNS was described by Stoller in the late 1990s [1]. PTNS device was approved by FDA in 2006. PTNS is performed by means of a 34-gauge needle electrode inserted 4–5 cm cephalad to the medial malleolus [1]. When current is applied, flexion of big toe or movement of other toes confirms correct electrode positioning. Current intensity is the highest level tolerated by patient. Generally, sessions last for 30 min and are done once a week for 10–12 weeks. However, a more frequent stimulation and/or a shortened treatment program seems to guarantee similar positive results in adult patients [1].

Mechanism of action of PTNS

Posterior tibial nerve is a peripheral mixed nerve (L4–S3), which also contributes to sensory and motor control of bladder–sphincter complex. Even if several studies have tried to better clarify mechanism of action, it still remains unclear. The main neurophysiological mechanism of PTNS could be bladder activity modulation by depolarizing somatic sacral and lumbar afferent fibers. Recently, Tai and coworkers [8] have found that irritation-induced bladder overactivity is suppressed by tibial nerve stimulation in cats. An effect on supraspinal centers has also been demonstrated by Finazzi-Agro' et al. [9] who found significant increase in long latency somatosensory evoked potentials amplitude after the end of PTNS program. This finding could reflect a modification in an elaborate mechanism of sensory stimuli, suggesting a possible reorganization of cortical excitability after PTNS. A peripheral effect on the bladder has also been hypothesized by Danisman who demonstrated reduction of mast cells count in an animal model [10].

PTNS in pediatric lower urinary tract dysfunction

Only prospective nonrandomized trials (level of evidence 2–3) are available for PTNS as treatment for refractory LUTD in children (Table 17.1).

In 2002, Hoebeke et al. published the first pilot study on PTNS in pediatric OAB [5]. The Authors found reasonable efficacy of PTNS and patient compliance (Table 17.1).

Successively, our group studied and confirmed the good tolerability of PTNS in children, evaluating the level and type of pain at needle insertion and during stimulation [4]. Relevant improvement rate was found in both children with OAB (80%) and DV (71%) who were investigated for PTNS tolerability.

Recently, we analyzed long-term results of PTNS in different types of pediatric refractory LUTD, comparing neurogenic with nonneurogenic LUTD and OAB

Table 17.1 PTNS in children with lower urinary tract dysfunction.

Reference	Stimulation	Treatment period	LUTD	pts	Improvement rate (%)	Follow-up
Hoebeke et al. [5]	30 min/session 1 session/week	12 weeks	OAB	31	87	3 months
De Gennaro et al. [4]	30 min/session 1 session/week	12 weeks	OAB	10	80	3 months
			DV	7	71	
Capitanucci et al. [6]	30 min/session 1 session/week	12 weeks + maintenance (1 session/month)	NB	7	14	2 years
			OAB	14	86	
			DV	14	100	

DV, dysfunctional voiding; NB, neurogenic bladder; OAB, overactive bladder.

with DV cases (Table 17.1) [6]. Improvement was significantly greater ($p < 0.002$) in nonneurogenic (78%) than in neurogenic (14%) patients [6]. Improvement in some patients with neurogenic LUTD due to spinal dysraphism could be explained by the heterogeneity and incompleteness of neurological lesions. A careful selection of neurogenic patients could improve PTNS effectiveness in this patient subset. In this view, changes of amplitude of long latency somatosensory evoked potential [9] could be particularly useful to identify neuropathic children who might be responders to PTNS. Cure rate at a 2-year follow-up in OAB and DV cases [6] is reported in Table 17.1: in the long-term, 50% of patients with OAB and 29% of those with DV needed of a chronic monthly PTNS session to maintain results. Whether such maintenance session has precise neurophysiological basis or is simply a placebo effect remains to be clarified.

Conclusions

Long-term results of PTNS in children with both OAB and DV indicate that PTNS should be a part of the pediatric urological armamentarium. Waiting for further randomized controlled trials that definitively confirm PTNS efficacy and safety, use of PTNS may be reasonably suggested in refractory cases of OAB and DV.

References

1 Gabriele G, Topazio L, Iacovelli V et al.: Percutaneous tibial nerve stimulation (PTNS) efficacy in the treatment of lower urinary tract dysfunctions: a systematic review. *BMC Urol.*, 2013, **13**:61–72.
2 De Gennaro M, Capitanucci ML, Mosiello G et al.: Current state of nerve stimulation technique for lower urinary tract dysfunction in children. *J. Urol.*, 2011, **185**(5):1517–7.

3 Lordelo P, Teles A, Veiga ML et al.: Transcutaneous electrical nerve stimulation in children with overactive bladder: a randomized clinical trial. *J. Urol.*, 2010,**184**(2):683–9.

4 De Gennaro M, Capitanucci ML, Mastracci P et al.: Percutaneous tibial nerve neuromodulation is well tolerated in children and effective for treating refractory vesical dysfunction. *J. Urol.*, 2004,**171**:1911–13.

5 Hoebeke P, Renon C, Petillon L et al.: Percutaneous electrical nerve stimulation in children with therapy resistant non-neuropathic bladder-sphincter dysfunction. *J. Urol.*, 2002, **168**:2605–7.

6 Capitanucci ML, Camanni D, Demelas F et al.: Long-term efficacy of percutaneous tibial nerve stimulation for different types of lower urinary tract dysfunction in children. *J. Urol.*, 2009,**182**(4): 2056–61.

7 Barroso U, Viterbo V, Bittencourt J et al.: Posterior tibial nerve stimulation vs parasacral transcutaneous neuromodulation for overactive bladder in children. *J. Urol.*, 2013, **190**(2):673–7.

8 Tai C, Chen M, Shen B et al.: Irritation induced bladder overactivity is suppressed by tibial nerve stimulation in cats. *J. Urol.*, 2011,**186**(1):326–30.

9 Finazzi-Agro' E, Rocchi C, Pachatz C et al.: Percutaneous tibial nerve stimulation produces effect on brain activity: study on the modifications of the long latency somatosensory evoked potentials. *Neurourol. Urodyn.*, 2009,**28**:320–4.

10 Danisman A, Kutlu O, Akkaya E, Karpuzoğlu G, Erdoğru T: Tibial nerve stimulation diminishes mast cell infiltration in the bladder wall induced by interstitial cystitis urine. *Scand. J. Urol. Nephrol.*, 2007,**41**(2):98–102.

CHAPTER 18

Sacral nerve stimulation therapy for the treatment of functional voiding problems

Alonso Carrasco Jr[1], Moira E. Dwyer[1] and Yuri E. Reinberg[2]

[1] Department of Urology, Mayo Clinic Rochester, Rochester, MN, USA
[2] Department of Urological Surgery, Children's Hospitals & Clinics of Minnesota, Pediatric Surgical Associates Ltd., Minneapolis, MN, USA

Introduction

Sacral nerve stimulation (SNS) therapy using the InterStim II® device (Medtronic, Minneapolis, MN; Figure 18.1) was first approved in 1997 for the treatment of urge incontinence in adults. Safety and effectiveness of InterStim therapy have not been established for pediatric use under the age of 16 for urinary control or under the age of 18 for bowel control. However, the off-label application of this device in children with bladder bowel dysfunction (BBD) emerged. BBD, a diagnosis of exclusion, is a well-recognized condition characterized by symptoms that include urinary incontinence, frequency, urgency, nocturnal enuresis, constipation, and encopresis [1]. BBD is currently the most common indication for SNS therapy in children. In this chapter, we provide a review of SNS therapy for treatment of BBD in children.

Mechanism of action of SSN

SSN originated from attempts to outline the complex micturition pathway. For a more detailed review of the neurophysiology of voiding and defecation, the reader is referred to Sections 1 and 3 of this book. It is well established that the integration and balance of inhibitory (sympathetic), excitatory (parasympathetic), somatic, and supratentorial signals result in continence and the voiding reflex. Typically, the periaqueductal gray (PAG) receives afferent input from the bladder (unconscious control) along with anterior cingulate cortex and prefrontal cortex input (conscious control) [2]. The PGA integrates these data and modulates the bladder accordingly (storage versus and emptying) via input to the pontine

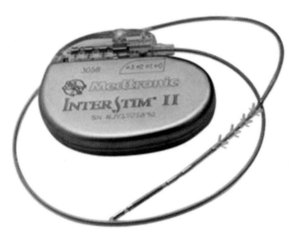

Figure 18.1 Implantable pulse generator of InterStim II® device (Medtronic, Minneapolis, MN) with quadripolar tined lead. Reprinted with the permission from Medtronic, Inc. © 2010.

micturition center (PMC) [2]. The PMC provides output signal to parasympathetic, sympathetic, and sphincter motor nuclei in the lumbosacral spinal cord to coordinate voiding reflexes via sacral nerve roots 2–4 [2]. Symptoms of BBD are likely to represent an imbalance or miscommunication between these complex signal pathways. Although the mechanisms underlying the neuromodulation and therapeutic effects of SNS are still unclear, functional brain imaging studies have demonstrated that SNS restores normal activity in the micturition pathway via afferent stimulation of the PAG, PMC, and cingulated cortex, rather than direct activation of efferent sacral nerves [3–5]. Neuromodulation of these areas is believed to result in alteration in the storage and emptying reflexes leading to the therapeutic effects of SNS [4, 5].

Patient selection for SSN

A full medical history, physical examination, basic laboratories, urinalysis, and functional/anatomic tests (abdominal radiograph, voiding cystourethrogram, renal ultrasound, and urodynamic studies) should be obtained to rule out other etiologies of voiding and bowel symptoms (neurologic or metabolic). One should consider obtaining a lumbosacral magnetic resonance imaging to rule out occult spinal cord abnormalities. Once other causes have been ruled out, the patient can be diagnosed with BBD.

Conservative therapies such as timed voiding, double voiding, and dietary modifications can result in symptom improvement in a large proportion of patients. Noninvasive therapies such as biofeedback, stool softeners, and antimuscarinic and/or alpha-adrenergic medications may be used as indicated. In our practice, in order to qualify for SNS therapy, the patients must have tried and failed at least 6 months of maximal medical and behavioral therapy as demonstrated with voiding/defecation diary. If a patient is a candidate for SNS therapy, a full discussion of the risks, benefits, and alternatives (e.g., percutaneous tibial nerve stimulation, biofeedback, intravesical Botox) must be undertaken. Risks that must be discussed include pain at site of device implantation, wound/device infection (9–13%), undesirable stimulation or sensations (<1%), device malfunction such as lead migration/breakage (40%), and ineffectiveness of therapy (7%).

Implantation technique

Physician training and certification is required prior InterStim II® implantation. For a more extensive review of the device itself and information on training/certification, the readers should consult Medtronic's website (www.medtronic.com). For a more detailed explanation and illustration of surgical technique, the reader is recommended to review the literature dedicated exclusively to this [6, 7].

Implantation consists of a two-step process under general anesthesia (holding use of paralytics), using prophylactic antibiotics, with the patient in the prone position and with the feet and buttocks exposed in order to assess the motor response to SNS (bellows and dorsiflexion of the great toe). Stage 1 consists of placing a 20 gauge 3.5 in. insulated foramen needle percutaneously under fluoroscopic guidance into the S3 foramen at a 60° angle relative to the skin. Stimulation is applied to confirm placement of needle looking for motor response. If there is poor motor response, the needle is reposition, inserted in the contralateral S3 foramina, and in extreme circumstances inserted in a different foramina. When adequate response is noted, the foramen needle is exchanged for a quadripolar tined lead (four electrodes numbered from most distal to proximal 0–3) over a guide wire and motor response is assed in each electrode (Figure 18.2). The tined lead is then connected to a lead extension and tunneled subcutaneously for external stimulation (Figure 18.3). If the patient has good response (≥50% improvement in symptoms) after a 2- to 4-week trial period, stage 2 of the procedure consists of placing a subcutaneous implantable pulse generator (IPG). This requires making a less than 4 cm incision over the lateral upper quadrant of the buttocks, removing the lead extension, and connecting the quadripolar lead to the IPG (Figure 18.4). Alternatively, patients can be offered a single stage procedure under which both tined lead and IPG are implanted in one step as long as a motor response to stimulation is elicited. In our experience, over 98% (86/88) of children go on to stage II, and single stage implantation carries no apparent increased risk of reoperation in the short term and equivalent symptom control. Single stage procedure is ideal for patients at high risk of lead dislodgement. Patients are typically prescribed a 7-day course of antibiotics to cover skin flora after each stage. Patient should avoid stretching and lifting heavy objects in the immediate post-op period (2 weeks), and any physical activities that may damage the lead or IPG in the long term.

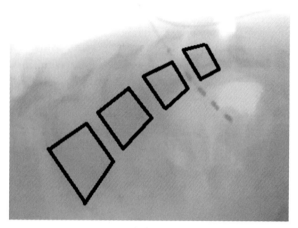

Figure 18.2 Fluoroscopic image of the sacrum with quadripolar tined lead in the S3 foramen and electrodes 2 and 3 straddle on the ventral surface of the sacrum.

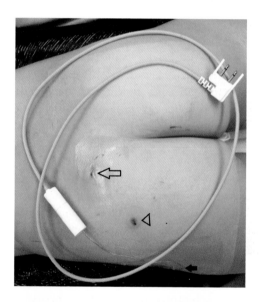

Figure 18.3 Postoperative picture of stage 1 with external extension lead coming out in the left lower buttocks (solid arrow). Hollow arrow points to percutaneous lead placement site, and arrow head points to blue inked site marking lead and lead extension connector, which is used as reference point for stage 2.

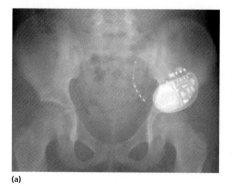

(a)

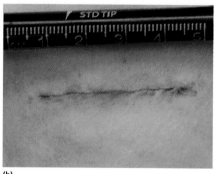

(b)

Figure 18.4 (a) Plain film X-ray of all implanted InterStim II® device components. **(b)** Postoperative incision (<4 cm) after stage 2.

Table 18.1 InterStim II® electrode programming.

	C1	C2	C3	C4
Initial	0–/3+	1–,3+	2–/0+	3–/0+
Secondary	0–/1+	1–/2+	2–/3+	3–/2+
Tertiary	0+/1–/2+ (guarded)	1+/2–/3+ (guarded)	Case+/0–/1–	Case+/1–/2–

Table 18.1 shows the initial Medtronic recommended electrode configuration using the standard device settings (pulse width of 210 and frequency of 14). However, all parameters (amplitude, pulse width, frequency, and electrode configuration) can be adjusted on a case-by-case basis to optimize symptom relief, minimize discomfort from stimulation, and target the pelvic area for stimulation sensation. Electrodes that resulted in stronger bellows motor response during lead placement should primarily be used during programming. Patients are provided with a transcutaneous remote, which can be preprogram by the clinician with four different stimulation settings. Adjustments to the programs can be done on an as needed basis, and can take approximately 6 weeks for patients to get used to the stimulation. Periodic visits (at 6 weeks, 6 months, and yearly) should be scheduled to verify programming parameters and fine-tuning of device to maximize battery life.

Outcomes of SSN

In 2006, we published the first outcome study of SNS for refractory BBD in children [8]. Since then, we have prospectively accumulated data on 105 children with a mean age of 8.8 years (range, 6–15) and median follow-up of 2.72 years (range, 0.01–9.63). Urinary incontinence, constipation, nocturnal enuresis, urgency and/or frequency, and constipation were improved or resolved in 88% (89/101), 66% (59/89), 67% (54/81), and 79% (73/92) of children, respectively. A total of 94% (99/105) of children experienced improvement of at least one symptom and 11% (12/105) had at least one symptom worsen. Complete resolution of all symptoms was achieved in 10% (10/105). Reoperation occurred in 50% (53/105) patients with device malfunction and infection accounting for 33% (35/105) and 9% (9/105), respectively. Therapy was ineffective in 7% (7/105) of patients.

Stephany et al. prospectively evaluated patients undergoing SNS for bladder dysfunction using a validated quality of life and bladder dysfunction questionnaire. Patients undergoing SNS had significant improvement in bladder dysfunction, psychosocial, and total quality of life scores at 1 month with persistence in improve bladder dysfunction scores at 4 months [9]. Outcomes of SNS in children with neurogenic bladder dysfunction (NBD) are limited. Recently, Haddad et al. reported that SNS showed significant increase in bladder capacity and overall positive clinical response of 81% for urinary and 78% for bowel function in patients with NBD [10]. Similarly, Groen et al. reported a 78% full or partial short-term response and 73% long-term response along with significant decrease in incontinence episodes in a cohort of patients with nonneurogenic and NBD [11].

Conclusions

SSN therapy is a minimally invasive alternative for the treatment of recalcitrant BBD. Our data, along with that of others, shows that SNS therapy is effective for the management of BBD in the appropriately selected patients with an understanding of the significant risk of reoperation secondary to device malfunction and infection. The role of biologic nervous system maturation in symptom improvement and resolution remains unknown. The application on SNS in NBD is limited but promising. Larger randomized studies with standardized objective outcome measures and longer follow-up are still necessary. In children, SNS should be given consideration before irreversible or more invasive surgical procedures are undertaken.

References

1 Hinman F, Baumann FW. Vesical and ureteral damage from voiding dysfunction in boys without neurologic or obstructive disease. *J Urol*. 1973 Apr;**109**(4):727–32.

2 de Groat WC, Wickens C. Organization of the neural switching circuitry underlying reflex micturition. *Acta Physiol (Oxf)*. 2013 Jan;**207**(1):66–84.

3 Zhang F, Zhao S, Shen B, Wang J, Nelson DE, Roppolo JR, et al. Neural pathways involved in sacral neuromodulation of reflex bladder activity in cats. *Am J Physiol Renal Physiol*. 2013 Mar;**304**(6):F710–7.

4 Dasgupta R, Critchley HD, Dolan RJ, Fowler CJ. Changes in brain activity following sacral neuromodulation for urinary retention. *J Urol*. 2005 Dec;**174**(6):2268–72.

5 Leng WW, Chancellor MB. How sacral nerve stimulation neuromodulation works. *Urol Clin North Am*. 2005 Feb;**32**(1):11–8. Research Support, U.S. Gov't, P.H.S. Review.

6 McGee SM, Routh JC, Granberg CF, Roth TJ, Hollatz P, Vandersteen DR, et al. Sacral neuromodulation in children with dysfunctional elimination syndrome: description of incisionless first stage and second stage without fluoroscopy. *Urology*. 2009 Mar;**73**(3):641–4; discussion 4.

7 Siegel SW. Management of voiding dysfunction with an implantable neuroprosthesis. *Urol Clin North Am*. 1992 Feb;**19**(1):163–70. Clinical Trial Multicenter Study.

8 Humphreys MR, Vandersteen DR, Slezak JM, Hollatz P, Smith CA, Smith JE, et al. Preliminary results of sacral neuromodulation in 23 children. *J Urol*. 2006 Nov;**176**(5):2227–31. Clinical Trial.

9 Stephany HA, Juliano TM, Clayton DB, Tanaka ST, Thomas JC, Adams MC, et al. Prospective evaluation of sacral nerve modulation in children with validated questionnaires. *J Urol*. 2013 Oct;**190**(4 Suppl):1516–22. Research Support, N.I.H., Extramural Research Support, Non-U.S. Gov't Validation Studies.

10 Haddad M, Besson R, Aubert D, Ravasse P, Lemelle J, El Ghoneimi A, et al. Sacral neuro-modulation in children with urinary and fecal incontinence: a multicenter, open label, randomized, crossover study. *J Urol.* 2010 Aug;**184**(2):696–701. Multicenter Study Randomized Controlled Trial Research Support, Non-U.S. Gov't.

11 Groen LA, Hoebeke P, Loret N, Van Praet C, Van Laecke E, Ann R, et al. Sacral neuromodu-lation with an implantable pulse generator in children with lower urinary tract symptoms: 15-year experience. *J Urol.* 2012 Oct;**188**(4):1313–7.

CHAPTER 19

Superficial stimulation therapy for the treatment of functional voiding problems

Ubirajara Barroso, Jr

Federal University of Bahia, Bahiana School of Medicine, Centro Médico Aliança, Salvador, Bahia, Brazil

Introduction

Children with overactive bladder (OAB) are in general initially treated with a variety of behavioral orientations (standard urotherapy). Those who fail this treatment are usually managed with anticholinergics. However, prolonged use of these medications in children brings on problems with compliance, worsens constipation, and yields others adverse side effects. It is in this scenario that transcutaneous electric nerve stimulation (TENS) emerged as a good alternative for treating lower urinary tract symptoms (LUTS). This chapter will discuss the results of the main works related to TENS and its applicability in the current context of the treatment of OAB in children.

For children with OAB, TENS was originally used by Hoebeke et al. and Bower et al. in 2001 [1, 2]. In these studies, the treatment was performed at home, usually for 3–6 months with 2 h sessions. Then in 2006, we described the results with a shorter period of treatment. The patients were treated with parasacral TENS in the outpatients clinic, with a maximum of 20 sessions, 20 min each, and a frequency current of 10 Hz [3]. For this treatment, two superficial electrodes are placed on each side of S3 and S2 (see Figure 19.1).

Currents with low frequency in the range of 2–20 Hz have an autonomic effect, whereas frequencies of 50 Hz stimulate skeletal muscle. The mechanism of action of neuromodulation in LUTS is not completely understood. Several mechanisms have been considered: stimulation may (i) reinnervate partly denervated muscle fibers in the bladder wall, (ii) inhibit C-fiber activation by possibly reducing c-fos gene expression [4], (iii) act on pudendal nerve acting on the urethral–bladder reflex, (iv) act on the reflexogenic pathways involved in the lower urinary tract (LUT) control, (v) modulate the inhibitory sympathetic

Pediatric Incontinence: Evaluation and Clinical Management, First Edition. Edited by Israel Franco, Paul F. Austin, Stuart B. Bauer, Alexander von Gontard and Yves Homsy.
© 2015 John Wiley & Sons, Ltd. Published 2015 by John Wiley & Sons, Ltd.

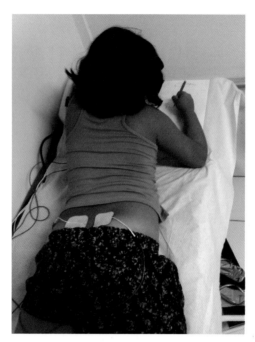

Figure 19.1 A child undergoing parasacral TENS.

neurons and inhibit the parasympathetic excitatory neurons that come and go to the bladder or interneurons in the spinal cord, and (vi) modulate at the supraspinal level. In a study of women with urinary retention by Dasgupta et al., the findings suggest that neuromodulation achieves its therapeutic effect at the level of functional interactions between the midbrain and limbic cingulate cortex [5]. Liao et al., after sacral root stimulation in six adult patients with idiopathic OAB, concluded that sacral root stimulation might reorganize the human brain and its ability to excite the motor cortex, in turn modulating LUT function [6].

Clinical results

In the Hoebeke et al. study, the electrodes were placed in the parasacral area at the level of sacral root S3 [1]. There were 15 girls and 26 boys evaluated with proved detrusor hyperactivity. Most children were nonrespondent to anticholinergic therapy. Stimulation of 2 Hz was applied for 2 h every day. They found that 76% had some response to the treatment and 56% had a complete response. They also noted improvement in the bladder capacity and reduction in the number of voiding frequency. Relapse was observed in seven patients (17%).

Bower et al. published their series with TENS for 17 children with OAB and no signs of dysfunctional voiding [2]. The current frequency was 10 Hz when parasacral TENS was used and 150 Hz for suprapubic stimulation. It was a home-based therapy, 2 h per day, and the duration of treatment ranged from 1 to 5 months. Daytime incontinence improved in 73.3% of children (41% became dry).

Malm-Buatsi et al. in 2007 used a similar protocol of Bower et al. but with sessions of 20 min to improve compliance [7]. They treated 18 children with OAB refractory to standard therapy. The mean length of TENS used was 8 ± 7 months. Of the 15 patients with incontinence, two became dry (13%), nine were significantly improved (60%), and four reported no improvement (27%).

We have described parasacral TENS of shorter duration [3]. Possible advantages of this scheme are as follows: (i) best children's compliance, (ii) the possibility to increase the current intensity until the maximum tolerated by the child in each session, and (iii) being conducted by a urotherapist, behavioral treatment can be reinforced during each session. In a first study, out of 19 children with OAB treated, 12 (63%) showed complete clinical improvement and no side effects were observed [3]. The effectiveness of this same protocol in the long term was investigated by evaluating 36 girls and 13 boys [8]. The rate of complete resolution of symptoms after 2 years of follow-up was, respectively, for daytime urgency and urinary incontinence, 84 and 73%. Recurrence of symptoms was seen in 10% of the cases.

We evaluated parasacral TENS in a randomized clinical trial [9]. The test group was stimulated in the parasacral area and the sham at the scapula. From a total of 37 patients, 61% reported complete resolution of symptoms in the test group compared with no patients that reported complete resolution of symptoms in the sham group ($p < 0.001$). The test group was also associated with a higher reduction in dysfunctional voiding score system (DVSS), higher increase in the voiding volume, as well as reduction in voiding frequency.

Hagstroem et al., using daily sessions for 2 h, with a current frequency of 10 Hz, in a randomized clinical trial of 27 children with OAB refractory to anticholinergics, also concluded that the parasacral TENS was superior to sham in the treatment of daytime urinary incontinence (61% vs. 21%, $p < 0.05$) [10]. Nevertheless, they did not notice any difference in the voided volume change.

Practical aspects

We use the device Dualpex Uro 961 (Quark, Piracicaba, São Paulo). The current is biphasic, with a pulse width of 700 μs and frequency 10 Hz. We place two 5×5 cm self-adhesive surface electrodes in the parasacral area between S2 and S4. The superior iliac spine is palpated, which is the reference of S1 vertebra. Therefore, S2 is the vertebra below.

Comparative studies with other methods

We compared the results of parasacral TENS and percutaneous tibial posterior nerve stimulation (PTNS) [11]. A total of 22 consecutive patients were treated with PTNS and 37 with parasacral TENS. Complete resolution of symptoms was seen in 70% of the group undergoing parasacral TENS and in 9% of the posterior tibial nerve stimulation group ($p = 0.02$). There was a significant decrease in DVSS scores after treatment in both groups, but not when the two groups were compared.

We compared children treated with parasacral TENS and oxybutynin in a randomized clinical trial [12]. In the sham group, there was stimulation through the electrodes on scapular area and the patients took oxybutynin. In the test group, the stimulation was sacral and patients took placebo. Twenty-eight children were analyzed. The study was conducted with the hypothesis that parasacral TENS was not inferior to oxybutynin. As a result, there was no difference regarding the improvement of the symptoms of OAB between groups after 3 months of therapy. However, constipation was resolved more often in the TENS group, and in more than half of the patients in the oxybutynin group, side effects were observed.

Tens for constipation

Clarke et al. performed a randomized clinical trial in which 26 children with functional constipation were randomized to receive either 12 real or sham interferential electrical stimulation sessions for a 4-week period [13]. Colonic transit was significantly faster only in children given real treatment.

Our group assessed the results of TENS parasacral 14 children with LUTS and constipation [14]. After treatment, 85.7% of constipation and LUTS symptoms in the children subsided. This demonstrates that one of the advantages of TENS is the combined treatment of these two conditions.

Enuresis

A possible indication of TENS would be the treatment of enuresis. Oliveira et al. performed a prospective randomized clinical trial included 29 girls and 16 boys older than 6 years with primary mono symptomatic enuresis [15]. Children were treated either with behavioral therapy or behavioral therapy plus 10 sessions of parasacral TENS. Rates of wet nights were 49.5 and 31.2%, respectively, at the end of treatment ($p = 0.02$). However, despite better results in the stimulation group, these patients saw the urotherapist more often than in the nonstimulation group (three times a week vs. once a month). Therefore, more visits to the office may act as a placebo effect or a more intensive behavioral therapy in the TENS group.

Lordêlo et al. evaluated the results with parasacral TENS for patients with non-monosymptomatic enuresis [16]. Nineteen children were studied prospectively. Enuresis resolved in 42% of the cases, was partially improved in 21%, and did not improve in 37%.

Conclusion

A recent systematic review by Barroso et al. showed that electroneuromodulation is a good alternative for children with nonneurogenic DTUI [17]. Less invasive methods of stimulation such as parasacral TENS or the PTNS are preferred.

TENS is a simple and effective method. It can be performed at home or in the office and has the great advantage of also managing constipation while relieving LUTS. Therefore, parasacral TENS, in my view, should be seen as a first-line treatment after or in combination with behavioral treatment. It can also be used after failure with anticholinergics. Those cases of failure with TENS may in many cases be redeemed with medication. However, there is a great way to research in the future. The mechanism of action of the stimulation, the ideal frequency current, the pulse width, as well as the number of sessions per week are not known. Furthermore, TENS could be tested also in the treatment of other conditions such as dysfunctional voiding and hypoactive bladder.

References

1 Hoebeke P, Van Laecke E, Everaert K, et al. Transcutaneous neuromodulation for the urge syndrome in children: a pilot study. *J Urol* 2001;**166**:2416–9.
2 Bower WF, Moore KH, Adams RD. A pilot study of the home application of transcutaneous neuromodulation in children with urgency or urge incontinence. *J Urol* 2001;**166**:2420–2.
3 Barroso U Jr, Lordêlo P, Lopes AA, et al. Nonpharmacological treatment of lower urinary tract dysfunction using biofeedback and transcutaneous electrical stimulation: a pilot study. *BJU Int* 2006;**98**:166–71.
4 Wang Y, Hassouna MM. Neuromodulation reduces C-fos gene expression in spinalized rats: a double-blind randomized study. *J Urol* 2000;**163**:1966–70.
5 Dasgupta R, Critcheley HD, Dolan RJ, et al. Changes in brain activity following sacral neuromodulation for urinary retention. *J Urol* 2005; **174**: 2268–72.
6 Liao KK, Chen JT, Lai KL, et al. Effect of sacral-root stimulation on the motor cortex in patients with idiopathic overactive bladder syndrome. *Clin Neurophysiol* 2008; **38**: 39–43.
7 Malm-Buatsi E, Nepple KG, Boyt MA, et al. Efficacy of transcutaneous electrical nerve stimulation in children with overactive bladder refractory to pharmacotherapy. *Urology* 2007;**70**: 980–3.
8 Lordêlo P, Soares PV, Maciel I, et al. Prospective study of transcutaneous parasacral electrical stimulation for overactive bladder in children: long-term results. *J Urol* 2009;**182**:2900–4.
9 Lordêlo P, Teles A, Veiga ML, et al. Transcutaneous electrical nerve stimulation in children with overactive bladder: a randomized clinical trial. *J Urol* 2010;**184**:683–9.
10 Hagstroem S, Mahler B, Madsen B, et al. Transcutaneous electrical nerve stimulation for refractory daytime urinary urge incontinence. *J Urol* 2009;**182**:2072–8.
11 Barroso U Jr, Viterbo W, Bittencourt J, Farias T, Lordêlo P. Posterior tibial nerve stimulation vs parasacral transcutaneous neuro modulation for overactive bladder in children. *J Urol.* 2013;**190**(2):673–7.
12 Barroso U Jr, Cunha C, Moraes M, et al. Parasacral transcutaneous electrical stimulation versus oxybutynin in the treatment of overactive bladder in children: a randomized clinical trial. Presented at the Society for Pediatric Urology's 62nd Annual Meeting, Orlando, FL.

13 Clarke MC, Chase JW, Gibb S, et al. Decreased colonic transit time after transcutaneous interferential electrical stimulation in children with slow transit constipation. *J Pediatr Surg* 2009;**44**:408–12.

14 Veiga ML, Lordêlo P, Farias T, et al. Evaluation of constipation after parasacral transcutaneous electrical nerve stimulation in children with lower urinary tract dysfunction—a pilot study. *J Pediatr Urol* 2013;**9**:622–6.

15 de Oliveira LF, de Oliveira DM, da Silva de Paula LI, et al. Transcutaneous parasacral electrical neural stimulation in children with primary mono symptomatic enuresis: a prospective randomized clinical trial. *J Urol* 2013;**190**:1359–63.

16 Lordêlo P Benevides I, Kerner EG, et al. Treatment of non-monosymptomatic nocturnal enuresis by transcutaneous parasacral electrical nerve stimulation. *J Pediatr Urol* 2010;**6**: 486–9.

17 Barroso U Jr, Tourinho R, Lordêlo P, et al. Electrical stimulation for lower urinary tract dysfunction in children: a systematic review of the literature. *Neurourol Urodyn* 2011; **30**:1429–36.

CHAPTER 20

Botulinum toxin in the treatment of the functional bladder

Luitzen-Albert Groen and Piet Hoebeke
Department of Pediatric and Reconstructive Urology, Ghent University Hospital, Ghent, Belgium

Use of botulinum toxin in children: Introduction

Despite the need for new minimally invasive treatments, there is a lack of clinical studies in pediatric urology and in pediatrics in general.

Appropriate and timely licensing of medication is even scarcer. Therefore, it is virtually impossible to practice modern pediatric urology without using off-label medication. To guide its clinical use, we cannot rely on AUA or EAU guidelines. In the 2015 EAU guidelines, the use of botulinum toxin is mentioned. It is stated that in cases of therapy resistance, reevaluation will be required, which may consist of video urodynamics and MRI of the LS spine. This can guide off-label treatment such as some of the nonlicensed drugs in children, botulinum toxin injection, and sacral nerve stimulation. Moreover, the guidelines suggest that it should only be offered in highly experienced centers [1]. However, clues or guidance as to when to start the use in daily clinical practice is still needed.

In this chapter, we give an overview of the existing literature that might be useful as a tool for clinicians in the field to plan individually tailored treatments for therapy-resistant overactive bladder (OAB) or dysfunctional voiding with the promising and remarkable poison: botulinum toxin A.

Use of botulinum toxin in children: Historical perspective

As early as in 1822, Justinus Kerner, who is nowadays considered the godfather of research on botulinum neurotoxin (BoNT), described in detail the effect of BoNT, at that time called "sausage poison" [2].

Kerner was unable to isolate the poison. He was however aware of its biological origin because of the development of the toxin under anaerobic conditions, and he suggested very correctly that sausages should be boiled long enough

---

Pediatric Incontinence: Evaluation and Clinical Management, First Edition. Edited by Israel Franco,
Paul F. Austin, Stuart B. Bauer, Alexander von Gontard and Yves Homsy.
© 2015 John Wiley & Sons, Ltd. Published 2015 by John Wiley & Sons, Ltd.

and stored under aerobic conditions. The possible therapeutic applications he mentioned at that time were visionary [3].

By examining the food and the victims on the occasion of an outbreak of botulism in 1895, Emile Van Ermengem (Ghent University) was able to isolate an anaerobic microorganism that was called *Bacillus botulinus* (botulus, Latin for sausage), later renamed *Clostridium botulinum* [4].

Botulinum toxin is a potent neurotoxin (potentially lethal). The interaction at a presynaptic level inhibits the release of acetylcholine and results in muscle paralysis. When used in a small dose injected in several spots, it results in decrease of muscle tension or muscle relaxation.

Eight subtypes of botulinum toxin have been discovered: botulinum toxin A–H.

Botulinum toxin A is commercially available as *onabotulinumtoxinA* (ona-BoNT-A, Botox®, Allergan), *abobotulinumtoxinA* (abo-BoNT-A, Dysport®, Ipsen), and *incobotulinumtoxinA* (inco-BoNT-A, Xeomin®, Merz), and botulinum toxin B as *rimabotulinumtoxinB* (rima-BoNT-B, Myobloc®, Solstice).

In urology, ona-BoNT-A and abo-BoNT-A are frequently used. In the United States, ona-BoNT-A is the product of choice because it has an FDA approval for use in bladder conditions in adults such as OAB or neurogenic detrusor overactivity (NDO).

The doses are expressed in IU, which reflects the median lethal dose (LD_{50}). This is the dose, if injected intraperitoneally in mice, needed to kill half of a mouse population. This ability to kill is an equivalent to the potency of different products. However, it is a measurement that is not completely reliable because of different reactions in different species. The different brands of BoNT used in (pediatric) urology are not identical; the dose–effect relation for ona-BoNT is approximately three times higher than that for abo-BoNT.

BoNT is used in a variety of pediatric specialties and indications. Its use has mainly expanded in neurogenic patients and in anatomic disorders: in orthopedic surgery (e.g., treatment of patients with cerebral palsy (CP), spastic equinus), ophthalmology (e.g., esotropia, blepharospasm), stomatology (e.g., treatment of drooling), and gastroenterology (e.g., treatment of achalasia).

The use of BoNT for nonneurogenic functional problems is rising, for example, the use of BoNT in palmar and axillary hyperhidrosis and treatment of anal fissures. It is nowadays even commonly used for bruxism.

Dennis Dykstra pioneered its use in urology in 1988, with his report on BoNT for detrusor–sphincter dyssynergia in spinal cord-injured patients [5].

The first report of the use of botulinum toxin in a pediatric bladder was for a functional indication in 1997 [6]. Steinhardt treated a 7-year-old girl for dysfunctional voiding by sphincter injection. This indication did not gain popularity, probably because of other less invasive alternatives (e.g., urotherapy, pelvic floor biofeedback training). However, it is still a valuable treatment option for therapy-resistant detrusor sphincter dyssynergia. BoNT has been used mainly for the treatment of NDO in children and neurogenic detrusor–sphincter dyssynergia. We reported the first series of its use in non-NDO in 2006 [7].

Biochemical

Mode of action

BoNT is a high molecular weight polypeptide chain of 150 kDa, which consists of two chains of 100 and 50 kDa, connected by a single disulfide bond.

BoNT induces muscle cell paralysis by cleaving the synaptosome-associated protein 25 (SNAP-25), which is essential for normal vesicular transport of Acetylcholine (ACh).

ACh is a neurotransmitter, which is important for muscle cell contraction.

After cleavage of the 150 kDa polypeptide chain into two shorter chains, by the toxin's zinc protease, the heavy part (100 kDa) binds to the nerve at the neuromuscular junction. The light part (50 kDa) is endocytosed and cleaves a specific site of the SNAP-25, which makes docking and releasing of neurotransmitter containing vesicles impossible.

The result is a reversible but long-lasting relaxation of the muscle fibers, which can be described as "chemical muscular denervation."

Associated effects

The main effect of BoNT in the bladder is attributed to the blockage of the pre-synaptic release of ACh, causing paralysis of some detrusor smooth muscle cells, analogous to the effect in skeletal muscle cells. The working mechanism of BoNT on the detrusor is much more complex compared to the effect on skeletal muscle cells, because of a more complex molecular and neurogenic function of the bladder compared to the skeletal muscles. The effect of BoNT on urgency, which is a sensory (afferent) phenomenon [8], can only be explained by other secondary (associated) working mechanisms. Ikeda et al. proved in an adult mice spinal cord transection model that BoNT-A suppresses NDO by targeting afferent as well as efferent pathways in the bladder [9].

Several receptors have been identified in the pathophysiology of OAB: the capsaicin receptor TRPV1, the purinergic receptors P2X2 and P2X3, as well as sensory neuropeptides such as substance P and calcitonin-related peptide (CGRP). These receptors and peptides may play a role as well in the mechanism of action of BoNT [10].

Lawrence et al. proved that atropine (desensitizer of P2X1 and P2X3 receptors) did not alter the rate at which muscle BoNT-A weakened contractions [11].

We can conclude that, although it has an effect on many pathways, the main effect of BoNT is related to blockage of the release.

Use of Botox in pediatric urology

Possible indications
1 NDO and/or low bladder compliance
2 Non-NDO
3 Detrusor–sphincter dyssynergia

Bladder
In 2006, we published our initial experience with ona-BoNT-A for nonneurogenic therapy-resistant detrusor overactivity [7]. All patients received a standard dose of 100 IU ona-BoNT-A; the injection was performed in 15 extratrigonal spots and without including the bladder dome. No systemic side effects were observed.

The included patients were true therapy resistant, meaning that all previous therapies, both urotherapy and medical treatment, were unsuccessful.

In this population, without other treatment options left, we achieved improvement in 73% and a full response in 60%. One boy had clinical signs of vesicoureteral reflux (pain at the costovertebral angle). Because of refusal of cystographic examination, the diagnosis was not confirmed and the symptoms persisted only 2 weeks.

One girl had a 10-day temporary retention. We suspect that in this patient the inability to void was caused by the combination of the botulinum toxin effect and severe dysfunctional voiding. However, we do count it as a local side effect of the BoNT injections. Analysis of the data of 200 consecutive BoNT detrusor injections in children (unpublished data) did not show a second case of retention. It is mandatory to avoid this treatment for patients with associated severe or untreated dysfunctional voiding.

In 2010, Marte et al. reported their experience with ona-BoNT-A for incontinence caused by idiopathic OAB refractory to anticholinergic drugs [12]. The dose that was used was 12.5 IU ona-BoNT-A/kg, without exceeding 200 IU. Full response was obtained in 38% (8/21) of their patients after one injection. In case of absence of response, a second injection was performed, leading to an additional partial response in 57% (12/21) of patients.

In 2012, McDowell et al. [13] reported their retrospective study on 57 subjects. The indication for all patients was bladder overactivity. Improvement of daytime LUT symptoms and daytime wetting were assessed. After the first injection, improvement (complete or partial success) was observed in 75% of the patients (complete success, 50%; partial success, 25%). No drug-induced side effects were observed. A mean duration of the effect that was observed was 8 months.

Blackburn et al. reported the first use of abo-BoNT-A for idiopathic detrusor overactivity in 2013. Their retrospective study included 27 patients, aged 6–16 years. Fifteen IU/kg abo-BoNT-A (Dysport) was administered (400–500 IU) uniformly throughout the bladder, sparing the trigone. Dryness was reported in 44% of the patients. One patient could not void spontaneously for 2 months. The authors suggest that this might be caused by too high a dose of BoNT (they did exceed 20 IU/kg abo-BoNT in this case). This study does not provide us with dose relation data that could suggest the ideal dose of abo-BoNT in children. However, the median dose in successful treatment was slightly higher (14 IU/kg) but not statistically different compared to the dose in unsuccessfully treated children (13 IU/kg). The best dose to choose for abo-BoNT is probably 15 IU/kg.

From these studies, it can be concluded that in therapy-resistant OAB complete control of symptoms can be obtained in approximately 50% of patients and another 25% show partial improvement. Because most of these studies are retrospective and noncontrolled, the level of evidence is low. The effect in naïve populations that had no former treatment is so far unknown.

Sphincter

Treatment of dysfunctional voiding by injection of BoNT in the sphincter has been described using both transperineal and endoscopic injection techniques.

Nine years after the initial report of Steinhardt, Radojicic published their results of transperineal (endoscopically assisted) sphincteric/pelvic floor BoNT injection. In boys, the level of the external urethral sphincter was localized by transillumination on the perineum, with the cystoscope at the level of the sphincter. In girls, BoNT was injected approximately 1.5–2 cm deep around the urethral meatus. The mean PVR decreased from 70 to 24 mL. In 80% of the patients, this was a normalization (≤20 mL). Eighty-eight percent of the children were cured of UTI.

Mokhless was the first to describe endoscopical BoNT injection at the urinary sphincter [14]. The population treated in this study consisted of very severe therapy-resistant dysfunctional voiders. Ten children were treated with 50 or 100 IU ona-BoNT-A. The mean PVR was reduced from 335 to 75 mL. In one patient with VUR grade III, this was downgraded to grade. I. In all patients with hydronephrosis (n=4), this was improved; in 2/4, complete normalization was observed.

Preoperatively, 9/10 children were on indwelling catheters or CIC, but 6 months after treatment, all were able to void spontaneously.

Franco et al. published in 2007 another study about endoscopic sphincter injection [15]. This group used a higher dose of 200–300 IU ona-BoNT-A. The average PVR was more drastically reduced—from 108 to 8 mL—leading to normalization of the PVR in all patients (13/13).

In the same year, Petronijeviv et al. [16] reported the first series with abo-BoNT injection in girls. The toxin was injected transperineally and periurethrally into the external urinary sphincter under EMG control. The authors stated that this was done because they considered their method less invasive than endourethral toxin injections.

Seventy-five percent of the children were cured of recurrent UTIs. The mean residual urine improved from 52 to 19 mL. The complete success rate for incontinence was 80% (4/5).

Recently, the pioneers of endoscopic sphincter injection in children did study the use of ona-BoNT injection in the hypertrophic bladder neck of urethral valve patients [17]. BoNT might indeed be a reversible alternative to bladder neck incisions, without long-term effects such as incontinence or retrograde ejaculation. 100 IU abo-BoNT was injected in 10 randomized study patients. Unfortunately, the RCT did not prove any significant improvement on UTI, hydronephrosis, vesicoureteral reflux, cystometric capacity, or voiding pressure. The results do not even show a favorable trend.

This might be explained by overestimation of the role of bladder neck hypertrophy in the pathophysiology of bladder dysfunction. However, both the study group and the control group were on CIC and anticholinergics. Moreover, insufficient dosage of BoNT might be as well an explanation. In 2014 Gino Vricella [18] from the group of Paul Austin described their experience with sphincteric injections of botulinum toxin A. A dose of 100 IU ona-BoNT diluted in 4 cc saline was used in all patients. In girls the injections were performed periurethrally and in boys endoscopically. Eight of the 12 children (67%) experienced significant improvement in voiding parameters. Forty-five percent had a normalized voiding pattern and 40% had improved voiding parameters. A repeated injection was performed in half of the patients on average 15 months later. In Rotterdam, Lisette 't Hoen and Jeroen Scheepe [19] described their experience with sphincteric injections for therapy-refractory dysfunctional voiding. Twenty patients were treated with 100 IU ona-BoNT-A diluted in 3 ml saline and injected into the sphincter at the 3, 9, and 12 o'clock positions. For their main outcome measure, the post-void residual urine volume, a significant decrease (75%) was observed. In 10 of 14 patients the PVR normalized.

Although with more limited numbers than for OAB, these studies indicate that there might be a place for BoNT injections in therapy-resistant sphincter overactivity. We also learn that a higher dose (200–300 IU ona-BoNT) might be mandatory to achieve excellent results. The level of evidence remains very low.

Median duration of positive effect

The principal advantage of BoNT is that the effect is reversible and temporary. This is reassuring, because even in the event of undesired effects (e.g., urinary retention in bladder injection or (increased) incontinence in sphincter injection), these side effects are limited in time as well. A possible disadvantage, however, is of course the need for repeated injections. In adults, this is not a major problem, because the procedure can be done under local anesthesia. In children, this is of course not feasible, because it could be a psychologically traumatizing event. A short sedation or general anesthesia is desirable.

The mean duration of the effect of BoNT in neurogenic patients has been studied by Kask et al.: median duration of the response was 15 months (range, 3–42 months) [20]. Schulte-Baukloh reported a study in which, with association of anticholinergic drugs, an even larger median efficacy was reported with a need for repeated injection up to 18 months [21].

The duration of action in nonneurogenic patients is unknown.

In contrast to the neurogenic patients, we observed that many functional patients do not need repeated treatments. It can be hypothesized that the duration of action can be influenced by the fact that in children the bladder function can still mature as part of development. Like the way anticholinergics can cure OAB, we can hypothesize that BoNT can be as effective and thus can cure OAB just with one injection. Prospective studies (which are on their way) will be needed to prove this concept.

We suppose that BoNT can overcome a delay in bladder maturation and that the extra bladder capacity that it offers can be easily maintained. In clinical practice, we observe that only patients with very severe detrusor overactivity need repeated injections. When BoNT effects are exhausted, this is usually very obvious for patients and parents. Their strong demand for repeating treatment, usually after long periods of cure, is an indication of efficacy and does encourage us to continue the use of BoNT in well-selected patients.

Technique of injection

The treatment of a dysfunctional bladder is typically performed by several injections with a small quantity of botulinum toxin A. The dose, dilution factor, injection depth, number of injection sites, and injection sites of preference are not yet well determined.

For discussion of the dose, we refer to the next part: "Dose, patient safety, and antibodies."

Dilution factor

The dilution factor might be crucial, as Ana Coelho et al. described in their experiments on a guinea pig model [22]. SNAP-25 is a synaptosome-associated protein, which is the target of the toxin. Its cleavage product, cSNAP-25, can be used as a marker of neurotoxin diffusion.

Interestingly, this group found that a single ona-BoNT could spread to the opposite site of the guinea pig bladder if diluted to achieve 0.1 IU/μL. When the same dose of 2 IU is injected at a 10 times lower dilution factor (1 IU/μL), the number of cleaved fibers and its spreading seems to be much lower.

If we dilute in clinical practice 100 IU in 15, 20, or 30 ML, we achieve easily an even lower dilution (0.006, 0.005, or 0.003 IU/μL).

Injection depth

A both interesting and practical question is whether BoNT injections should be performed at the level of the urothelium or into the detrusor. In a pilot study, Krhut et al. revealed in a multicenter RCT of 32 adult patients no statistically different results with injection at the level of the urothelium or of the detrusor [23].

Number of bladder injections

Since there are no RCTs comparing different injection protocols, we do provide in the table below the protocols used in the available studies. Probably, the number of injections is not the most determining factor for treatment success.

	Number of injections (cc)
Hoebeke	15 × 1
Marte	20 × 0.5
McDowell	n/k × 0.1
Blackburn	n/k × 0.5–1

Site preference

Because the trigone is much more innervated, it seems to be logical to inject there. Recent data in adult females [24] did show subjective superior outcome (overactive bladder symptom score (OABSS)). However, because of the unavailability of long-term data on the future effect of this (fear for neurogenic damage) and because of the possibility to evoke iatrogenically vesicoureteral reflux, most pediatric urologists prefer to avoid the trigone.

Intravesical instillation

Intravesical instillation has been proposed by Kajbafzadeh et al. [25, 26].

The permeability of the intact urothelium for the BoNT molecules is doubtful because of their high molecular weight; therefore, they proposed an electromotive drug administration. These studies have not so far been reproduced.

Dose, patient safety, and antibodies

General considerations, legal aspects, and warnings

The need for new minimally invasive treatments is often much higher than the availability of clinical studies in pediatric urology and in pediatrics in general. Appropriate and timely licensing of medication is even scarcer. Therefore, it is virtually impossible to practice modern pediatric urology without using off-label medication.

As science evolves, insights in drug safety can change over time. Therefore, it is mandatory for each physician to follow the current literature and changing knowledge.

Local and leading international websites of different governmental and scientific institutions are easily reachable (e.g., Medline, FDA, etc.).

A decision about every indication and treatment has to be made based on the individual patient, balancing possible benefits and risks (e.g., individual risk of general anesthesia).

Knowledge about the potency and differences of the commercially available botulinum toxin preparations is mandatory, as botulinum toxin products cannot be interchanged.

Possible general side effects

The toxin causes general side effects if it spreads beyond the site where it was injected, and symptoms of botulism occur.

General muscle weakness is the most feared sign; this can lead to respiratory failure and has to be treated immediately by mechanical ventilation.

Local side effects are caused by unadapted dosage. Profound investigations are mandatory to determine the individually adapted dose. Urodynamics can reveal the degree of detrusor overactivity and give an impression of coexisting detrusor–sphincter dyssynergia, which might be a risk factor for urinary retention.

On the other hand, when used for sphincter injection, local side effects (overtreatment) are less hazardous, and incontinence might be temporarily increased instead of cured.

Recommended dosage for detrusor injection

No specific dose–effect studies are available concerning the use in nonneurogenic functional bladder dysfunction. We can only rely on the data that has been published by four experienced centers. The doses used are relatively low. In neurologically normal children, we have, in contrary to neurogenic patients on CIC, the obligation to keep the doses low enough to avoid urinary retention.

	Dose used	Side effects (%)
Hoebeke	100 IU ona-BoNT	5 (1/21)
Marte	12, 5 IU ona-BoNT	0
McDowell	12 IU/kg abo-BoNT	4 (1/27)
Blackburn	15 IU/kg abo-BoNT	4 (1/27)

Recommended dosage for sphincter injection

No specific dose–effect studies are available concerning the use in nonneurogenic sphincter dysfunction. As stated earlier, we do not risk bladder retention, only the worsening of incontinence. Dose limits are therefore less restrictive.

Some honest authors provide detailed data about increased incontinence, usually temporary. It is difficult to objectify, to compare the different studies, and to determine whether it is caused by de BoNT injections itself or not.

Dose limitation

To avoid generalized toxin-related side effects, a safe dose interval has to be respected.

Because data on functional pediatric urologic usage is rare, data on other pediatric usage can be useful. Thousands of children have been treated in orthopedic surgery, mainly for spastic limb problems caused by CP. International consensus has been reached, thanks to pooling of data of more than 10,000 patients and over 45,000 treatments [27]. In urological practice, we have a low risk on generalized side effects as, according to the current available literature, the recommended doses are below 20 IU/kg in order to avoid local side effects.

	Ona-BoNT	Abo-BoNT
Range (U/kg bw)	1–20 (–25)	1–20 (–25)
Max total dose (U)	400 (–600)	500–1000

Consensus use of botulinum toxin CP dose ranges [U, 1/4 units; kg bw, 1/4 kg body weight]

Age limitation

The use of botulinum toxin can be considered safe. A large meta-analysis of Naumann and Jankovic that included 2309 patients form 23 studies showed an overall adverse event (AE) rate of 25%. All the AEs were mild or moderate.

However, the drug is obviously a potentially lethal drug and can cause death if used at high doses [28].

An interesting question is whether we could determine a minimum age for which the use of BoNT is safe.

Probably, we cannot. There is some evidence that side effects of the use of Botox are not age related [29]. In orthopedic surgery, there are several reasons to treat infants under the age of 2 years or ever under 1 year old. The prognosis of spastic hip in CP is improved if treated early, because subluxation can be prevented. In case of obstetric brachial palsy, treatment is even performed in the first month of life to prevent shoulder joint limitation. The data of this study shows interestingly that in the treatment of 74 infants, no excess AEs were observed. No serious AEs were observed.

Antibodies

Schulte-Baukloh summarizes in his study very carefully the causes of therapeutic failure and the role of antibodies [30] in neurogenic patients. However, most of the causes of therapeutic failure are probably identical in nonneurogenic patients. He suggests that therapeutic failure can be primary or secondary. When it is primary, it might be patient related or technique related. Patient-related primary failure could be caused by an initial bad indication for the use of BoNT because the condition is not BoNT sensible or has reduced sensibility to BoNT. Technique-related primary failure could be caused by improper dosing of BoNT, improper handling of the pharmacon (e.g., transport, storage), or poor injection technique.

Secondary failure might be caused by patient-related changes such as upregulation of receptors or the presence of Botox antibodies.

The role of BoNT antibodies is so far not very well determined.

In the study of Schulte-Baukloh, 6/17 (35%) patients had detection (clearly positive or borderline) of ona-BoNT antibodies. They all had objective (urodynamic) therapy failure. Mann–Whitney test and Spearman's test could not reveal correlation with the number of previous Botox injections, total dose injected, interval since the last Botox injection, or age of the patient.

In contrary, Kajbafzadeh et al. [31] concluded in a study of abo-BoNT-A a high incidence of antibody formation (71%). Nevertheless, a high (partial) improvement rate was observed.

A relation between recurrent UTI or latex allergy and the formation of BoNT antibodies has not yet been proven.

Conclusion

From the studies presented in this chapter, it can be concluded that BoNT seems to be effective in reducing OAB and dysfunctional voiding symptoms; however, the level of evidence today is too low, and further prospective multicenter studies are needed to prove this concept.

At this time, reasonable amount of data are available to consider the usage of Botox by well-trained medical specialists safe. However, as science evolves, insights in drug safety can change. It is therefore mandatory for each physician to follow the current literature and changing knowledge.

References

1 Tekgul S, Riedmiller H, Dogan HS, Hoebeke PB, Kocvara R, NIJMAN R, et al. Chapter; members of the European Association of Urology (EAU) Guidelines Office. Guidelines on Paediatric Urology. In: EAU Guidelines, edn. presented at the EAU Annual Congress Milan 2013; **10**: 1–126, ISBN. 90-70244-37-3. Available at http://www.uroweb.org/gls/pdf/22%20 Paediatric%20Urology_LR.pdf (accessed March 16, 2015).

2 Hanchanale VS, Rao AR, Martin FL, Matanhelia SS. The unusual history and the urological applications of botulinum neurotoxin. *Urol Int*. 2010;**85**(2):125–30.

3 Erbguth FJ. Historical notes on botulism, *Clostridium botulinum*, botulinum toxin, and the idea of the therapeutic use of the toxin. *Mov Disord*. 2004 Mar;**19**(Suppl 8):S2–6.

4 van Ermengem E. Classics in infectious diseases. A new anaerobic bacillus and its relation to botulism. E. van Ermengem. Originally published as "Ueber einen neuen anaëroben Bacillus und seine Beziehungen zum Botulismus" in Zeitschrift für Hygiene und Infektionskrankheiten 26: 1–56, 1897. *Rev Infect Dis*. 1979 Jul–Aug;**1**(4):701–19.

5 Dykstra DD, Sidi AA, Scott AB, Pagel JM, Goldish GD. Effects of botulinum A toxin on detrusor-sphincter dyssynergia in spinal cord injury patients. *J Urol*. 1988 May;**139**(5):919–22.

6 Steinhardt GF, Naseer S, Cruz OA. Botulinum toxin: novel treatment for dramatic urethral dilatation associated with dysfunctional voiding. *J Urol*. 1997 Jul;**158**(1):190–1.

7 Hoebeke P, De Caestecker K, Vande Walle J, Dehoorne J, Raes A, Verleyen P, et al. The effect of botulinum-A toxin in incontinent children with therapy resistant overactive detrusor. *J Urol*. 2006 Jul;**176**(1):328–30. Discussion 330–1.

8 Popat R, Apostolidis A, Kalsi V, Gonzales G, Fowler CJ, Dasgupta P. A comparison between the response of patients with idiopathic detrusor overactivity and neurogenic detrusor overactivity to the first intradetrusor injection of botulinum-A toxin. *J Urol*. 2005 Sep;**174**(3):984–9.

9 Ikeda Y, Zabbarova IV, Birder LA, de Groat WC, McCarthy CJ, Hanna-Mitchell AT, et al. Botulinum neurotoxin serotype A suppresses neurotransmitter release from afferent as well as efferent nerves in the urinary bladder. *Eur Urol*. 2012 Dec;**62**(6):1157–64.

10 Apostolidis A, Dasgupta P, Fowler CJ. Proposed mechanism for the efficacy of injected botulinum toxin in the treatment of human detrusor overactivity. *Eur Urol*. 2006 Apr;**49**(4):644–50.

11 Lawrence GW, Aoki KR, Dolly JO. Excitatory cholinergic and purinergic signaling in bladder are equally susceptible to botulinum neurotoxin a consistent with co-release of transmitters from efferent fibers. *J Pharmacol Exp Ther*. 2010 Sep;**334**(3):1080–6.

12 Marte A, Borrelli M, Sabatino MD, Balzo BD, Prezioso M, Pintozzi L, et al. Effectiveness of botulinum-A toxin for the treatment of refractory overactive bladder in children. *Eur J Pediatr Surg*. 2010 May;**20**(3):153–7.

13 McDowell DT, Noone D, Tareen F, Waldron M, Quinn F. Urinary incontinence in children: botulinum toxin is a safe and effective treatment option. *Pediatr Surg Int*. 2012 Jan;**28**(3):315–20.

14 Mokhless I, Gaafar S, Fouda K, Shafik M, Assem A. Botulinum a toxin urethral sphincter injection in children with nonneurogenic neurogenic bladder. *J Urol.* 2006 Oct;**176**(4 Pt 2):1767–70. Discussion 1770.

15 Franco I, Landau-Dyer L, Isom-Batz G, Collett T, Reda EF. The Use of botulinum toxin a injection for the management of external sphincter dyssynergia in neurologically normal children. *J Urol.* 2007 Oct;**178**(4):1775–80.

16 Petronijevic V, Lazovic M, Vlajkovic M, Slavkovic A, Golubovic E, Miljkovic P. Botulinum toxin type A in combination with standard urotherapy for children with dysfunctional voiding. *J Urol.* 2007 Dec;**178**(6):2599–602; discussion 2602–3. Epub 2007 Oct 22.

17 Mokhless I, Zahran A-R, Saad A, Yehia M, Youssif ME. Effect of Botox injection at the bladder neck in boys with bladder dysfunction after valve ablation. *J Pediatr Urol.* 2014 Feb;**10**(5):899–904.

18 Vricella GJ, Campigotto M, Coplen DE, Traxel EJ,Austin PF. Long-term efficacy and durability of botulinum-A toxin for refractory dysfunctional voiding in children. *J Urol.* 2014 May;**191**(5 Suppl):1586–1591.

19 't Hoen LA, van den Hoek J, Wolffenbuttel KP, van der Toorn F, Scheepe JR. Breaking the vicious circle: Onabotulinum toxin A in children with therapy-refractory dysfunctional voiding. *J Pediatr Urol.* 2015 Jun;**11**(13 Suppl):119.e1–6.

20 Kask M, Rintala R, Taskinen S. Effect of onabotulinumtoxinA treatment on symptoms and urodynamic findings in pediatric neurogenic bladder. *J Pediatr Urol.* 2014 Apr;**10**(2):280–3.

21 Schulte-Baukloh H, Knispel HH, Stolze T, Weiss C, Michael T, Miller K. Repeated botulinum-a toxin injections in treatment of children with neurogenic detrusor overactivity. *Urology.* 2005 Oct;**66**(4):865–70.

22 Coelho A, Cruz F, Cruz CD, Avelino A. Spread of onabotulinumtoxinA after bladder injection. Experimental study using the distribution of cleaved SNAP-25 as the marker of the toxin action. *Eur Urol.* 2012 Jun;**61**(6):1178–84.

23 Krhut J, Samal V, Nemec D, Zvara P. Intradetrusor versus suburothelial onabotulinumtoxinA injections for neurogenic detrusor overactivity: a pilot study. *Spinal Cord.* 2012 Dec;**50**(12):904–7.

24 Manecksha RP, Cullen IM, Ahmad S, McNeill G, Flynn R, McDermott TED, et al. Prospective randomised controlled trial comparing trigone-sparing versus trigone-including intradetrusor injection of abobotulinumtoxinA for refractory idiopathic detrusor overactivity. *Eur Urol.* 2012 May;**61**(5):928–35.

25 Kajbafzadeh A-M, Ahmadi H, Montaser-Kouhsari L, Sharifi-Rad L, Nejat F, Bazargan-Hejazi S. Intravesical electromotive botulinum toxin type A administration—part II: clinical application. *Urology.* 2011 Feb;**77**(2):439–45.

26 Kajbafzadeh A-M, Montaser-Kouhsari L, Ahmadi H, Sotoudeh M. Intravesical electromotive botulinum toxin type A administration: part I—experimental study. *Urology.* 2011 Jun;**77**(6):1460–4.

27 Heinen F, Desloovere K, Schroeder AS, Berweck S, Borggraefe I, van Campenhout A, et al. The updated European consensus 2009 on the use of botulinum toxin for children with cerebral palsy. *Eur J Paediatr Neurol.* 2010 Jan;**14**(1):45–66.

28 Beseler-Soto B, Sánchez-Palomares M, Santos-Serrano L, Landa-Rivera L, Sanantonio-Valdearcos F, Paricio-Talayero JM. Iatrogenic botulism: a complication to be taken into account in the treatment of child spasticity. *Rev Neurol.* 2003 Sep 1–15;**37**(5):444–6. Spanish. PubMed PMID: 14533094.

29 Pascual-Pascual SI, Pascual-Castroviejo I. Safety of botulinum toxin type A in children younger than 2 years. *Eur J Paediatr Neurol.* 2009 Nov;**13**(6):511–5.

30 Schulte-Baukloh H, Herholz J, Bigalke H, Miller K, Knispel HH. Results of a BoNT/A antibody study in children and adolescents after onabotulinumtoxin A (Botox®) detrusor injection. *Urol Int.* 2011;**87**(4):434–8.

31 Kajbafzadeh AM, Nikfarjam L, Mahboubi AH, Dianat SS. Voiding function and dysfunction. *Urology.* 2010 Jul;**76**(1):233–7.

CHAPTER 21

Psychological management of BBD

Monika Equit[1] and Alexander von Gontard[2]

[1] Department of Clinical Psychology and Psychotherapy, University of Saarland, Saarbrucken, Germany
[2] Department of Child and Adolescent Psychiatry, Saarland University Hospital, Homburg, Germany

Introduction

According to the International Children's Continence Society (ICCS), the term "daytime incontinence" (or daytime urinary incontinence, DUI) refers to when a child wets while awake [1]. DUI can be organic or—in most cases—functional [1]. The following common subtypes can be differentiated [2]: *urge incontinence* is characterized by urge symptoms, increased micturition frequency, and small voided volumes. Typical signs of *voiding postponement* are a low voiding frequency and postponement of micturition. In d*ysfunctional voiding*, the sphincter muscle is contracted paradoxically during voiding (instead of relaxation), leading to straining and an interrupted urine stream.

According to ICD-10 and DSM-5, encopresis is defined as both voluntary and involuntary passages of feces in inappropriate places in a child aged 4 years or older after ruling out organic causes. The more exact Rome III criteria [3] propose the neutral term of *fecal incontinence* (FI) instead of encopresis. In this classification, *functional constipation*, which can be accompanied by FI, and *nonretentive FI*, which denotes children who soil without any signs of constipation, are differentiated.

The ICCS suggests the term "bladder and bowel dysfunction" (BBD) to describe children with a combination of functional bladder and bowel disturbances [1].

Psychological aspects in evaluation of BBD

The basic steps in the assessment of BBD are identical with those of nocturnal enuresis (NE) (see Chapter 27). As the rate of comorbid behavioral disorders is much higher in FI (30–50%) and DUI (20–40%) than in NE (20–30%) [2],

Pediatric Incontinence: Evaluation and Clinical Management, First Edition. Edited by Israel Franco,
Paul F. Austin, Stuart B. Bauer, Alexander von Gontard and Yves Homsy.
© 2015 John Wiley & Sons, Ltd. Published 2015 by John Wiley & Sons, Ltd.

special care is needed to identify co-occurring psychological factors and disturbances. Screening in all cases and detailed assessment (when problems are present) is recommended.

Psychological management of BBD

Treatment guidelines for the psychological management of BBD differ regarding quality and level of evidence. Systematic reviews and randomized controlled trials are rare for the treatment of DUI or FI [4].

General treatment principles

Most interventions can be provided in primary care on an outpatient basis. General principles should be followed [5]:

- Children should be at least 4 years old for a treatment of FI and 5 years for a treatment of DUI.
- Treatment should be symptom oriented.
- Comorbid emotional and behavioral disorders should be treated separately.
- In combined disorders, FI and constipation should be treated first, as many children will stop wetting once these problems have been dealt with.
- DUI should be treated second, as many children will stop wetting at night once the daytime problems have been treated.

Following assessment, counseling and psychoeducation of the parents and the child are the basis for all subsequent interventions [2, 6, 7]. Counseling is an active process engaging both parents and children. It can be defined as a professional provision of assistance and guidance in resolving personal, social, medical, or psychological difficulties. Counseling is part of everyday practice, and many doctors are well acquainted in giving advice regarding feeding, sleeping, and other aspects of child care. To ensure that advice is followed, that is, if parents and child adhere to the recommended instructions, the implementation should be checked (e.g., by filling out charts) and can be reinforced positively (with rewards). Psychoeducation can be understood as provision of information in a wider context including subjective views and attributions of patients. A related term is demystification, that is, clarification of dysfunctional and inappropriate opinions. Sometimes, it can be useful not just to provide information on a verbal level but to actively coach and demonstrate suggested behaviors (e.g., how to sit on the toilet in a relaxed way, how to use toilet paper, how to apply an alarm, etc.). Additionally, enhancing motivation and a good therapeutic relationship are relevant factors of treatment. Feelings of guilt, parental frustration, as well as ineffective parental interventions (e.g., punishment) should be verbalized [7].

Management of FI

In the treatment of FI or functional constipation, psychoeducation includes demystification, provision of information about bowel function, instruction in proper toilet posture, encouragement of fiber-rich foods, and normalization of fluid intake [7, 8].

The main treatment approach is a regular toilet training. Children are asked to sit on the toilet in a relaxed way three times a day for 5–10 min after the main mealtimes. The aim of toilet training is not necessarily micturition or defecation, but a regulation of defecation behavior. Toilet training is the *basic therapy* for all types of FI and the main treatment component in nonretentive FI. The toilet sessions should be documented in charts and can be combined with reward systems for compliance [7]. Toilet training is significantly more efficient than pharmacological treatment alone or biofeedback treatment [9].

In functional constipation with or without FI, laxatives are combined with toilet training [7]. Successful treatment of constipation includes four steps: education, disimpaction, prevention of reaccumulation of feces, and follow-up [10]. Biofeedback training does not provide additional benefit to conventional treatment of FI, and the combination of behavioral treatment components (toilet training, dietary advice, etc.) and laxatives is more successful than laxative therapy alone.

Management of DUI

Standard urotherapy (including demystification, perception of bladder function, proper toilet posture, fluid intake, self-observation via voiding schedule, etc.) is the first-choice treatment of DUI [2]. If necessary, these treatment components can be combined with cognitive behavioral reinforcement systems for compliance. Cognitive behavioral therapy (CBT) is a subtype of psychotherapy that has shown to be effective for many disorders, including BBD. CBT comprises two components that are usually combined, but can be implemented separately: cognitive therapy and behavioral therapy. Cognitive therapy focuses on irrational, dysfunctional presumptions, thoughts, and beliefs. After identifying dysfunctional cognitions, these can be modified by techniques such as "self-monitoring" (observation and registration), "activity scheduling" (organization of activities), and "labeling" (using positive suggestive statements). Behavioral therapy concentrates on observable behavior. Techniques include "classical conditioning" (based on linking of stimulus and behavior), "operant conditioning" (learning by positive and aversive reinforcement), "shaping" (achieving changes step by step), and many others.

Urge incontinence

For the treatment of urge incontinence, standard urotherapy and a symptom-oriented cognitive behavioral approach are effective [11]. Children are instructed to perceive urgency, to go to the toilet immediately and to note voidings and wet episodes in a chart. Incontinence is reduced in many children by these simple techniques, while others need a combination with anticholinergics [2]. Effects of standard urotherapy were significantly improved when using a programmable timer watch [12].

Voiding postponement

In the treatment of voiding postponement, a symptom-oriented cognitive behavioral approach is indicated [2]. Children are instructed to go to the toilet at least seven times a day and to note each micturition in a voiding chart. By this timed voiding, micturition frequency is increased and postponement behavior is reduced. It is often necessary to combine the approach with positive reinforcement, especially in children with low compliance or oppositional behavior.

Reminders to go to the toilet by programmed watches (or cell phones) can be helpful [12].

Dysfunctional voiding

In dysfunctional voiding, a combination of cognitive behavioral elements, relaxation, drinking, and toileting advice is indicated, but the most effective treatment is biofeedback, using either uroflow or pelvic floor EMG [6]. Child-appropriate animations are available. Biofeedback training improves the effects of cognitive behavioral standard urotherapy [13].

Complex cognitive behavioral training programs

Special cognitive behavioral trainings (for individual or group setting) have been developed to treat children who do not respond to standard therapy [14]. Bladder and/or bowel trainings contain a combination of different treatment components, including providing information, psychoeducation and counseling, biofeedback, as well as components of cognitive behavioral and body-related therapies [14–17]. Body-related therapies include relaxation techniques (such as progressive muscle relaxation (PMR)) and measures to enhance body perception (such as body imagery techniques) [14]. Overall, high success rates were reported [17]. As a result of one bladder training, wetting frequency and comorbid psychological problems decreased [14].

Conclusion

Psychological screening and assessment in FI, constipation, and DUI are the same as in NE. Simple and complex psychological treatments, especially with a cognitive behavioral focus, are the most effective components in the treatment of BBD. They can be combined with laxatives and anticholinergics, when indicated. Randomized controlled treatment trials are lacking as most recommendations are still based on a low level of evidence.

References

1 Austin PF, Bauer S, Bower W, Chase J, Franco I, Hoebeke P, et al. The standardization of terminology of bladder function in children and adolescents: update report from the Standardization Committee of the International Children's Continence Society (ICCS). *J Urol* 2014;**191**(6):1863–1865.e13.

2 von Gontard A. Enuresis. In: Rey JM (ed), IACAPAP Textbook of Child and Adolescent Mental Health, online, 2012. Available at http://iacapap.org/iacapap-textbook-of-child-and-adolescent-mental-health (accessed March 17, 2015).

3 Rasquin A, Di Lorenzo C, Forbes D, Guiraldes E, Hyams JS, Staiano A, Walker LS. Childhood functional gastrointestinal disorders: child/adolescent. *Gastroenterology* 2006;**130**:1527–37.

4 Brazzelli M, Griffiths PV, Cody JD, Tappin D. Behavioural and cognitive interventions with and without other treatments for the management of faecal incontinence in children. *Cochrane Database Syst Rev* 2011;(**12**):CD002240.

5 von Gontard A. The impact of DSM-5 and guidelines for assessment and treatment of elimination disorders. *Eur Child Adolesc Psychiatry* 2013;**22**(suppl. 1):S61–S67.

6 Chase J, Austin P, Hoebeke P, McKenna P. The management of dysfunctional voiding in children: a report from the Standardisation Committee of the International Children's Continence Society. *J Urol* 2010;**183**(4):1296–1302.

7 von Gontard A. Encopresis. In: Rey J (ed), IACAPAP Textbook of Child and Adolescent Mental Health, online, 2012b. Available at http://iacapap.org/iacapap-textbook-of-child-and-adolescent-mental-health (accessed March 17, 2015).

8 Burgers RE, Mugie SM, Chase J, Cooper CS, Von Gontard A, Rittig CS, et al. Management of functional constipation in children with lower urinary tract symptoms: report from the standardization committee of the international children's continence society. *J Urol* 2013;**190**(1):29–36.

9 Borowitz SM, Cox DJ, Sutphen JL, Kovatchev B. Treatment of childhood encopresis: a randomized trial comparing three treatment protocols. *J Pediatr Gastroenterol Nutr* 2002; **34**: 378–84.

10 Tabbers MM, Boluyt N, Berger MY, Benninga MA. Clinical practice—diagnosis and treatment of functional constipation. *Eur J Pediatr* 2011;**170**:955–63.

11 Vijveberg MAW, Elzinga-Plomb A, Messer AP, van Gool JD, de Jong TPVM. Bladder rehabilitation, the effect of a cognitive training programme on urge incontinence. *Eur Urol* 1997; **31**: 68–72.

12 Hagstroem S, Rittig S, Kamperis K, Djurhuus JC. Timer watch assisted urotherapy in children: a randomized controlled trial. *J Urol* 2010;**184**(4):1482–8.

13 Vesna ZD, Milica L, Stanković I, Marina V, Andjelka S. The evaluation of combined standard urotherapy, abdominal and pelvic floor retraining in children with dysfunctional voiding. *J Pediatr Urol* 2011;**7**(3):336–41.

14 Equit M, Sambach H, Niemczyk J, von Gontard A. *Urinary and fecal incontinence. A training program for children and adolescents*. Boston/Göttingen, Hogrefe Publishing, 2015.

15 van Dijk M, Benninga MA, Grootenhuis MA, Onland-van Nieuwenhuizen AM, Last BF. Chronic childhood constipation: a review of the literature and the introduction of a protocolized behavioural intervention program. *Patient Educ Couns* 2007;**67**:63–77.

16 Mulders MM, Cobussen-Boekhorst H, De Gier RPE, Feitz WFJ, Kortmann BBM. Urotherapy in children: quantitative measurements of daytime urinary incontinence before and after treatment: according to the new definitions of the international children's continence society. *J Pediatr Urol* 2011; **7**: 213–8.

17 Hoebeke P. Twenty years of urotherapy in children: what have we learned? *Eur Urol* 2006;**49**:426–8.

SECTION 5

Nocturnal enuresis

Israel Franco

Introduction

Nocturnal enuresis (NE) is a pervasive and disturbing problem for many children and their families. This is a worldwide problem where in some cultures the problem can lead to major issues for the child that is beyond their control. NE originally was thought to be a psychiatric/psychological problem, and the pendulum then swung heavily to it being a somatic problem with issues in excessive urine production at night. We are starting to see the pendulum swing back to a more central position that is beginning to recognize this is possibly due to one or more issues. Arousal and/or nocturnal overproduction of urine appear to be the main factors in NE. In NMNE, we are aware that the bladder is playing a role as well. As all things in medicine, the answers are not as simple as first thought to be.

Through this section of the book, we are graced with four authors who have had extensive experience in the field of NE. Each provides their unique knowledge to lead the reader to the most up-to-date data available on the topic. We have omitted a chapter on the management of the patient with NMNE since management of the day issues is covered in the rest of the book and containing this problem first is critical to the success in NMNE.

In Chapter 22, Dr.'s Rittig and Kamperis elucidate the pathogenesis of nocturnal polyuria and include some new work on circadian rhythms. Their discussion of reduced bladder reservoir function is critical for the reader to understand and plays a central role in the patient with NMNE.

In Chapter 23, Dr. Neveus takes us through the intake of a patient with NE and gives us a nice step-by-step means of evaluating these patients in a detailed

Pediatric Incontinence: Evaluation and Clinical Management, First Edition. Edited by Israel Franco, Paul F. Austin, Stuart B. Bauer, Alexander von Gontard and Yves Homsy.
© 2015 John Wiley & Sons, Ltd. Published 2015 by John Wiley & Sons, Ltd.

plan. All care providers can use this chapter as a road map to begin the evaluation of their patients with NE.

In Chapter 24, Dr. Johan Vande Walle provides us with the management of the patient with NE. Johan rightfully goes on to discuss the need for uniformity in how we should classify our patients so that, in the future, studies can be implicitly compared one to another. The rest of the chapter takes us through all the means of managing this problem available to the reader at this present time.

Finally, Chapter 25 by Dr.'s Baeyens and von Gontard delve into the psychologic aspects of NE, for example, how to evaluate such patients, and they outline three types of patients that are at increased risk for NE. This is done in a concise manner that is helpful to the reader and provides the reader with the appropriate tools to evaluate these patients.

It is this editor's own personal belief that when the volume of urine which elicits the first sensation of filing is reached, primitive micturition reflexes that normally should be suppressed by the centers involved with continuous monitoring of bladder activity are not suppressed. Impaired communication and arousability in the appropriate centers that are needed to suppress spontaneous reflex bladder emptying are not adequately recruited fast enough or never recruited in some cases, leading to enuresis. This lack of arousal, for lack of a better term, most likely plays a role in the patients with NE due to all causes. In the disturbed bladder of patients with NMNE, the reduced stretch capabilities lead to a lower threshold volume that in turn leads to repetitive NE at lower than normal volumes. Obviously, this is all speculation on my part based on a CNS-centric way of thinking, and further work needs to be done to better understand the exact CNS processes in these patients. Due to the limitations imparted on the use of fMRI because of its low spatial resolution and the need to perform tasks repetitively to allow identifying brain centers involved in this surveillance scheme, it will be a hard task to prove these theories with present-day modalities. It is such a CNS-centric scheme that can explain the psychological, somatic, and nocturnal urine production theories and marry them together. Only time will tell what the true mechanisms are in NE.

CHAPTER 22

Pathophysiology of nocturnal enuresis

Søren Rittig and Konstantinos Kamperis

Department of Pediatrics, Aarhus University Hospital, Aarhus, Denmark

Introduction

The perception of the pathogenesis of enuresis has undergone marked changes over the past 30 years from a psychiatric/psychological background to a more somatic model where nighttime urine production and bladder capacity are main components together with an arousal dysfunction that prevents the enuretic child from waking up to the signals of a full bladder (Figure 22.1). Furthermore, it has become very clear that several pathogenic mechanisms exist either alone or in combination explaining the variety of clinical subtypes with different responses to treatment. In this chapter, we will review the current evidence behind today's perception of enuresis pathogenesis.

Nocturnal polyuria

Increased nighttime urine production was proposed as a causative factor and named "relative nocturnal polyuria" already in the early 1950s [1, 2]. However, such a hypothesis was not tested further until the early 1980s where standardized *inpatient* circadian studies demonstrated that enuresis patients showed an abnormally large nocturnal urine production that exceeded the cystometric bladder capacity [3, 4]. Also, pointing toward a possible role of nocturnal urine output were a few placebo-controlled studies reporting the positive effect of antidiuretic therapy with the synthetic AVP analogue desmopressin [5, 6]. Since then, nocturnal polyuria at least in a subpopulation of enuresis patients was confirmed using home recording methods, either by diaper weighing [7] or timed urine collections [8]. Furthermore, it was shown that nocturnal urine

Pediatric Incontinence: Evaluation and Clinical Management, First Edition. Edited by Israel Franco, Paul F. Austin, Stuart B. Bauer, Alexander von Gontard and Yves Homsy.

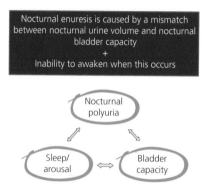

Figure 22.1 The box (upper panel) expresses a general consensus of enuresis pathogenesis involving nocturnal urine production and bladder capacity together with an inability to awaken. Thus, enuresis pathogenesis can be condensed into a "three-factor model" highlighting the main pathogenic elements (lower panel).

production is significantly larger during wet nights than dry nights and is larger in patients who respond positively to desmopressin treatment [9]. In 2006, international consensus was obtained regarding the definition of nocturnal polyuria in children (nocturnal urine volume on a wet night greater than 130% of expected bladder capacity for age) [10].

Underlying pathogenic mechanisms

Since the documentation of nocturnal polyuria as a causative factor, research has been directed toward the underlying pathogenic mechanisms (Figure 22.2).

Renal factors
Detailed circadian studies have revealed several mechanisms behind nocturnal polyuria in enuresis. Firstly, a proportion of enuretic children with nocturnal polyuria have an abnormally low urinary osmolality during nighttime, indicating a problem in antidiuretic function [4, 11, 12]. Secondly, some children show increased osmotic excretion due to decreased tubular reabsorption of particularly sodium, potassium, and urea during night [8, 13]. Such patients are characterized by nocturnal polyuria with relatively high urine osmolality and treatment resistance to desmopressin. Thirdly, some but not all studies have implicated an increased nocturnal GFR estimated by fractional creatinine clearance measurements [14, 15]. Also, increased nocturnal urinary excretion of prostaglandin E2 has pointed toward a possible role of the prostaglandin system [13].

Hormones
A number of hormone systems participate in the normal regulation of water and salt balance and several of these have been investigated in enuresis. Of these, only vasopressin (AVP) has been attributed a pathogenic role. Several independent

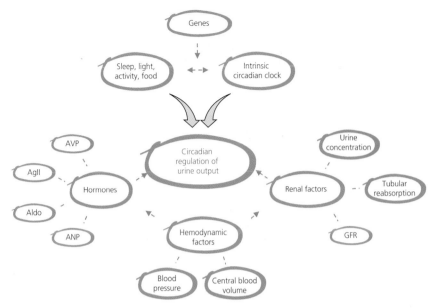

Figure 22.2 Schematic drawing of some important factors involved in the regulation of the circadian rhythm of urine output. For explanation of abbreviations: AgII, angiotensin II; Aldo, aldosterone; ANP, Atrial natriuretic peptide; AVP, arginine vasopressin; GFR, glomerular filtration rate.

studies of the circadian rhythm of plasma AVP have demonstrated a lack of the normal nocturnal rise seen in healthy children [3, 4, 16, 17]. Furthermore, nocturnal plasma AVP levels are lower during wet than dry nights and lower in patients who respond positively to desmopressin [9]. Thus, a circadian defect in AVP seems to play a role in patients with polyuria due to increased free water excretion. The role of the renin–angiotensin–aldosterone system has been investigated as a possible mechanism behind the increased nocturnal solute excretion, but so far, there is little evidence to support this hypothesis [13, 18]. Also, no pathogenic role has been attributed plasma atrial natriuretic peptide in enuresis [14].

Hemodynamic factors

Blood pressure is an important factor behind the renal excretion of sodium and other solutes and recent studies have stimulated increased focus on the importance of high nocturnal blood pressure levels behind nocturnal polyuria and natriuresis. Thus, elevated nocturnal blood pressure has been associated with concomitant polyuria in both nocturnal enuresis [19] and other conditions with nocturnal polyuria, that is, nocturia in the elderly [20], elderly males with benign prostatic hyperplasia [21], and renal transplant patients [22].

The role of the baroregulatory response to the increase in central blood volume seen when going to bed at night has been investigated in enuresis. During daytime, however, such positional change is associated with a comparable suppression of baroregulatory hormones in normal subjects and enuretics contradicting a pathogenic role of central blood volume changes [23].

Intrinsic circadian rhythms

Urine output has a well-known circadian rhythm with a marked reduction during night [24, 25]. A central factor behind such rhythms is the suprachiasmatic nuclei (SCN) that are considered the central coordinators of a plethora of tissue based, autonomously active cellular clocks dispersed across the body. By virtue of their retinal innervation and efferent connections, the SCN have the unique role of maintaining appropriate synchrony between these local clocks and the local metabolic rhythms dependent upon solar time, thereby ensuring that physiology across the entire organism is temporally integrated [26]. Since 1997, the importance of molecular mechanisms behind circadian rhythms was emphasized with the characterization of mammalian clock genes [27–30]. Today, a long list of genes (e.g., PER1-3, CRY1-2, Clock, and Bmal1) [31] form different sets of interlocking transcriptional feedback loops that interact within the cell to either up- or downregulate gene expression in an oscillatory manner. A significant mediator of many of these functions is believed to be an influence of SCN on the autonomic nervous system, that is, the balance between sympathetic and parasympathetic nervous outflows [32, 33]. The exact role of the intrinsic circadian regulatory machinery behind enuresis pathogenesis is not fully understood but in theory circadian rhythm dysregulation could be the primary pathogenic mechanism not only for urine output mechanisms but also for nocturnal bladder function (Figure 22.3) [34, 35]. The close proximity between SCN centers controlling AVP release, sleep/arousal, micturition, and baroregulation could provide the basis for a defect circadian rhythm in one or more of these biological functions.

Reduced nocturnal bladder reservoir function

The function of the urinary bladder is to store urine as well as to facilitate its complete emptying at will and on socially acceptable occasions. Any disturbances in bladder function may lead to nocturnal enuresis with or without daytime symptoms. In children with the nonmonosymptomatic form of the disorder, bladder dysfunction is a common denominator.

Reduced bladder capacity

The most common finding in children with MNE related to bladder function concerns its ability to accommodate urine and there is substantial evidence that one of the main etiological factors of enuresis is a reduced bladder capacity (Figure 22.1). It is still unclear, however, which types of bladder dysfunction are implied by the term "small bladder." The term does not refer to anatomical but

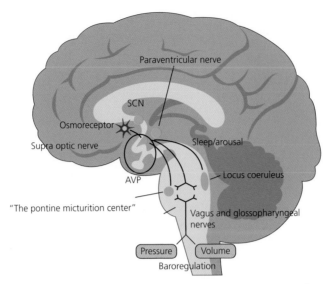

Figure 22.3 Location of CNS centers and mechanisms involved in enuresis pathogenesis and illustrates the close proximity between central brain centers controlling AVP release, sleep/arousal, micturition, and baroregulation. The locus coeruleus receives connections from the anterior cingulate gyrus and the prefrontal cortex where these are processed by the frontal lobes, thereby making the frontal lobes a player in the nocturnal enuresis process. AVP, arginine vasopressin; SCN, suprachiasmatic nucleus.

rather functional abnormalities. Since urodynamic evaluation is rarely indicated in MNE patients, studies of bladder function in children with MNE are sparse and we do lack experimental data that could unambiguously cover the issue.

Urodynamic studies in enuresis are to be found in the literature. In a number of studies, nocturnal detrusor overactivity has been related to nocturnal enuresis in the majority of patients [36–38]. These early studies were performed during daytime, using invasive techniques and the recruited patients suffered daytime symptoms such as frequency, urgency, and daytime incontinence. Thus the validity of any conclusions on nocturnal bladder function in children with monosymptomatic nocturnal enuresis is questionable. In a landmark study on bladder function in enuresis, Nørgaard et al. performed nighttime cystometric investigations and continuous overnight detrusor pressure recordings through suprapubic catheters in 31 patients with nocturnal enuresis and no daytime incontinence [38]. The studies revealed normal cystometric capacities in these children and nocturnal bladder contractions that, however, did not lead to enuresis episodes. Yeung and colleagues studied children with enuresis refractory to treatment with the enuresis alarm and desmopressin [39] demonstrating patterns of bladder dysfunction typically in the form of detrusor instability evident either solely at night or both during daytime and nighttime. The reduced bladder capacities in children with enuresis are typically reflected in home recordings [7] where the maximal voided volumes achieved are well below the expected for age [40]. The current definition of reduced bladder capacity is less than 65% of the expected for age [41, 42]. It is, however, debatable to what extent daytime and nighttime bladder functions are related. It seems that some children with enuresis who present with normal bladder reservoir function during the day share reduced bladder capacities only during sleep. Molecular studies have identified the expression of genes in the bladder with circadian regulation patterns such as connexin 43, a gene associated with the regulation of bladder capacity [43].

Although initially considered as a normal voiding with full bladder emptying, a study in children with monosymptomatic enuresis revealed that the majority of the enuresis episodes are interrupted voidings leading to incomplete bladder emptying [44]. Despite that, children with monosymptomatic enuresis do not share abnormalities in the voiding phase of the bladder function during daytime as evaluated by uroflowmetry [45]. Such abnormalities may, however, be seen when daytime symptoms are present and include dysfunctional voiding with or without detrusor sphincter dyssynergia typically revealed by staccato or interrupted voiding in uroflowmetry with or without residual urine. The prevalence of dysfunctional voiding in enuresis is considerably higher when comorbidity such as constipation is present.

Disturbed sleep/arousal function

For many years, it has been a common belief both among mothers and health-care providers that enuresis is caused by deep sleep. However, conventional sleep studies analyzing sleep EEG failed to show any convincing abnormalities in sleep architecture of enuretic children [46, 47]. Thus, enuresis occurs during all sleep stages, and cystometric sleep studies showed no difference between sleep stages with regard to the occurrence of enuresis during bladder filling [38]. As a fundamental problem in enuresis seems to be an inability to wake up to the signal from a full bladder, the role of arousal function has been investigated. Although one study was able to demonstrate reduced ability to arouse to an acoustic stimulus [48], there is little evidence of a specific arousal defect in enuresis. Also, a significant proportion of normal nonenuretic children were also unable to wake up when bladder overfilling was induced contradicting an arousal defect as the primary factor in enuresis [49].

Recently, a new pathogenic theory was proposed suggesting that signals from an overactive bladder causes increased arousal levels during sleep [50]. This may be in line with the finding that sleep latency was increased and sleep efficiency reduced in enuretics indicating a poor sleep quality [51]. Also supportive of this theory was the demonstration of concomitant increased sleep fragmentation and abnormally increased "periodic limb movements" during sleep in treatment resistant enuresis [52]. The demonstration of increased blood pressure levels and increased urine production and natriuresis in both children and adults during acute sleep deprivation may indicate a role of sleep behind nocturnal polyuria [53, 54]. Thus, a new pathogenesis paradigm may be developing stating that sleep in children with enuresis may in fact be too "light" and inefficient and currently focus is directed toward possible daytime consequences of a disturbed sleep.

Genetic factors

Family studies assessing the incidence of bed wetting among relatives of children affected by the disorder have repeatedly shown that nocturnal enuresis is highly familial. Thus, approximately 65–75% of first-degree relatives have a positive history of enuresis [55]. It has further been noted from family studies that the phenotypes within families are often heterogeneous, for example, coexistence of primary and secondary enuresis as well as mono- and nonmonosymptomatic nocturnal enuresis [56]. Even cases where family members are affected by two different conditions, for example, urge incontinence and nocturnal enuresis, simultaneously or at different times during development have been described [57]. Several twin studies showed higher concordance rates in monozygotic twins compared to dizygotic strongly indicating a substantial genetic component of the disease etiology [58].

Analysis of the segregation of nocturnal enuresis within families has revealed several different modes of inheritance implying genetic heterogeneity. The most frequent mode of inheritance seems to be autosomal dominant with high penetrance. This inheritance pattern was, for example, identified in a study by Eiberg in 1995 in which he analyzed a total of 430 Danish families among which 11 families had primary nocturnal enuresis in at least two generations or more [59]. Less frequent is autosomal dominant inheritance with reduced penetrance [55] and autosomal recessive transmission [60].

Linkage studies in nocturnal enuresis have predominantly been performed in large families with autosomal dominant inheritance of the disease [59–61]. These studies led to the identification of nocturnal enuresis loci on five different chromosomes as summarized in Figure 22.4. The first study was a linkage study including 11 families with primary nocturnal enuresis and autosomal dominant inheritance [59]. In five of these families, there was evidence for linkage to chromosome 13q (13q13-13q14.2) with positive LOD scores for microsatellite markers D13S291 and D13S263 of respectively, $Z=3.77$ and $Z=2.9$. The most recent linkage study in nocturnal enuresis is a study of a large four-generation family with a phenotype of combined urge incontinence and nocturnal enuresis [62]. In conclusion, nocturnal enuresis is clearly a complex disease involving both environmental and genetic factors, and it includes both locus heterogeneity and no clear phenotype–genotype correlation. The lack of positive findings for markers in the already identified loci in some families clearly implies that

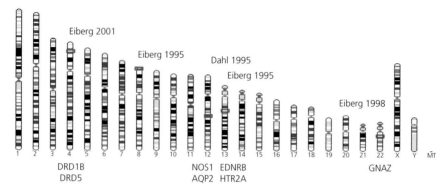

Figure 22.4 Location of five different linkage areas for nocturnal enuresis so far identified on human chromosomes (red boxes). Above is indicated the author and publication year for each locus and below are listed proposed candidate genes in these areas. To date, no specific enuresis gene has been documented.

additional loci exists and remains to be identified. Although a number of candidate genes have been identified, no specific gene variants have yet been confirmed in nocturnal enuresis.

References

1 Poulton, E. M.: Relative nocturnal polyuria as a factor in enuresis. *Lancet*, **2**: 906, 1952.

2 Poulton E. M.: The classification of enuresis. *Arch Dis Child*, **28**: 392, 1953.

3 Nørgaard, J. P., Pedersen, E. B., and Djurhuus, J. C.: Diurnal anti-diuretic-hormone levels in enuretics. *J Urol*, **134**: 1029, 1985.

4 Rittig, S., Knudsen, U. B., Norgaard, J. P., Pedersen, E. B., and Djurhuus, J. C.: Abnormal diurnal rhythm of plasma vasopressin and urinary output in patients with enuresis. *Am J Physiol*, **256**: F664, 1989.

5 Tuvemo, T.: DDAVP in childhood nocturnal enuresis. *Acta Paediatr Scand*, **67**: 753, 1978.

6 Terho, P. and Kekomaki, M.: Management of nocturnal enuresis with a vasopressin analogue. *J Urol*, **131**: 925, 1984.

7 Hansen, M. N., Rittig, S., Siggaard, C., Kamperis, K., Hvistendahl, G., Schaumburg, H. L. et al.: Intra-individual variability in nighttime urine production and functional bladder capacity estimated by home recordings in patients with nocturnal enuresis. *J Urol*, **166**: 2452, 2001.

8 Dehoorne, J. L., Raes, A. M., Van, L. E., Hoebeke, P., and Vande Walle, J. G.: Desmopressin resistant nocturnal polyuria secondary to increased nocturnal osmotic excretion. *J Urol*, **176**: 749, 2006.

9 Rittig, S., Schaumburg, H. L., Siggaard, C., Schmidt, F., and Djurhuus, J. C.: The circadian defect in plasma vasopressin and urine output is related to desmopressin response and enuresis status in children with nocturnal enuresis. *J Urol*, **179**: 2389, 2008.

10 Neveus, T., Von, G. A., Hoebeke, P., Hjalmas, K., Bauer, S., Bower, W. et al.: The standardization of terminology of lower urinary tract function in children and adolescents: Report from the Standardisation Committee of the International Children's Continence Society. *J Urol*, **176**: 314, 2006.

11 Vande, W. J., Vande, W. C., Van, S. P., De, G. A., Raes, A., Donckerwolcke, R. et al.: Nocturnal polyuria is related to 24-hour diuresis and osmotic excretion in an enuresis population referred to a tertiary center. *J Urol*, **178**: 2630, 2007.

12 Pomeranz, A., Abu-Kheat, G., Korzets, Z., and Wolach, B.: Night-time polyuria and urine hypo-osmolality in enuretics identified by nocturnal sequential urine sampling: Do they represent a subset of relative ADH-deficient subjects? *Scand J Urol Nephrol*, **34**: 199, 2000.

13 Kamperis, K., Rittig, S., Jorgensen, K. A., and Djurhuus, J. C.: Nocturnal polyuria in monosymptomatic nocturnal enuresis refractory to desmopressin treatment. *Am J Physiol Renal Physiol*, **291**: F1232, 2006.

14 Rittig, S., Knudsen, U. B., Norgaard, J. P., Gregersen, H., Pedersen, E. B., and Djurhuus, J. C.: Diurnal variation of plasma atrial natriuretic peptide in normals and patients with enuresis nocturna. *Scand J Clin Lab Invest*, **51**: 209, 1991.

15 De, G. A., Vande, W. C., Van, S. P., Raes, A., Donckerwolcke, R., Van, L. E. et al.: Nocturnal polyuria is related to absent circadian rhythm of glomerular filtration rate. *J Urol*, **178**: 2626, 2007.

16 Aikawa, T., Kasahara, T., and Uchiyama, M.: The arginine–vasopressin secretion profile of children with primary nocturnal enuresis. *Eur Urol*, **33** (Suppl 3): 41, 1998.

17 AbdelFatah, D., Shaker, H., Ismail, M., and Ezzat, M.: Nocturnal polyuria and nocturnal arginine vasopressin (AVP): A key factor in the pathophysiology of monosymptomatic nocturnal enuresis. *Neurourol Urodyn*, **28**: 506, 2009.

18 Rittig, S., Matthiesen, T. B., Pedersen, E. B., and Djurhuus, J. C.: Circadian variation of angiotensin II and aldosterone in nocturnal enuresis: Relationship to arterial blood pressure and urine output. *J Urol*, **176**: 774, 2006.

19 Kruse, A., Mahler, B., Rittig, S., and Djurhuus, J. C.: Increased nocturnal blood pressure in enuretic children with polyuria. *J Urol*, **182**: 1954, 2009.

20 Graugaard-Jensen, C., Rittig, S., and Djurhuus, J. C.: Nocturia and circadian blood pressure profile in healthy elderly male volunteers. *J Urol*, **176**: 1034, 2006.

21 Matthiesen, T. B., Rittig, S., Norgaard, J. P., Pedersen, E. B., and Djurhuus, J. C.: Nocturnal polyuria and natriuresis in male patients with nocturia and lower urinary tract symptoms. *J Urol*, **156**: 1292, 1996.

22 Alstrup, K., Graugaard-Jensen, C., Rittig, S., and Jorgensen, K. A.: Abnormal diurnal rhythm of urine output following renal transplantation: The impact of blood pressure and diuretics. *Transplant Proc*, **42**: 3529, 2010.

23 Rittig, S.: Neuroendocrine response to supine posture in healthy children and patients with nocturnal enuresis. *Clin Endocrinol (Oxf)*, **72**: 781, 2010.

24 Roberts, W. M..: Observations on some of the daily changes of the urine. *Edinb Med J*, **5**: 817, 1859.

25 Quincke, H.: Über tag- und nachtharn. *Arch Exp Pathol Pharmakol*, **32**: 211, 1893.

26 Hastings, M. H., Reddy, A. B., and Maywood, E. S.: A clockwork web: Circadian timing in brain and periphery, in health and disease. *Nat Rev Neurosci*, **4**: 649, 2003.

27 Antoch, M. P., Song, E. J., Chang, A. M., Vitaterna, M. H., Zhao, Y., Wilsbacher, L. D. et al.: Functional identification of the mouse circadian clock gene by transgenic BAC rescue. *Cell*, **89**: 655, 1997.

28 King, D. P., Zhao, Y., Sangoram, A. M., Wilsbacher, L. D., Tanaka, M., Antoch, M. P. et al.: Positional cloning of the mouse circadian clock gene. *Cell*, **89**: 641, 1997.

29 Tei, H., Okamura, H., Shigeyoshi, Y., Fukuhara, C., Ozawa, R., Hirose, M. et al.: Circadian oscillation of a mammalian homologue of the drosophila period gene. *Nature*, **389**: 512, 1997.

30 Sun, Z. S., Albrecht, U., Zhuchenko, O., Bailey, J., Eichele, G., and Lee, C. C.: RIGUI, a putative mammalian ortholog of the drosophila period gene. *Cell*, **90**: 1003, 1997.

31 Reppert, S. M. and Weaver, D. R.: Coordination of circadian timing in mammals. *Nature*, **418**: 935, 2002.

32 Buijs, R. M., La Fleur, S. E., Wortel, J., Van, H. C., Zuiddam, L., Mettenleiter, T. C. et al.: The suprachiasmatic nucleus balances sympathetic and parasympathetic output to peripheral organs through separate preautonomic neurons. *J Comp Neurol*, **464**: 36, 2003.

33 Scheer, F. A., Kalsbeek, A., and Buijs, R. M.: Cardiovascular control by the suprachiasmatic nucleus: Neural and neuroendocrine mechanisms in human and rat. *Biol Chem*, **384**: 697, 2003.

34 Negoro, H., Kanematsu, A., Doi, M., Suadicani, S. O., Matsuo, M., Imamura, M. et al.: Involvement of urinary bladder Connexin43 and the circadian clock in coordination of diurnal micturition rhythm. *Nat Commun*, **3**: 809, 2012.

35 Noh, J. Y., Han, D. H., Kim, M. H., Ko, I. G., Kim, S. E., Park, N. et al.: Presence of multiple peripheral circadian oscillators in the tissues controlling voiding function in mice. *Exp Mol Med*, **46**: e81, 2014.

36 Palmtag, H., Heering, H., and Ziegler, G.: Functional abnormality of "non-provocative" bladder instability in children. *Urol Int*, **34**: 176, 1979.

37 Mahony, D. T., Laferte, R. O., and Blais, D. J.: Studies of enuresis. VIII. Detrusor and sphincter instability caused by overactivity of integral voiding reflexes. *Urology*, **9**: 590, 1977.

38 Norgaard, J. P., Hansen, J. H., Wildschiotz, G., Sorensen, S., Rittig, S., and Djurhuus, J. C.: Sleep cystometries in children with nocturnal enuresis. *J Urol*, **141**: 1156, 1989.

39 Yeung, C. K., Chiu, H. N., and Sit, F. K.: Bladder dysfunction in children with refractory monosymptomatic primary nocturnal enuresis. *J Urol*, **162**: 1049, 1999.

40 Koff, S. A.: Estimating bladder capacity in children. *Urology*, **21**: 248, 1983.

41 Neveus, T., Eggert, P., Evans, J., Macedo, A., Rittig, S., Tekgul, S. et al.: Evaluation of and treatment for monosymptomatic enuresis: A standardization document from the International Children's Continence Society. *J Urol*, **183**: 441, 2010.

42 Austin, P. F., Bauer, S. B., Bower, W., Chase, J., Franco, I., Hoebeke, P. et al.: The standardization of terminology of lower urinary tract function in children and adolescents: Update report from the Standardization Committee of the International Children's Continence Society. *J Urol*, **19**: 1863, 2014.

43 Negoro, H., Kanematsu, A., Yoshimura, K., and Ogawa, O.: Chronobiology of micturition: Putative role of the circadian clock. *J Urol*, **190**: 843, 2013.

44 Hagstroem, S., Kamperis, K., Rittig, S., Rijkhoff, N. J., and Djurhuus, J. C.: Monosymptomatic nocturnal enuresis is associated with abnormal nocturnal bladder emptying. *J Urol*, **171**: 2562, 2004.

45 Rittig, N., Hagstroem, S., Mahler, B., Kamperis, K., Siggaard, C., Mikkelsen, M. M. et al.: Outcome of a standardized approach to childhood urinary symptoms-long-term follow-up of 720 patients. *Neurourol Urodyn*, **33**: 475, 2014.

46 Norgaard, J. P., Hansen, J. H., Nielsen, J. B., Petersen, B. S., Knudsen, N., and Djurhuus, J. C.: Simultaneous registration of sleep-stages and bladder activity in enuresis. *Urology*, **26**: 316, 1985.

47 Bader, G., Neveus, T., Kruse, S., and Sillen, U.: Sleep of primary enuretic children and controls. *Sleep*, **25**: 579, 2002.

48 Wolfish, N. M., Pivik, R. T., and Busby, K. A.: Elevated sleep arousal thresholds in enuretic boys: Clinical implications. *Acta Paediatr*, **86**: 381, 1997.

49 Kirk, J., Rasmussen, P. V., Rittig, S., and Djurhuus, J. C.: Provoked enuresis-like episodes in healthy children 7 to 12 years old. *J Urol*, **156**: 210, 1996.

50 Yeung, C. K., Diao, M., and Sreedhar, B.: Cortical arousal in children with severe enuresis. *N Engl J Med*, **358**: 2414, 2008.

51 Ertan, P., Yilmaz, O., Caglayan, M., Sogut, A., Aslan, S., and Yuksel, H.: Relationship of sleep quality and quality of life in children with monosymptomatic enuresis. *Child Care Health Dev*, **35**: 469, 2009.

52 Dhondt, K., Baert, E., Van, H. C., Raes, A., Groen, L. A., Hoebeke, P. et al.: Sleep fragmentation and increased periodic limb movements are more common in children with nocturnal enuresis. *Acta Paediatr*, **103**: e268, 2014.

53 Kamperis, K., Hagstroem, S., Radvanska, E., Rittig, S., and Djurhuus, J. C.: Excess diuresis and natriuresis during acute sleep deprivation in healthy adults. *Am J Physiol Renal Physiol*, **299**: F404, 2010.

54 Mahler, B., Kamperis, K., Schroeder, M., Frokiaer, J., Djurhuus, J. C., and Rittig, S.: Sleep deprivation induces excess diuresis and natriuresis in healthy children. *Am J Physiol Renal Physiol*, **302**: F236, 2012.

55 von Gontard, A., Schaumburg, H., Hollmann, E., Eiberg, H., and Rittig, S.: The genetics of enuresis: A review. *J Urol*, **166**: 2438, 2001.

56 Schaumburg, H. L., Kapilin, U., Blasvaer, C., Eiberg, H., Von, G. A., Djurhuus, J. C. et al.: Hereditary phenotypes in nocturnal enuresis. *BJU Int*, **102**: 816, 2008.

57 von Gontard, A., Eiberg H., Schaumburg H., and Rittig S.: Enuresis-associations of phenotype and genotype. *Mol Psychiatry*, **4**: S57, 1999.

58 Hublin, C., Kaprio, J., Partinen, M., and Koskenvuo, M.: Nocturnal enuresis in a nationwide twin cohort. *Sleep*, **21**: 579, 1998.

59 Eiberg, H., Berendt, I., and Mohr, J.: Assignment of dominant inherited nocturnal enuresis (ENUR1) to chromosome 13q. *Nat Genet*, **10**: 354, 1995.

60 Arnell, H., Hjalmas, K., Jagervall, M., Lackgren, G., Stenberg, A., Bengtsson, B. et al.: The genetics of primary nocturnal enuresis: Inheritance and suggestion of a second major gene on chromosome 12q. *J Med Genet*, **34**: 360, 1997.

61 Loeys, B., Hoebeke, P., Raes, A., Messiaen, L., De, P. A., and Vande, W. J.: Does monosymptomatic enuresis exist? A molecular Genetic exploration of 32 families with enuresis/incontinence. *BJU Int*, **90**: 76, 2002.

62 Eiberg, H., Shaumburg, H. L., von Gontard, A., and Rittig, S.: Linkage study of a large Danish 4-generation family with urge incontinence and nocturnal enuresis. *J Urol*, **166**: 2401, 2001.

CHAPTER 23

Evaluation of the enuretic child

Tryggve Nevéus

Pediatric Nephrology Unit, Department of Women's and Children's Health, Uppsala University, Uppsala University Children's Hospital, Uppsala, Sweden

The primary evaluation of children with enuresis is usually uncomplicated: a good case history and a bladder diary will be enough [1]. If a few warning signs are kept in mind, the health-care provider will find the few children who need extra evaluation. In this chapter, we will first list the relevant tools, after which guidelines for the suggested evaluation will be provided.

Tools

History

No amount of tests can substitute for a good case history. There are three crucial things we need to know: (i) are there signs of underlying conditions that call for extra evaluation, (ii) is there significant comorbidity, and (iii) are there clues to guide the choice of therapy? The focus of the history taking is outlined in Table 23.1.

When gathering these data, we have to remember to talk to the child. It is his or her problem, not the parents', and it is the child's collaboration that will be needed.

Physical examination

The physical status of enuretic children without warning signs in the case history is usually completely normal. If the child has had recurrent UTIs, or if there is a history of voiding difficulties such as weak stream, interrupted micturitions or the need to strain to void, signs of occult spinal dysraphism need to be looked for. These include exaggerated lower limb reflexes, a positive Babinski sign, asymmetrical buttocks or legs or tell-tale signs on the lumbar spine such as

Pediatric Incontinence: Evaluation and Clinical Management, First Edition. Edited by Israel Franco, Paul F. Austin, Stuart B. Bauer, Alexander von Gontard and Yves Homsy.
© 2015 John Wiley & Sons, Ltd. Published 2015 by John Wiley & Sons, Ltd.

Table 23.1 Case history at first appointment.

Field of interest	Topics/questions	Reasons for asking
Growth and development	Has psychomotor development been normal? Adequate growth? Previous urinary tract infections?	The psychomotor status of the child will influence therapy Motor problems means neurogenic bladder may have to be excluded Poor growth in renal tubular disorders UTIs often caused by bladder or bowel dysfunction
General health	Weight loss or nausea? Excessive thirst with a need to drink at night?	These symptoms, if present, mean that diabetes or renal tubular disorder need to be excluded
The enuresis	Primary or secondary enuresis? Wet every night or sporadically?	Underlying conditions or relevant comorbidity more common in secondary enuresis Long-term prognosis poor if wet every night, response to alarm therapy probably poor if enuresis is infrequent
Micturition habits and symptoms	Daytime incontinence and/or urgency? Voiding postponement? Weak stream, interrupted voidings, or need to strain to void?	Urgency and/or daytime incontinence indicates underlying detrusor overactivity Daytime symptoms need to be addressed before the enuresis The presence of weak stream, interrupted voidings, or the need to strain to void means that urodynamic investigations are needed
Bowel habits	Defecation every day or more seldom? Stool consistency? Fecal incontinence?	Constipation needs to be treated before antienuretic therapy and may solve the problem
Sleep	Is the child difficult to arouse from sleep? If awakened at night, does he/she become fully awake? Is there snoring or sleep apneas?	If the child is extremely difficult to awaken from sleep, alarm therapy may be difficult Heavy snoring or sleep apneas may cause enuresis
Psychosocial factors	Are there behavior issues at home or at school? Does the child view the enuresis as a big problem?	Neuropsychiatric comorbidity may need to be addressed The child needs to be motivated for therapy

dimples or tufts of hair. Palpation of the abdomen in many cases can readily pick up large amounts of stool in the left lower quadrant and at times extending into the left upper quadrant. These would be an indication of constipation. In some cases, a rectal examination will be valuable if there is any suspicion of constipation, but it cannot be confirmed with abdominal palpation, since the presence of stool in the rectum in a child who does not have a present urge to defecate indicates that the child is indeed constipated. The advisability of rectal examinations varies between different cultures and health-care traditions, but it can usually be done quickly and without much discomfort to the child, some teenagers excepted. General symptoms such as weight loss, fatigue, or nausea indicate that a full physical examination needs to be done.

Bladder diaries: Frequency volume charts

There are several reasons to have the child and family complete a bladder diary as a part of initial evaluation:

1 It will increase the child's awareness of his/her body functions.
2 It will objectivize history data.
3 It will give pathognomonic clues. Frequent micturitions with small voided volumes indicate detrusor overactivity. Nocturnal urine production greater than 130% of expected bladder capacity for age means nocturnal polyuria.
4 Contraindications to therapy may be detected. The child with habitual polydipsia should not be given desmopressin.
5 It gives prognostically valuable information. Nocturnal polyuria with normal daytime voided volumes indicates that desmopressin will probably work.
6 It detects family's low compliance. If the family cannot complete the bladder diary adequately, adherence to labor-intensive therapies will be low.

The ideal bladder diary will document wet and dry nights as well as daytime symptoms such as incontinence or urgency for at least one week and the following data for at least 48 h: the number and volume of daytime voidings, fluid intake, and nocturnal urine production (assessed by measuring the weight of diapers) [2]. Examples of bladder diaries can be found in Chapter 13.

Laboratory tests

Apart from a simple dipstick urine test, blood or urine sampling is usually not indicated. And even the value of the urine dipstick test can be questioned in children with primary monosymptomatic enuresis. The reason in performing this test is to exclude diabetes mellitus and UTI.

Of course, if glucosuria is present blood sugar needs to be measured without delay. Children with enuresis caused by diabetes mellitus usually have other symptoms as well (excessive thirst, weight loss, stomach pains), and their enuresis is of the secondary type. If enuresis is caused by UTI, there will usually be concurrent daytime symptoms, such as urgency, daytime incontinence and, above all, dysuria. Asymptomatic bacteriuria is probably more common than enuresis due to UTI [3]. Thus, a positive urine culture does not automatically mean that antibiotics should be given.

General symptoms such as unexplained weight loss, nausea, or excessive thirst with a need to drink at night indicate that renal function needs to be screened. The latter symptom may also warrant further evaluation of renal concentrating capacity.

Urodynamic investigations

No urodynamic investigations are normally needed in the initial investigation. Flowmetry, with assessment of residual urine, is indicated if anticholinergic medication is considered. These examinations are also indicated if the child experiences voiding difficulties as described earlier, as well as in boys with UTIs or girls with recurrent UTIs.

Invasive urodynamic investigations are only indicated if flowmetry shows consistent clear pathology or if neurogenic bladder is for other reasons suspected.

Radiology

If there are general symptoms suggesting renal failure or pathological polyuria, an ultrasonographical examination of the kidneys is warranted, and imaging is also indicated if there are recurrent UTIs or symptoms suggesting obstruction. But enuresis per se, even if it proves to be therapy resistant, constitutes no reason to evaluate the kidneys or the urinary tract radiologically.

The most valuable radiological examination of the enuretic child is probably the ultrasonographical evaluation of the horizontal rectal diameter behind the bladder. If this measure is greater than 30–35 mm, then constipation is very likely. Sometimes, the rectum may even be seen to compress the bladder [4].

Evaluation strategy

Primary evaluation

Any health-care professional with a basic understanding of enuresis pathogenesis and therapy can be the first one to assess the enuretic child, as long as he or she knows which warning signs to look out for. The two cornerstones of primary evaluation are history and a bladder diary [1].

The focus of the history taking is described in Table 23.1. If any of the warning signs listed in Table 23.2 is present, serious underlying disorders need to be excluded without delay.

If daytime incontinence is present, this needs to be addressed before the enuresis. If constipation is present, this needs to be addressed before the

Table 23.2 Warning signs that may indicate serious underlying conditions.

Warning sign	Possible background	Action
Secondary enuresis	Rarely diabetes mellitus, kidney disease, or UTI	Urine dipstick test
Excessive thirst with a need to drink at night	Diabetes or kidney disease	Urine dipstick test Creatinine
Nausea, weight loss, fatigue	Diabetes or kidney disease	Urine dipstick test Creatinine
Voiding difficulties	Neurogenic bladder? Anatomic or functional obstruction?	Uroflow and residual urine measurement. Consult pediatric urologist

bladder-related problems. Children with heavy snoring or sleep apneas may need to see an otorhinolaryngologist. If there are significant behavior issues, a screening questionnaire should be completed and psychiatric assistance may be considered.

Combined with the results of a bladder diary, the history usually gives enough information for the health-care provider to be able to start therapy. The choice of primary therapy—the enuresis alarm or desmopressin—will depend on history and bladder diary data, as well as family preferences.

Secondary evaluation

Children who have without success tried standard treatment need the services of a pediatrician or pediatric urologist. The history needs to be penetrated once again, a physical examination needs to be done and a bladder diary, including measurements of nocturnal urine production, needs to be completed.

In addition to the topics listed in Table 23.1, we need extra information regarding how the antienuretic therapy was used and why it did not work. Perhaps the parents were not properly instructed about how to use the enuresis alarm or were not able to follow the instructions? One common reason for failure is that the parents have not been told to help the child to wake up from sleep when the alarm sounds. Desmopressin therapy is easier to manage, but errors occur. The drug may, for instance, have been given immediately before going to bed, instead of the appropriate 30–60 min earlier.

We also recommend that the urodynamic function of these children be examined with uroflow and residual urine assessment, since anticholinergic medication will often be considered. Constipation is common in this group, so rectal examination (if feasible), and/or ultrasonographic measurement of rectal diameter, will often be indicated. Still, therapy-resistant enuresis as such is no reason for invasive examinations or even blood tests [5].

References

1 Nevéus T, Eggert P, Evans J, Macedo A, Rittig S, Tekgül S, et al. Evaluation and treatment of monosymptomatic enuresis—a standardisation document from the International Children's Continence Society (ICCS). *J Urol.* 2010;**183**:441–447.

2 Nevéus T, von Gontard A, Hoebeke P, Hjälmås K, Bauer S, Bower W, et al. The standardization of terminology of lower urinary tract function in children and adolescents: report from the standardisation committee of the International Children's Continence Society (ICCS). *J Urol.* 2006;**176**(1):314–324.

3 Hansson S, Martinell J, Stokland E, Jodal U. The natural history of bacteriuria in childhood. *Inf Dis Clin North Am.* 1997;**11**(3):499–512.

4 Joensson IM, Siggaard C, Rittig S, Hagstroem S, Djurhuus JC. Transabdominal ultrasound of rectum as a diagnostic tool in childhood constipation. *J Urol.* 2008;**179**(5):1997–2002.

5 Nevéus T. The evaluation and treatment of therapy-resistant enuresis: a review. *Ups J Med Sci.* 2006;**111**(1):61–72.

CHAPTER 24

Management of monosymptomatic nocturnal enuresis (enuresis)

Johan Vande Walle

Pediatric Nephrology, University Hospital, Ghent, Belgium

Introduction

Despite the high prevalence of enuresis [1], the professional training of doctors in the management of this condition is often insufficient and routinely not evidence based [2–4], additionally, in many instances these guidelines are inadequately followed [3–5]. Literature search results often end with disappointing outcomes, since characterization of the patients is often inappropriately done and/or described, thereby not allowing for proper differentiation between monosymptomatic nocturnal enuresis (MNE) and nonmonosymptomatic enuresis (NMNE) [5]. The majority of studies in MNE, selected in the different Cochrane meta-analyses were from an era when the new ICCS standardization of terminology was not yet accepted, resulting in high contamination of NMNE in the MNE study groups, making extrapolation of those observations to clinical practice with strict MNE definitions very difficult today [6–16]. This lack of hard evidence in the "true" MNE patients has forced us to follow a strategy that is practical, mainly experience based and pathophysiology driven [5].

The pathophysiology of enuresis is complex, involving both the central and peripheral nervous systems (several neurotransmitters and receptors), circadian rhythm (sleep vasoactive hormones), hemodynamic and kidney function, diuresis, and bladder (dys)function [3, 17–24]. A simplified screening process [1], as mentioned in the previous chapters, enables identification of two archetypes of enuresis: the first archetype is the underlying nocturnal polyuria classically associated with low overnight vasopressin levels [18, 19], decreased urinary osmolality, and high desmopressin response rate. The second archetype is the "small for age" bladder volume associated with OAB (overlaps with subtype of NMNE—patients with lower urinary tract symptoms), reduced desmopressin

Pediatric Incontinence: Evaluation and Clinical Management, First Edition. Edited by Israel Franco, Paul F. Austin, Stuart B. Bauer, Alexander von Gontard and Yves Homsy.

response, and higher rates of response to the enuresis alarm [5]. A combination of both forms is possible, and such patients generally respond well to combined therapy with desmopressin and an alarm [5]. In addition to these urinary/ bladder storage characteristics, all children with enuresis experience impaired arousal from sleep which prevents waking to void in the toilet [25, 26].

Who should start the treatment?

A variety of caregivers "claim" that they are the first-line of treatment for children with MNE. It is obvious that many subspecialities can play a role, as long as they identify (i) that MNE is a complex multidisciplinary disorder, where not a single treatment regimen will fit for every patient. (ii) The caregivers should be dedicated enough to spend enough time with the individual patient and his parents during the intake as well as the follow-up. (iii) They should properly differentiate NMNE from MNE and (iv) choose the optimal treatment regimen for the individual patient, titrated to the characteristics registered during the noninvasive screening. (v) The choice may be to some extent country and insurance dependent and might include GPs, nurse practitioners, urotherapists, pediatricians, pediatric nephrologists, and urologists.

In primary care, "trial and error" treatment for enuresis is often the rule rather than the exception, but is no longer defendable. This approach is a waste of time and money and increases frustration among families and doctors. It may also have an adverse psychological effect on the child [27]. We believe that the rational therapeutic approach outlined in the ICCS standardization document [4, 5] would lead to higher success rates and is the optimal way to proceed.

When to start the treatment?

In children aged greater than or equal to 5 years, enuresis is considered abnormal. Reasons for proactive management include the distress caused to child and family, difficulty with "sleeping over" on holiday or at friends' houses, social withdrawal, reduced self-esteem [27, 28], and potential disturbance of the child's and the parents' sleep architecture that may have an impact on daytime functioning and health [28–33]. Moreover, untreated enuresis (especially if severe) can persist indefinitely, with prevalence rates in adulthood of 2–3% [34–36]. Spontaneous resolution is low in children greater than 5 years with severe bedwetting, making a wait-and-see attitude no longer defendable. The impact on child and family cannot be neglected: risk for intolerance of some parents [25–27], the burden [37], and costs associated with frequent laundering of bedsheets and clothing [29, 38]. Children with severe enuresis are likely to benefit from appropriately timed treatment. Whether the 2–3% who continue to wet into early adulthood without early intervention would benefit from early intervention remains to be reported [36, 39–42].

Treatment

Step 1: Demystification

A keystone to the success of this process is an explanation on the pathophysiological mechanisms that are involved to the children and families. It should be explained that bedwetting is a common problem and that they should not be embarrassed. They should understand that this definitely not a primary psychological problem. Patients should understand that the primary cause is a mismatch between nocturnal diuresis volume and functional bladder volume overnight (the bottle and the glass). Patients with high arousability may overcome this problem, by developing nocturia. But nocturia, although frequent and increasing with age in adults, remains infrequent as a spontaneous cure method in enuresis. Nocturia tends to develop after a child has achieved continence, rarely does it serve as a mechanism for continence. Empathetic support should be provided if enuresis persists, and both parents and children should be warned that success rates of monotherapy vary from 30 to 60%, leaving one-third of the children with persistent enuresis after 1 year. This message is obligatory to prevent early frustration during therapy [3–5]. Recently practical guidelines were published: These recommendations have been reviewed and endorsed by committees representing the American Academy of Pediatrics, European Society for Paediatric Urology (ESPU), European Society for Paediatric Nephrology, and ICCS. This guideline is intended as a practical supplement to the recent ICCS standardization report [4].

It is imperative that we mention that two alternative strategies to determine the most appropriate course of treatment are available [5]. The first is a basic assessment covering only the essential components of diagnostic investigation, which can be carried out in one office visit. The second strategy includes several additional evaluations including completion of a voiding diary, which requires extra time during the initial consultation and two office visits before treatment or specialty referral is provided. This approach should yield greater success than first-line treatment of enuresis. This second strategy should be mentioned to parents who want to reduce the failure risk to the maximum (see Figure 24.1).

Step 2: Urotherapy

Urotherapy [35, 43, 44] has been extensively described in Chapter 13 and includes all nonspecific advices, including toilet habits, frequency, fluid intake, and nutrition advice. This is a well-accepted first-line therapy in children with enuresis, although it remains to be elucidated if it is of value as monotherapy in the subpopulation of true MNE patients. The effect of urotherapy has mainly been demonstrated in children with bladder dysfunction or those with NMNE.

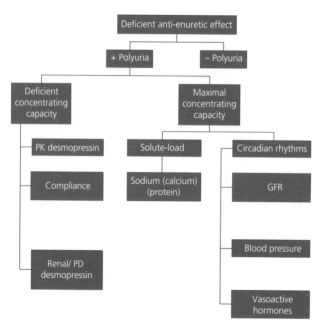

Figure 24.1 Therapeutic approach.

Fluid and nutritional intake

Fluid and nutritional intake, although often considered as a part of common urotherapy, might be of special interest in children with MNE. It is evident that changing lifestyle, nutritional and drinking habits might result in higher nocturnal diuresis volume overnight. Many children have their maximum fluid intake at home in the evening, at a moment that their vasopressin system is probably maximally stimulated, since they are virtually fluid deprived during school time. This has to result in higher diuresis rate in the early night. The main meal, including high sodium and protein load has shifted from noon to the evening meal, resulting in higher osmotic stimulus to vasopressin, but also increased solute excretion, and secondary NP overnight. This has been extensively demonstrated in children with desmopressin refractory polyuria. Experts advice that fluid and nutritional intake should be normalized through-out the day, with more fluid intake, spread along the whole day, avoiding caffeinated beverages and high water intake in the evening [3–5], although most of these recommendations are not supported by empirical evidence. This should be accompanied with healthy food intake in the evening, avoiding high protein and sodium load, and therefore osmotic diuresis [45, 46].

Sleep-related factors

Sleep-related factors are gaining increased interest since there appears to be an association between disrupted sleep, nocturnal polyuria, and enuresis, although they are often neglected in questionnaires on enuresis. Children should have good sleep practices, including set sleep times and duration. Hyperstimulation of the brain (light flashes, computer games, television, music) should be tempered before sleeping, since this has profound influence on melatonin circadian rhythm and sleep pattern. Children should not forget to void, and all lights should go out, once in bed light. Children should not drink during the night [47, 48].

Step 3: Medical management

If urotherapy and lifestyle advice are unsuccessful, medical treatment is mandatory: The alarm and/or desmopressin are the only two evidence-based medicine (EBM) IA recommendations. We strongly believe that the choice between the two options should be individualized, titrated to the patient's characteristics, which can be identified during the screening [5]. An increasing amount of evidence is supporting that the response to these treatments in MNE depends to a large extent on the underlying mechanism:

1 The alarm would be the treatment of choice in the archetype with low nocturnal urine production, high urinary osmolality, and small functional bladder volume and where desmopressin resistance is to be expected.

2 Whereas patients with large nocturnal urine production, low urinary osmolality, and normal functional bladder volume will likely not respond to the alarm, without developing nocturia.

In general, desmopressin and alarm treatments should not be regarded as competing modalities but as supplementary to each other and targeting different patient archetypes. If, however, initial evaluation of the underlying enuresis mechanism is not possible, or the clinical pattern is in between the two archetypes, other factors such as family motivation and preferences, availability of close follow-up, costs, and frequency of enuretic episodes should all be included in the decision process.

Enuresis alarms

Enuresis alarms have a level 1, grade A International Consultation on Incontinence (ICI) recommendation [3–5, 49]. Although different variations of alarm exist, the common factor is a sensor in the sheets or night clothes triggered when it becomes wet, setting off an auditory or vibration signal causing the child to wake, cease voiding, and arise to void. Parents are advised to wake their child when the alarm is activated—otherwise, children are prone to turn it off and go back to sleep. The alarm should be worn every night. Response is not immediate and treatment should be continued for 2–3 months or until the child is dry for 14 consecutive nights (whichever comes first). The aim is that the child is able to sleep through the night by suppressing the need to void during the sleep, and not to develop nocturia. Often compared to Pavlov training mechanisms, the true mechanism remains poorly understood. There may be cultural differences in its acceptability, as it may be highly disruptive for the household and may require a significant commitment of time and effort. The family must be motivated and adhere to this therapy if it is to be successful so they should be preemptively apprised of likely difficulties. They should be assured that the first few weeks are the most troublesome. Doctors should monitor the child's progress early to address any problems and facilitate adherence. The response rate is high in families who continue treatment for a sufficient period, with relatively low relapse rates (though lasting cure rate is still <50%) [9].

Poor compliance and early withdrawal from treatment are common [50, 51], which may exacerbate parental intolerance. Identifying the right motivated patient in the right family is essential in cases where the child or his or her family is reluctant to accept the alarm; desmopressin is the alternative [52]. Alarm therapy has high failure rates when the buzzer went off early in the night or two or more times a night [53].

Desmopressin therapy [15, 54–57]

Desmopressin is a synthetic analog of arginine vasopressin, the naturally occurring antidiuretic hormone. One of its major actions on the V2 receptor is to reduce the volume of urine produced overnight to within normal limits. Since the demonstration of nocturnal polyuria in patients with MNE and the lack of the normal rise in plasma AVP levels during night, the use of dDAVP became a logical choice [18, 19, 24]. Apart from its well-established effect on free water reabsorption, it has been suggested that dDAVP has additional effects in enuresis, that is, on detrusor muscle, central control of micturition, sleep or arousal function. The effect on sleep and arousal, however, has been contradicted both by other studies and by the fact that dDAVP does not seem to pass the blood–brain barrier. Recently, the effect of dDAVP on sodium excretion has been emphasized and it is possible that besides the marked effects on water reabsorption it has additional tubular effects [58].

Desmopressin has a level 1, grade A recommendation from the ICI in 2009 [49]. Several formulations are on market: a nasal solution, desmopressin nasal spray, desmopressin oral tablet, and the desmopressin oral lyophilisate (sublingual), all characterized by rather low biodisponibility, with large intraindividual variability (0.08–0.16% in adults), but only the last two formulations are labeled for the indication of enuresis in children. The low biodisponibility is largely related to the peptide structure, making oral /intestinal reabsorption very difficult, although pharmacodynamic (PD) effects remain very predictable [59], and, when used regularly, rarely is associated with serious adverse effects. It is available for the indication of enuresis as a tablet (dosage, 0.2–0.6 mg) or a fast-melting oral lyophilisate (dosage, 120–360 μg). The latter is a recommended formulation for all children and is preferred by children under 12 years [60–63]. It is not affected by nasal congestion or gastrointestinal transit and does not require fluid intake. Since tablets can require up to 200 ml of fluid intake, which is approximately 25% of a 7-year-old's bladder capacity, the fastmelting oral lyophilisate formulation is more suited to the antidiuretic indication of desmopressin. Good PD data are available for the Melt and its dosing in children with enuresis [60].

The efficacy of desmopressin in the treatment of enuresis is well documented. In a Cochrane Library analysis of 17 controlled trials, all showed superiority of desmopressin compared to placebo regardless of the route of administration [15]. An estimated 70% of the enuresis population has full or partial response to the drug [62] and the response to desmopressin is highly dependent on factors such as nocturnal urine production and bladder capacity. The few studies that have tried to compare different doses of the drug reveal comparable efficacies [64, 65]. Several key issues should be taken into consideration, when the drug is prescribed. 200 to 400 mg tablets are considered bioequivalent to 120–240 µg fastmelting oral lyophilisate and are the therapeutical range for children with MNE from 7 to 18 years. The recent documented size relationship suggests that higher doses might be needed in larger children [63]. Medication should be taken 1 h before the last void before bedtime to allow timely enhanced concentration of urine to occur. Fluid intake should be reduced from 1 h before desmopressin administration and for 8 h subsequently to encourage optimal concentrating capacity and treatment response, as well as to reduce the risk of hyponatremia/water intoxication [60, 62].

Desmopressin is only effective on the night of administration; therefore, it must be taken on a daily basis. Full adherence is required to avoid wet nights. Desmopressin acts immediately, but in our expert opinion, the initial duration of treatment should be for 2–6 weeks to ascertain its antienuretic effect [5]. If a sufficient degree of improvement is experienced, then treatment can be continued for an additional 3 months—where appropriate, country-specific regulations regarding treatment breaks should be followed. If patients are dry on treatment after this initial period, breaks are recommended to ascertain whether the problem has resolved and therapy is no longer necessary. If the child does not achieve complete dryness, or if wetting resumes once treatment is withdrawn, it should be continued/resumed. There is some evidence that structured withdrawal of medication may reduce relapse rates following its discontinuation [37, 66]. Desmopressin is well tolerated, but clinicians should be aware that it is a potent antidiuretic and families must be educated regarding the rare possibility of patients developing hyponatremia/water intoxication with symptoms including headache, nausea, and vomiting [55]. Self-titration of medication should be avoided.

Importance of adherence to the management plan, especially for a drug whose action covers only the night after intake, is critical. It is estimated that approximately 30% of nonresponders are not taking the medication correctly [67, 68]. Nonadherence to recommendations regarding timing of medication, voiding before bedtime, and limitation of evening fluids can increase treatment success [69]. Moreover, compliance is often overestimated, both by patients and MDs; therefore, it should be documented in a diary. Regular contacts between caregivers and the patient are necessary to keep up compliance. Patients who appear treatment-resistant should be advised of the importance of full adherence and asked if they have had any difficulty with complying with recommendations. We may also neglect, that in divorced families, information has to be given to both parents, so that the treatment is appropriately given on daily basis.

Desmopressin has higher success rates in children with large bladder and nocturnal polyuria [69]. The response rate in the initial studies was greater than 70% but has been decreasing in more recent studies to as low as 20–30%, since the prevalence of occult OAB patients with small bladder volume and low nocturnal diuresis volume was high in these populations [70].

There are several unanswered questions regarding desmopressin therapy. It is still unclear whether desmopressin treatment leads to better long-term outcome than the spontaneous cure rate. The long-term cure rate of 15–30% annually is higher than the spontaneous cure rate [71–73]. Long-term follow-up showed persistent LUTS in the patients with NMNE and not in the MNE patients [36]. The suggestion that tapering of the dose and the structured withdrawal program should be beneficial is still unproven [66, 74] but suggested in the opinion of the editor.

Tricyclic antidepressants

Tricyclic antidepressants have been the first drugs widely used in enuresis, but in a phase where NMNE and MNE patients were largely mixed up [75–80]. They act on adrenergic and serotonergic receptors in the central nervous system. Although the exact mechanism remains unclear, imipramine reduces both sodium and the overall osmolar excretion in the kidney, decreasing the nocturnal urine output in children with nocturnal polyuria. Imipramine also has the potential to modulate sleep and increase arousability. It has some anticholinergic like effect on the detrusor, and an alpha-mimetic activity on the bladder neck, mechanisms that are beyond the bladder can also increase arousability. Side effects are the major drawback of the treatment of enuresis with imipramine spanning from postural hypotension, mouth dryness, and constipation to considerable hepatotoxicity and cardiotoxicity in large doses [81]. The agent is currently not recommended in primary enuresis treatment. It is not longer defendable as first-line therapy prior to the alarm or desmopressin.

Antimuscarinic therapy

Antimuscarinic therapy (e.g., oxybutynin, tolterodine, propiverine, solifenacin) has not been proven to have a place as effective monotherapy for patients with MNE, although there is increasing interest [82, 83]. These drugs are widely prescribed in children with NMNE for the daytime symptoms and are accepted to have beneficial effect on the enuresis episodes [83], but prospective RCTs failed to document it. They might be indicated in the subgroup of patients with MNE (=without daytime symptoms), with small for age functional bladder volume (FBV), past history of LUTS, and appearance of daytime symptoms during fluid load, indicating a missed overactive bladder, or the subgroup with OAB only overnight [84]. They have been used with some success in children with small for age FBV but often as add-on therapy to DDAVP and urotherapy [85]. The level of evidence of monotherapy remains rather weak. Antimuscarinic therapy might be considered in the subgroup of patients with small FBV and no NP as rescue therapy (opinion).

Cognitive training and psychotherapy

Cognitive training and psychotherapy received a lot of interest in the decades where desmopressin was not available, and when medical doctors were less involved in the treatment. They still have a value as an adjuvant to conventional therapy, but they have lost their monopoly, more because they are so time-consuming than because of efficiency. Most of studies are performed in patient groups according to the DMS IV criteria, but unfortunately, these criteria do not differentiate between MNE and NME. Also many of the patients treated with psychotherapy have a higher incidence of psychopathology [5].

Alternative treatments

There are multiple claims for some effect of alternative treatments but there is little evidence: sometimes no better than placebo, less effective than desmopressin, almost always with poor subtyping of patients, and as such not reaching enough level of EBM. Hypnosis [86–88] *chiropractic [89–91] and reflexology have no evidence to support their use. There are some weak scientific indices of a benefit from traditional acupuncture [92, 93]. Variations such as manual acupressure, electroacupuncture, and laser acupuncture [94] have been tried, but evidence remains insufficient.* The effect of TENS neuromodulation on enuresis was promising but mainly in a NMNE population [95, 96].

Refractory MNE

The major reasons that patients with MNE are subsequently proven to be non-responders or partial responders are (i) that the initial intake was not performed appropriately and (ii) that patients according to the new ICCS standardization should be considered as NMNE. Therefore, it is essential to **redo** THE FULL SCREENING with history of daytime incontinence (DI), daytime symptoms after the age of 3.5 years, high/low frequency, postponing during normalized fluid intake are very suggestive for bladder dysfunction, as well as small enuresis volumes early in the night. Spontaneous low fluid intake is suggestive for a defense mechanism and may mask the OAB symptoms. These symptoms are often not mentioned by parents and deserve repeated questioning or documentation in a bladder diary during standardized fluid intake ($10.5\,ml/1.73\,m^2/day$) and can give additional information. Uroflow and bladder ultrasonography can give additional information in this phase.

But in the absence of any bladder dysfunction, one should concentrate on the desmopressin effect in differentiating different pathophysiologic characteristics that might be involved: (i) antienuretic effect (=number of wet nights), (ii) the antidiuretic effect (=nocturnal dieresis rate), and (iii) concentrating capacity (=urinary osmolality).

Partial response to desmopressin in MNE (antienuretic effect) is related to persistent nocturnal polyuria on the wet nights [97].

Poor compliance should be excluded [67], such as not taking the drug (consider letting the patient fill in a drug diary; register the number of prescriptions/compliance).

Other causes are as follows:

1 The child forgets to void before sleeping and starts already with a filled bladder.
2 Exclude drinking overnight, since fluid intake overnight or even the hour before desmopressin administration reduces both maximal and duration of antidiuretic effect and the concentrating capacity significantly.
3 Intermittent polyuria might as well be related to the pharmacokinetic (PK)/PD characteristics of desmopressin [60, 62, 63]:
   (a) The three formulations (tablet, melt, spray) have a poor biodisponibility, ranging, respectively, from 00.2 to 2% and to 4%, but with a rather large SD = intraindividual variability. Only for the melt, dose–response data and proper PD and PK data in children are available. The melt showed superior PK and PD profile, better compliance, and some indices of higher response rates. Prior to concluding that there is a desmopressin resistance, it is wise to switch to the melt.
   (b) Make sure that the child takes the drug just before bedtime (the time to reach maximum concentrating capacity and antidiuretic effect is 1–3 h, and therefore, the drug should be taken at least one hour before the last void before sleeping) [60].
   (c) Interference with absorption of the tablet (the tablet should be given on an empty stomach: at least 2 h after the last meal [61, 63] but 1 h before sleep. In some cases, this is not realistic in children and is a consideration that favors the melt above the tablet).
   (d) The melt study has demonstrated that, even in the therapeutic range of 120–240 µg, there are large standard deviations in maximal concentrating capacity and antidiuresis, as well as duration of action. Better understanding of this PK/PD dynamics can lead to more personalized medicine, with individualized dose schemes. The PK/PD data demonstrates that at least 25% of patients might benefit from higher doses. These patients can be identified by PD testing in an ambulatory setting (24 h concentration profile); this is especially beneficial in the older patients. Increasing the dose without this test is not defendable, because of the risk for toxicity.

Desmopressin refractory nocturnal polyuria with low urinary osmolality

In desmopressin refractory nocturnal polyuria with low urinary osmolality, we should exclude renal diabetes insipidus. The X-linked DI in boys does not present as enuresis patients solely. The female carriers might have a more fruste pattern with enuresis as major symptom. Many renal diseases (CKD, tubulopathies, renal dysplasia, uropathy) can present with enuresis. Hypertension, especially nighttime hypertension, coincides with nocturnal polyuria and should be considered in refractory patients. Although there might be some antidiuretic effect of desmopressin, these patients never reach maximum concentrating capacity. A desmopressin /vasopressin concentration test may be helpful if conventional diagnostic tools (ultrasound, lab) fail. We cannot deny that the majority of studies on desmopressin in children with MNE demonstrate that up to 25% of patients do not reach >850 mosmol/L after desmopressin. Although these patients do not fulfill the criteria of DI, there is an increased prevalence of patients at the lower end of the normal range of concentrating capacity in these children. A 20% decrease in concentrating capacity results in 20% increase in diuresis, which is the difference between continence and enuresis in many patients.

Desmopressin-resistant nocturnal polyuria with high urinary osmolality

Desmopressin-resistant nocturnal polyuria might be associated/correlated with high urinary osmolality overnight. This can be caused by an increased solute load only in the evening or during 24 h [45, 46]. Sodium is the major osmotic agent [46, 98–101]. Although nutritional intake plays a major role, abnormalities of several circadian rhythms such as **prostaglandins** [99, 100, 102], GFR [103], blood pressure [104], and sleep pattern [105, 106] have a significant impact in selected tertiary care patient populations. Extrapolation into the primary care enuresis patients remains premature. But these findings offer indices for future treatment options. Some pilot studies had promising results, such as sodium-restricted diet, diuretics (furosemide) [101], NSAIDs, treatment of sleep disturbances, and melatonin [107–110]. A lot of attention was placed on the role of a calcium-restricted diet that might be effective [111, 112], but the hypercalciuria might be a rather secondary phenomenon to differences in diet.

Therapy resistance to conventional therapy can not only be related to underlying bladder dysfunction and renal response to desmopressin but also to the **association of comorbidities** [5]. Identifying these and tacking them if possible might increase the response rate. Constipation and fecal incontinence should be treated before the treatment of MNE but are often underestimated and underreported. Psychological comorbidities, as well internalizing and externalizing disorders, are frequent in enuresis patients. Attention deficit disorders and autism are well studied and seem to have common pathways. A structured therapeutic approach is mandatory. Renal dysfunction, hypertension, diabetes mellitus, and sleep disturbances are already mentioned but should be treated appropriately. Many drugs interfere with circadian rhythm of several biorhythms these include diuretics, steroids, cyclosporine A, neurotropic drugs and might be a possible cause for failure to respond to treatment.

Conclusion

In children with MNE, two first-line treatment options are available—desmopressin and an enuresis alarm, as monotherapy. If we do not guide our choice to the characteristics of the patients, the success rate in monotherapy might not exceed 30%, with up to 50% relapse rate.

Their optimal strategy is to follow these simple guidelines:

The initial selection should be guided by the family's level of motivation and their preference. Based on the information from diaries:

1 Identify subtypes of MNE what should allow further fine-tuning of treatment according to the child's characteristics and family motivation.
2 Children with a normal urine output during the night and normal bladder capacity can be given either the alarm or desmopressin.
3 Children with smaller than expected bladder capacity for age will likely be desmopressin-resistant and more sensitive to the alarm.
4 Children with NP and normal bladder volume will be more sensitive to desmopressin.
5 Children with both excessive urine output and reduced bladder capacity may find combined therapy of alarm and desmopressin to be successful. (This strategy lessens the burden of alarm treatment as the alarm is triggered several times per night. But even then, up to 30% will be therapy resistant.)
6 Individualize therapy on pathophysiologic mechanisms, bladder, kidney; sleep and comorbidities, in a multidisciplinary setting.

References

1 Differences in characteristics of nocturnal enuresis between children and adolescents: a critical appraisal from a large epidemiological study. Yeung CK, Sreedhar B, Sihoe JD, Sit FK, Lau J. *BJU Int.* 2006 May;**97**(5):1069–73.
2 Evidence based management of nocturnal enuresis. Evans JH. *BMJ.* 2001;**323**(7322):1167–9.
3 Nocturnal enuresis: an international evidence based management strategy. Hjalmas K, Arnold T, Bower W, Caione P, Chiozza LM, von Gontard A, Han SW, Husman DA, Kawauchi A, LAckgren G, Lottmann H, Mark S, Rittig S, Robson L, Walle JV, Yeung CK. *J Urol.* 2004 Jun;**171**(6 Pt 2):2545–61.
4 Evaluation of and treatment for monosymptomatic enuresis: a standardization document from the International Children's Continence Society. T Neveus, P Eggert, J Evans, A Macedo, S Rittig, S Tekgül, J Vande Walle, CK Yeung and L Robson. *J Urol.* 2010;**183**:441–7.
5 Practical consensus guidelines for the management of enuresis. Vande Walle J, Rittig S, Bauer S, Eggert P, Marschall-Kehrel D, Tekgul S, American Academy of Pediatrics, European Society for Paediatric Urology, European Society for Paediatric Nephrology, International Children's Continence Society. *Eur J Pediatr.* 2012 Jun;**171**(6):971–83. doi: 10.1007/s00431-012-1687-7.
6 The standardization of terminology of lower urinary tract function in children and adolescents: report from the Standardisation Committee of the International Children's Continence Society (ICCS). Nevéus T, von Gontard A, Hoebeke P, et al. *J Urol.* 2006;**176**(1):314–24.
7 Treating nocturnal enuresis in children: review of evidence. Glazener CM, Evans JH, Peto RE. *J Wound Ostomy Continence Nurs.* 2004 Jul–Aug;**31**(4):223–34. Review.

8 Complementary and miscellaneous interventions for nocturnal enuresis in children. Glazener CM, Evans JH, Cheuk DK. *Cochrane Database Syst Rev.* 2005 Apr **18**;(2):CD005230. Review. Update in: Cochrane Database Syst Rev. 2011;(12):CD005230.

9 Alarm interventions for nocturnal enuresis in children. Glazener CM, Evans JH, Peto RE. *Cochrane Database Syst Rev.* 2005 Apr; **18**(2):CD002911. Review.

10 Simple behavioural and physical interventions for nocturnal enuresis in children. Glazener CM, Evans JH. *Cochrane Database Syst Rev.* 2004;(2):CD003637. Review. Update in: Cochrane Database Syst Rev. 2013;7:CD003637.

11 Complex behavioural and educational interventions for nocturnal enuresis in children. Glazener CM, Evans JH, Peto RE. *Cochrane Database Syst Rev.* 2004;(1):CD004668.

12 Drugs for nocturnal enuresis in children (other than desmopressin and tricyclics). Glazener CM, Evans JH, Peto RE. *Cochrane Database Syst Rev.* 2003;(4):CD002238. Review. Update in: Cochrane Database Syst Rev. 2012;12:CD002238.

13 Tricyclic and related drugs for nocturnal enuresis in children. Glazener CM, Evans JH, Peto RE. *Cochrane Database Syst Rev.* 2003;(3):CD002117. Review.

14 Alarm interventions for nocturnal enuresis in children. Glazener CM, Evans JH, Peto RE. *Cochrane Database Syst Rev.* 2003;(2):CD002911. Review. Update in: Cochrane Database Syst Rev. 2005;(2):CD002911.

15 Desmopressin for nocturnal enuresis in children. Glazener CM, Evans JH. *Cochrane Database Syst Rev.* 2002;(3):CD002112.

16 Simple behavioural and physical interventions for nocturnal enuresis in children. Glazener CM, Evans JH. *Cochrane Database Syst Rev.* 2002;(2):CD003637. Review.

17 The standardization of terminology of lower urinary tract function in children and adolescents: update report from the Standardization Committee of the International Children's Continence Society. Austin PF, Bauer SB, Bower W, Chase J, Franco I, Hoebeke P, Rittig S, Walle JV, von Gontard A, Wright A, Yang SS, Nevéus T. *J Urol.* 2014;191(6):1863–5.

18 Abnormal diurnal rhythm of plasma vasopressin and urinary output in patients with enuresis. Rittig S, Knudsen UB, Nørgaard JP, Pedersen EB, Djurhuus JC. *Am J Physiol.* 1989 Apr;**256**(4 Pt 2):F664–71.

19 The circadian defect in plasma vasopressin and urine output is related to desmopressin response and enuresis status in children with nocturnal enuresis. Rittig S, Schaumburg HL, Siggaard C, Schmidt F, Djurhuus JC. *J Urol.* 2008;**179**(6):2389–95.

20 Polyuric and non-polyuric bedwetting—pathogenic differences in nocturnal enuresis. Hunsballe JM, Hansen TK, Rittig S, Nørgaard JP, Pedersen EB, Djurhuus JC. *Scand J Urol Nephrol Suppl.* 1995;**173**:77–8.

21 Nocturnal enuresis: an approach to treatment based on pathogenesis. Nørgaard JP, Rittig S, Djurhuus JC. *J Pediatr.* 1989 Apr;**114**(4 Pt 2):705–10.

22 Adult enuresis. The role of vasopressin and atrial natriuretic peptide. Rittig S, Knudsen UB, Jønler M, Nørgaard JP, Pedersen EB, Djurhuus JC. *Scand J Urol Nephrol Suppl.* 1989;**125**: 79–86.

23 Enuresis—background and treatment. Nevéus T, Läckgren G, Tuvemo T, Hetta J, Hjälmås K, Stenberg A. *Scand J Urol Nephrol Suppl.* 2000;(206):1–44. Review: 2389–2395.

24 The circadian defect in plasma vasopressin and urine output is related to desmopressin response and enuresis status in children with nocturnal enuresis. Rittig S, Schaumburg HL, Siggaard C, Schmidt F, Djurhuus JC. *J Urol.* 2008 Jun;**179**(6):2389–95.

25 Sleep and arousal in adolescents and adults with nocturnal enuresis. Hunsballe JM, Rittig S, Djurhuus JC. *Scand J Urol Nephrol Suppl.* 1995;**173**:59–60.

26 Depth of sleep and sleep habits among enuretic and incontinent children. Neveus T, Hetta J, Cnattingius S, et al. *Acta Paediatr.* 1999;**88**(7):748–52.

27 Self-image and performance in children with nocturnal enuresis. Theunis M, Van Hoecke E, Paesbrugge S, Hoebeke P, Vande Walle J. *Eur Urol.* 2002;**41**(6):660–7.

28 Sleep deprivation: health consequences and societal impact. Carskadon MA. *Med Clin North Am*. 2004;**88**(3):767–76.

29 Quality of life and self-esteem for children with urinary urge incontinence and voiding postponement. Natale N, Kuhn S, Siemer S, Stöckle M, von Gontard A. *J Urol*. 2009 Aug;**182**(2):692–8. doi: 10.1016/j.juro.2009.04.033. Epub 2009 Jun 17.

30 Relationship of sleep quality and quality of life in children with monosymptomatic enuresis. Ertan P, Yilmaz O, Caglayan M, Sogut A, Aslan S, Yuksel H. *Child Care Health Dev*. 2009 Jul;**35**(4):469–74.

31 Secondary insomnia in the primary care setting: review of diagnosis, treatment, and management. Culpepper L. *Curr Med Res Opin*. 2006;**22**(7):1257–68.

32 Sleepers wake! The gendered nature of sleep disruption among mid-life women. Hislop J, Arber S. *Sociology*. 2003;**37**:695–711.

33 Cortical arousal in children with severe enuresis. Yeung CK, Diao M, Sreedhar B. *N Engl J Med*. 2008;**358**(22):2414–5.

34 Characteristics of primary nocturnal enuresis in adults: an epidemiological study. Yeung CK, Sihoe JD, Sit FK, Bower W, Sreedhar B, Lau J. *BJU Int*. 2004;**93**(3):341–5.

35 Differences in characteristics of nocturnal enuresis between children and adolescents: a critical appraisal from a large epidemiological study. Yeung CK, Sreedhar B, Sihoe JD, Sit FK, Lau J. *BJU Int*. 2006;**97**(5):1069–73.

36 Long-term followup of children with nocturnal enuresis: increased frequency of nocturia in adulthood. Goessaert A-S, Schoenaers B, Opdenakker O, Hoebeke P, Everaert K, Vande Walle J. *J Urol*. 2014;**191**:1866–71.

37 Problem behavior, parental stress and enuresis. De Bruyne E, Van Hoecke E, Van Gompel K, Verbeken S, Baeyens D, Hoebeke P, Vande Walle J. *J Urol*. 2009 Oct;**182**(4 Suppl): 2015–20.

38 Self-esteem in 6- to 16-year-olds with monosymptomatic nocturnal enuresis. Kanaheswari Y, Poulsaeman V, Chandran V. *J Paediatr Child Health*. 2012;**48**(10):E178–82.

39 Nocturnal enuresis: economic impacts and self-esteem preliminary research results. Pugner K, Holmes J. *Scand J Urol Nephrol Suppl*. 1997;**183**:65–9.

40 The burden of nocturnal enuresis. Schulpen TW. *Acta Paediatr*. 1997;**86**(9):981–4.

41 Self-esteem before and after treatment in children with nocturnal enuresis and urinary incontinence. Hagglof B, Andren O, Bergstrom E, Marklund L, Wendelius M. *Scand J Urol Nephrol Suppl*. 1997;**183**:79–82.

42 Behavioral and self-concept changes after six months of enuresis treatment: a randomized, controlled trial. Longstaffe S, Moffatt ME, Whalen JC. *Pediatrics*. 2000;**105**(4 Pt 2): 935–40.

43 The management of childhood urinary incontinence. Maternik M, Krzeminska K, Zurowska A. *Pediatr Nephrol*. 2015;**30**(1):41–50.

44 National Institute for Health and Clinical Excellence (2010). *Nocturnal enuresis: the management of bedwetting in children and young people*. NICE, London, UK.

45 Nocturnal polyuria is related to 24-hour diuresis and osmotic excretion in an enuresis population referred to a tertiary center. Vande Walle J, Vande Walle C, Van SP, et al. *J Urol*. 2007;**178**(6):2630–4.

46 Desmopressin resistant nocturnal polyuria secondary to increased nocturnal osmotic excretion. Dehoorne JL, Raes AM, Van LE, Hoebeke P, Vande Walle JG. *J Urol*. 2006;**176**(2):749–53.

47 Evaluation and management of primary nocturnal enuresis. Riley KE. *J Am Acad Nurse Pract*. 1997;**9**(1):33–9.

48 Evidence of partial anti-enuretic response related to poor pharmacodynamic effects of desmopressin nasal spray. De Guchtenaere A, Raes A, Vande Walle C, Hoebeke P, Van Laecke E, Donckerwolcke R, Vande Walle J. *J Urol*. 2009 Jan;**181**(1):302–9.

49 Diagnosis and management of urinary incontinence in childhood. Report from the 4th International Consultation on Incontinence. Tekgul S, Nijman R, Hoebeke P, Canning D, Bower W, von Gontard A (2009) Health Publication Ltd, Paris, France.

50 Childhood nocturnal enuresis: the prediction of premature withdrawal from behavioral conditioning. Wagner WG, Johnson JT. *J Abnorm Child Psychol*. 1988;**16**(6):687–92.

51 Sleep/arousal and enuresis subtypes. Wolfish NM. *J Urol*. 2001;**166**(6):2444–7.

52 Randomized comparison of long-term desmopressin and alarm treatment for bedwetting. Evans J, Malmsten B, Maddocks A, Popli HS, Lottmann H. *J Pediatr Urol*. 2011;**7**(1):21–9.

53 Enuresis alarm treatment as a second line to pharmacotherapy in children with monosymptomatic nocturnal enuresis. Woo SH, Park KH. *J Urol*. 2004;**171**(6 Pt 2):2615–7.

54 Desmopressin in the treatment of severe nocturnal enuresis in adolescents—a 7-year follow-up study. Läckgren G, Lilja B, Nevèus T, Stenberg A. *Br J Urol*. 1998;**81**(3):17–23.

55 Desmopressin 30 years in clinical use: a safety review. Vande Walle J, Stockner M, Raes A, Nørgaard JP. *Curr Drug Saf*. 2007 Sep;**2**(3):232–8. Review.

56 Long-term treatment of nocturnal enuresis with desmopressin. A follow-up study. Knudsen UB, Rittig S, Nørgaard JP, Lundemose JB, Pedersen EB, Djurhuus JC. *Urol Res*. 1991;**19**(4):237–40.

57 Clinical practice. Evaluation and management of enuresis. Robson WL. *N Engl J Med*. 2009 Apr;360(14):1429–36.

58 The effect of desmopressin on renal water and solute handling in desmopressin resistant monosymptomatic nocturnal enuresis. Kamperis K, Rittig S, Radvanska E, Jørgensen KA, Djurhuus JC. *J Urol*. 2008 Aug;**180**(2):707–13; discussion 713–4. 63.

59 Effect of food intake on the pharmacokinetics and antidiuretic activity of oral desmopressin (DDAVP) in hydrated normal subjects. Rittig S, Jensen AR, Jensen KT, Pedersen EB. *Clin Endocrinol (Oxf)*. 1998 Feb;48(2):235–41.

60 A new fast-melting oral formulation of desmopressin: a pharmacodynamic study in children with primary nocturnal enuresis. Vande Walle JG, Bogaert GA, Mattsson S, Schurmans T, Hoebeke P, Deboe V, Norgaard JP, Desmopressin Oral Lyophilisate PD/PK Study Group. *BJU Int*. 2006 Mar;**97**(3):603–9.

61 A randomised comparison of oral desmopressin lyophilisate (MELT) and tablet formulations in children and adolescents with primary nocturnal enuresis. Lottmann H, Froeling F, Alloussi S, El-Radhi AS, Rittig S, Riis A, Persson BE. *Int J Clin Pract*. 2007 Sep;**61**(9):1454–60. Epub 2007 Jul 26.

62 Oral lyophylizate formulation of desmopressin: superior pharmacodynamics compared to tablet due to low food interaction. De Guchtenaere A, Van Herzeele C, Raes A, Dehoorne J, Hoebeke P, Van Laecke E, Vande Walle J. *J Urol*. 2011 Jun;**185**(6):2308–13.

63 Pharmacokinetics of desmopressin administered as tablet and oral lyophilisate formulation in children with monosymptomatic nocturnal enuresis. De Bruyne P, De Guchtenaere A, Van Herzeele C, Raes A, Dehoorne J, Hoebeke P, Van Laecke E, Vande Walle J. *Eur J Pediatr*. 2014 Feb;**173**(2):223–8.

64 Efficacy, safety, and dosing of desmopressin for nocturnal enuresis in Europe Hjalmas, K, Bengtsson, B. *Clin Pediatr*. Spec No:19-24.

65 Enuresis treated with minirin (DDAVP). A controlled clinical study. Kjoller, SS, Hejl, M, Pedersen, PS *Ugeskr Laeger*. 1984;**146**:3281.

66 Examination of the structured withdrawal program to prevent relapse of nocturnal enuresis. Butler RJ, Holland P, Robinson J. *J Urol*. 2001;**166**(6):2463–6.

67 Poor compliance with primary nocturnal enuresis therapy may contribute to insufficient desmopressin response. Van Herzeele C, Alova I, Evans J, Eggert P, Lottmann H, Nørgaard JP, Vande Walle J. *J Urol*. 2009 Oct;**182**(4 Suppl):2045–9.

68 Adherence in children with nocturnal enuresis. Baeyens D, Lierman A, Roeyers H, Hoebeke P, Walle JV. *J Pediatr Urol*. 2009;**5**(2):105–9.

69 Predictors of response to desmopressin in children and adolescents with monosymptomatic nocturnal enuresis. Rushton HG, Belman AB, Skoog S, Zaontz MR, Sihelnik S. *Scand J Urol Nephrol Suppl.* 1995;**173**:109–10.

70 Long-term desmopressin response in primary nocturnal enuresis: open-label, multinational study. Lottmann H, Baydala L, Eggert P, Klein BM, Evans J, Norgaard JP. *Int J Clin Pract.* 2009 Jan;**63**(1):35–45.

71 Long-term double-blind crossover study of DDAVP intranasal spray in the management of nocturnal enuresis. Rittig S, Knudsen UB, Sorensen S, et al. In: SR Meadow, ed., *Desmopressin in nocturnal enuresis.* Horus Medical Publications, Sutton Coldfield, England, 1989, 43.

72 Desmopressin in the treatment of severe nocturnal enuresis in adolescents—a 7-year follow-up study. Lackgren G, Lilja B, Neveus T, et al. *Br J Urol.* 1998;**81**(Suppl 3):17–23.

73 Long-term treatment with desmopressin in children with primary monosymptomatic nocturnal enuresis: an open multicentre study. Hjalmas K, Hanson E, Hellstrom AL, Swedish Enuresis Trial (SWEET) Group, et al. *Br J Urol.* 1998;**82**:704.

74 Structured desmopressin withdrawal improves response and treatment outcome for monosymptomatic enuretic children. Marschall-Kehrel D, Harms TW. *J Urol.* 2009;**182** (4 Suppl):2022–6.

75 Acute effects of atypical antidepressants on various receptors in the rat brain. Hall H, Sallemark M, Wedel I. *Acta Pharmacol Toxicol.* 1984;**54**:379.

76 The action of imipramine on the bladder musculature. Labay P, Boyarsky S. *J Urol* 1973; **109**:385.

77 Single dose imipramine reduces nocturnal urine output in patients with nocturnal enuresis and nocturnal polyuria. Hunsballe JM, RittigS, Pedersen EB, et al. *J Urol* 1997;**158**:830.

78 Effects of imipramine on enuretic frequency and sleep stages. Kales A, Kales JD, Jacobson A, et al. *Pediatrics* 1977;**60**:431.

79 Nocturnal enuresis: comparison of the effect of imipramine and dietary restriction on bladder capacity. Esperanca M, Gerrard JW. *Can Med Assoc J.* 1969;**101**:65.

80 Increased urinary antidiuretic hormone excretion by imipramine. Puri VN. *Exp Clin Endocrinol* 1986;**88**:112.

81 Imipramine toxicity. Rohner TJ Jr., Sanford EJ. *J Urol* 1975;**114**:402–3.

82 Desmopressin and Oxybutynin in monosymptomatic nocturnal enuresis: a randomized, double-blind, placebo-controlled trial and an assessment of predictive factors. Montaldo P, Tafuro L, Rea M, Narciso V, Iossa AC, Del Gado R. *BJU Int.* 2012;**110**(8 pt B):E381–6.

83 Combination therapy with desmopressin and an anticholinergic medication for nonresponders to desmopressin for monosymptomatic nocturnal enuresis: a randomized, double-blind, placebo-controlled trial. Austin PF, Ferguson G, Yan Y, Campigotto MJ, Royer ME, Coplen DE. *Pediatrics* 2008;**122**:1027–32.

84 Reduction in nocturnal functional bladder capacity is a common factor in the pathogenesis of refractory nocturnal enuresis. Yeung CK, Sit FK, To LK, Chiu HN, Sihoe JD, Lee E, Wong C. *BJU Int.* 2002 Aug;**90**(3):302–7.

85 Long-term efficacy and predictive factors of full spectrum therapy for nocturnal enuresis. Van Kampen M, Bogaert G, Akinwuntan EA, Claessen L, Van Poppel H, De Weerdt W. *J Urol.* 2004 Jun;**171**(6 Pt 2):2599–602.

86 Hypnotherapy as a treatment for enuresis. Edwards SD, van der Spuy HI. *J Child Psychol Psychiatry.* 1985 Jan;**26**(1):161–70.

87 Secondary diurnal enuresis treated with hypnosis: a time-series design. Iglesias A, Iglesias A. *Int J Clin Exp Hypn.* 2008 Apr;**56**(2):229–40.

88 Treatment of primary nocturnal enuresis: a randomized clinical trial comparing hypnotherapy and alarm therapy. Seabrook JA, Gorodzinsky F, Freedman S. *Paediatr Child Health.* 2005 Dec;**10**(10):609–10.

89 Chiropractic care of children with nocturnal enuresis: a prospective outcome study. Leboeuf C, Brown P, Herman A, Leembruggen K, Walton D, Crisp TC. *J Manipulative Physiol Ther.* 1991 Feb;**14**(2):110–5.

90 Chiropractic management of primary nocturnal enuresis. Reed WR, Beavers S, Reddy SK, Kern G. *J Manipulative Physiol Ther.* 1994 Nov–Dec;**17**(9):596–600.

91 Chiropractic treatment for primary nocturnal enuresis: a case series of 33 consecutive patients. van Poecke AJ, Cunliffe C. *J Manipulative Physiol Ther.* 2009 Oct;**32**(8):675.

92 Complementary and miscellaneous interventions for nocturnal enuresis in children. Huang T, Shu X, Huang YS, Cheuk DK. *Cochrane Database Syst Rev.* 2011 Dec;(12):CD005230.

93 Acupuncture as a treatment for nocturnal enuresis. Bower WF, Diao M. *Auton Neurosci.* 2010 Oct;**157**(1–2):63–7.

94 Effect of laser acupuncture for monosymptomatic nocturnal enuresis on bladder reservoir function and nocturnal urine output. Radvanska E, Kamperis K, Kleif A, Kovács L, Rittig S. *J Urol.* 2011 May;**185**(5):1857–61.

95 Treatment of non-monosymptomatic nocturnal enuresis by transcutaneous parasacral electrical nerve stimulation. Lordêlo P, Benevides I, Kerner EG, Teles A, Lordêlo M, Barroso U Jr. *J Pediatr Urol.* 2010 Oct;**6**(5):486–9.

96 Nonpharmacological treatment of lower urinary tract dysfunction using biofeedback and transcutaneous electrical stimulation: a pilot study. Barroso U Jr, Lordêlo P, Lopes AA, Andrade J, Macedo A Jr, Ortiz V. *BJU Int.* 2006 Jul;**98**(1):166–71.

97 Partial response to intranasal desmopressin in children with monosymptomatic nocturnal enuresis is related to persistent nocturnal polyuria on wet nights. Raes A, Dehoorne J, Van Laecke E, Hoebeke P, Vande Walle C, Vansintjan P, Donckerwolcke R, Vande Walle J. *J Urol.* 2007 Sep;**178**(3 Pt 1):1048–51.

98 Abnormal circadian rhythm of diuresis or nocturnal polyuria in a subgroup of children with enuresis and hypercalciuria is related to increased sodium retention during daytime. Raes A, Dehoorne J, Hoebeke P, Van Laecke E, Donckerwolcke R, Vande Walle J. *J Urol.* 2006 Sep;**176**(3):1147–51.

99 Effect of indomethacin on desmopressin resistant nocturnal polyuria and nocturnal enuresis. Kamperis K, Rittig S, Bower WF, Djurhuus JC. *J Urol.* 2012 Nov;**188**(5):1915–22. doi: 10.1016/j.juro.2012.07.019. Epub 2012 Sep 19.

100 Nocturnal polyuria in monosymptomatic nocturnal enuresis refractory to desmopressin treatment. Kamperis K, Rittig S, Jørgensen KA, Djurhuus JC. *Am J Physiol Renal Physiol.* 2006 Dec;**291**(6):F1232–40. Epub 2006 Jun 27.

101 Desmopressin resistant nocturnal polyuria may benefit from furosemide therapy administered in the morning. De Guchtenaere A, Vande Walle C, Van Sintjan P, Donckerwolcke R, Raes A, Dehoorne J, Van Laecke E, Hoebeke P, Vande Walle J. *J Urol.* 2007 Dec;**178**(6):2635–9; discussion 2639.

102 The circadian rhythm of urine production, and urinary vasopressin and prostaglandin E2 excretion in healthy children. Kamperis K, Hansen MN, Hagstroem S, Hvistendahl G, Djurhuus JC, Rittig S. *J Urol.* 2004 Jun;**171**(6 Pt 2):2571–5.

103 Nocturnal polyuria is related to absent circadian rhythm of glomerular filtration rate. De Guchtenaere A, Vande Walle C, Van Sintjan P, Raes A, Donckerwolcke R, Van Laecke E, Hoebeke P, Vande Walle J. *J Urol.* 2007 Dec;**178**(6):2626–9.

104 Increased nocturnal blood pressure in enuretic children with polyuria. Kruse A, Mahler B, Rittig S, Djurhuus JC. *J Urol* 2009 Oct;**182**(4 Suppl):1954–60.

105 Abnormal sleep architecture and refractory nocturnal enuresis. Dhondt K, Raes A, Hoebeke P, Van Laecke E, Van Herzeele C, Vande Walle J. *J Urol.* 2009.

106 Sleep fragmentation and increased periodic limb movements are more common in children with nocturnal enuresis. Dhondt K, Baert E, Van Herzeele C, Raes A, Groen LA, Hoebeke P, Vande Walle J. *Acta Paediatr.* 2014 Jun;**103**(6):e268–72.

107 Melatonin treatment in children with therapy-resistant monosymptomatic nocturnal enuresis. Merks BT, Burger H, Willemsen J, van Gool JD, de Jong TP. *J Pediatr Urol.* 2012 Aug;**8**(4):416–20. doi: 10.1016/j.jpurol.2011.

108 Enuretic children with obstructive sleep apnea syndrome: should they see otolaryngology first?Kovacevic L, Jurewicz M, Dabaja A, Thomas R, Diaz M, Madgy DN, Lakshmanan Y. *J Pediatr Urol.* 2013 Apr;**9**(2):145–50.

109 Respiration during sleep in children with therapy-resistant enuresis. Nevéus T, Leissner L, Rudblad S, Bazargani F. *Acta Paediatr.* 2014 Mar;**103**(3):300–4.

110 Orthodontic widening of the palate may provide a cure for selected children with therapy-resistant enuresis. Nevéus T, Leissner L, Rudblad S, Bazargani F. *Acta Paediatr.* Accepted.

111 Enuresis subtypes based on nocturnal hypercalciuria: a multicenter study. Aceto G, Penza R, Coccioli MS, Palumbo F, Cresta L, Cimador M, Chiozza ML, Caione P. *J Urol.* 2003 Oct;**170**(4 Pt 2):1670–3.

112 Low-calcium diet in hypercalciuric enuretic children restores AQP2 excretion and improves clinical symptoms. Valenti G, Laera A, Gouraud S, Pace G, Aceto G, Penza R, Selvaggi FP, Svelto M. *Am J Physiol Renal Physiol.* 2002.

CHAPTER 25

Psychological aspects in evaluation and management of nocturnal enuresis (NE)

Dieter Baeyens[1] and Alexander von Gontard[2]

[1] *Psychology and Educational Sciences, Research Unit Parenting and Special Education, Leuven University, Leuven, Belgium*
[2] *Department of Child and Adolescent Psychiatry, Saarland University Hospital, Homburg, Germany*

Introduction

Epidemiological representative studies indicate that 20–30% of all children with enuresis show clinically relevant behavioral problems at rates 2–4 times higher than children without enuresis [1, 2]. As these psychological behavioral problems affect the (medical) evaluation and management of nocturnal enuresis, basic knowledge and screening of psychological issues in all settings with enuresis are necessary.

Different types of nocturnal enuresis and different types of psychological problems

Subtyping enuresis into primary versus secondary enuresis and monosymptomatic versus nonmonosymptomatic enuresis is not just important from a urological perspective (in terms of specific medical treatment and long-term prognosis) but also from a psychological point of view. The rates of comorbid psychiatric disorders are increased in samples characterized by secondary and nonmonosymptomatic subtypes and by older age, male gender, low socio-economic status, and admission to specialized clinics [3]. Children with primary nocturnal enuresis are not more deviant than controls in epidemiological studies [2]. In contrast, secondary nocturnal enuresis is associated with a higher rate of weighted life events and psychiatric and psychological problems [2]. Similarly, children with monosymptomatic nocturnal enuresis have fewer behavioral symptoms, especially fears and anxieties, than those with nonmonosymptomatic forms [4].

Pediatric Incontinence: Evaluation and Clinical Management, First Edition. Edited by Israel Franco, Paul F. Austin, Stuart B. Bauer, Alexander von Gontard and Yves Homsy.

Children with special needs

Psychological issues encompass both subclinical symptoms (e.g., reduced self-esteem) and comorbid psychiatric disorders (e.g., depression). Subclinical symptoms are common and understandable emotional and behavioral reactions toward bedwetting. Psychiatric disorders are the result of a detailed diagnostic process, based on the criteria of a standardized classification system (e.g., DSM-5 or ICD-10). It is important to note that both subclinical symptoms and psychiatric disorders have an impact on the course, treatment, and prognosis of enuresis and need to be dealt with adequately.

The general rate of clinically relevant psychiatric disorders in children and adolescents lies between 10 and 15%. However, the rate of comorbid disorders is significantly increased in children with enuresis [2]. We provide a short overview of three disorders frequently associated with nocturnal enuresis. Each of these disorders is characterized by high levels of comorbid psychiatric disorders itself, hereby further complicating diagnostics and treatment.

Attention deficit hyperactivity disorder

The most studied psychiatric disorder associated with enuresis in children is attention deficit hyperactivity disorder (ADHD). ADHD is characterized by pervasive and impairing symptoms of inattention, hyperactivity, and impulsivity [5] and has a worldwide-pooled prevalence of 5.29% in childhood [6]. The disorder typically emerges during preschool years and is associated with functional disability across the lifespan, with functional remission by young adulthood as low as 10% [7]. Although complex gene–environment interactions have been implicated, polygenic genetic factors contribute 70–80% to its etiology. At the phenotypical level, three subtypes emerge: the predominantly inattentive presentation, the predominantly hyperactive–impulsive presentation, and the combined presentation [6]. In a clinic setting, the comorbidity rate for ADHD and nocturnal enuresis was reported to be 28.3% versus 10.3% in the community [8]. At 2-year follow-up, ADHD continued to be present in 72.5% of the children [9]. More importantly, ADHD was associated with a more negative outcome for enuresis: enuretic children with ADHD continued to wet the bed much more often (65%) than enuretic children without ADHD (37%, OR 3.17).

Autism spectrum disorder

Criteria for DSM-5's autism spectrum disorder (ASD) changed considerably from DSM-IV's autistic disorder. ASD is a broader diagnostic category (e.g., it also includes the Asperger syndrome) and is represented by two dimensions: social communication and repetitive behaviors [5]. ASD is a severe, incapacitating lifelong disorder with a strong genetic predisposition. The prevalence of ASD is estimated at 1.16% and in half of the cases accompanied by intellectual disability [10]. Although systematic research on incontinence in children with ASD is scarce, increased rates of nocturnal enuresis have been reported: in a retrospective study, 18 out of 20 children with ASD had nocturnal enuresis (90%) [11]. Specific training programs for ASD are available [12], but the impact of ASD on the course of enuresis needs further investigation.

Intellectual disability

Intellectual disability is defined by an IQ of less than 70. It is a heterogeneous condition with many different genetic and neurobiological etiologies. Intellectual disability is a major risk factor for enuresis, BBD, LUTS, and comorbid psychological disorders. The higher the rates of enuresis and incontinence, the lower the IQ. Children with specific syndromes such as Fragile X and Rett syndromes are at special risk. IQ-adapted treatment programs have been developed [13].

Reliable and early screening of these comorbid psychiatric disorders is important as their presence may negatively affect the outcome of enuresis treatment and lead to lower adherence and motivation rates [14].

Psychological aspects in evaluation

When admitted for wetting problems, psychological symptoms should be screened in every child as part of a routine assessment. A stepwise procedure can be followed [15].

Step 1: History, observation, and exploration

Besides a detailed history on the wetting problem, special needs should be addressed: current as well as past symptoms of emotional and behavioral dysfunctioning should be explored in a clinical interview with the child and his/ her parents. Observation of the child's behavior and interaction can provide valuable information on relevant domains of functioning (e.g., social communication). Based on all available information at this stage, a more detailed psychological/psychiatric assessment may be indicated.

Step 2: Screening questionnaires

In order to screen the whole range of frequent emotional and behavioral symptoms in childhood, we advise strongly to use broadband screening questionnaires. Several of these parent-informant questionnaires with excellent psychometric values been translated into many languages (e.g., the Child Behavior Checklist [16] and the Strengths and Difficulties Questionnaire [17]). These broadband questionnaires are highly informative and give clear, comprehensive indications for subclinical problems as well as psychiatric disorders. Shorter screening instruments derived from the CBCL such as the SSIPPE questionnaire have been validated [18] (see Appendix). However, if one chooses a short screening questionnaire first, then problem items should be followed by a more detailed evaluation with the CBCL (or similar) questionnaire.

Step 3: Full psychiatric/psychological assessment

If broadband questionnaires show indications of the presence of emotional and behavioral problems, a full psychiatric/psychological assessment is necessary. This detailed assessment is best performed by a multidisciplinary team of trained professionals including a child psychiatrist, with the goal of determining whether a diagnosis is present or not (according to a standardized classification system). Also, profiles of psychological strengths and weaknesses of the child and his/her environment are derived from specific tests, diagnostic interviews, and questionnaires (e.g., IQ, parent–child interactions).

Information gathered in steps 1 to 3 will be taken into account when planning treatment goals and interventions.

Psychological aspects of treatment

Treatment of enuresis

The general management of nocturnal enuresis has been outlined in Chapter 26 and is to a great degree nonmedical and nonsurgical, that is, psychological. Psychological aspects play an important role in creating a therapeutic relationship with the child and the parents [2]. Counseling, provision of information, encouragement, and reduction of distress are important first steps in treatment. Observation, self-monitoring, and registration of wet and dry nights (i.e., "simple" cognitive behavioral techniques) alone can lead to dryness in a minority of children. Alarm treatment, the most effective therapy of enuresis, is a behavioral therapy, that is, an operant conditioning including positive and negative reinforcers. Other cognitive behavioral additions (such as arousal training) can enhance the effectiveness of alarm treatment [2].

Treatment of comorbid disorders

The NICE guidelines conclude that subclinical emotional and behavioral problems in children with enuresis can be dealt with in the context of counseling, provision of information, and urotherapy [19]. Once continence is attained, the subclinical problems will often resolve. The treatment of enuresis in children with comorbid psychiatric disorders is more complex, and often, these clinical problems will not resolve when continence is attained. As such, professional treatment of comorbid psychiatric disorders is necessary and requires multidisciplinary expertise and experience [19, 20]. Treatment should be evidence based and follow standard guidelines. The sequence is based on clinical judgment. In most cases, enuresis and comorbid disorders can be treated simultaneously. In mild disturbances, enuresis can be treated first. In severe disorders such as ADHD and ASD, these have to be treated first to ensure sufficient compliance.

Conclusions

Psychological problems are present in up to 30% of all children with enuresis. As these problems may negatively affect the course of and the adherence to enuresis treatment, careful attention to psychological issues in the evaluation and management of enuresis is recommended. Initial screening of psychological problems and subsequent counseling of mild cases can be performed at the setting (after training). In severe cases, full psychological and psychiatric assessment and treatment are necessary and require the expertise of a multidisciplinary team, including a child psychiatrist.

Appendix 25.A Short screening instrument for psychological problems in enuresis (SSIPPE)

From: Van Hoecke, Baeyens, Vanden Bossche, Hoebeke, Braet and Vande Walle [18].
* Parental questionnaire
* Validated, based on the Child Behavior Checklist (CBCL) [16]
* Seven items for emotional problems
* Three items for attention symptoms
* Three items for hyperactivity/impulsivity symptoms
* YES/NO format
* If more than two YES answers are given for any of the three problem areas (emotional, attention, hyperactivity/impulsivity), this should be followed by a more detailed questionnaire such as the CBCL. If the CBCL T-scores are in clinical range (or many problem items are answered with a "2"), then a detailed child psychiatric assessment should follow.

Short screening instrument for psychological problems in enuresis (SSIPPE)

Name	Date of birth		
Emotional problems			
If more than two positive items, full screening required			
1. Does your child **sometimes have** the feeling that others are reacting negatively?		YES	NO
2. Does your child **sometimes** feel worthless and less confident?		YES	NO
3. Does your child **sometimes** have headaches?		YES	NO
4. Does your child **sometimes** feel sick?		YES	NO

5. Does your child **sometimes** have abdominal pain?   YES   NO

6. Is your child **sometimes** little active or lacking energy?   YES   NO

7. Does your child **sometimes** feel unhappy, sad, or depressive?   YES   NO

Inattention symptoms
If more than two positive items, full screening required

1. Does your child **frequently** pay insufficient attention to details or make   YES   NO
   careless defaults in schoolwork?

2. Does your child **frequently** have difficulties with organizing tasks and   YES   NO
   activities?

3. Does your child **frequently** forget in daily practice?   YES   NO

Hyperactivity/impulsivity symptoms
If more than two positive items, full screening required

4. Does your child **frequently** talk continuously?   YES   NO

5. Is your child **frequently** busy?   YES   NO

6. Does your child **frequently** run or climb in situations in which this is
   inappropriate?   YES   NO

Strengths and difficulties questionnaire (SDQ)

The Strengths and Difficulties Questionnaire (SDQ) is a brief behavioral screening questionnaire about 3–16-year-olds. It exists in several versions to meet the needs of researchers, clinicians, and educationalists. Official translations are available in 77 languages.

All versions of the SDQ ask about 25 attributes, some positive and others negative. These 25 items are divided between five scales:

1. Emotional symptoms (5 items)		(1) to (4) added together to
2. Conduct problems (5 items)	}	generate a total difficulties score
3. Hyperactivity/inattention (5 items)		(based on 20 items)
4. Peer relationship problems (5 items)		
5. Prosocial behavior (5 items)		

The Strengths and Difficulties Questionnaires, whether in English or in translation, are copyrighted documents that may not be modified in any way. Paper versions may be downloaded and subsequently photocopied without charge by individuals or nonprofit organizations provided they are not making any charge to families.

The questionnaires, scoring instructions, norms, and related articles can be downloaded free of charge at the following website: www.sdqinfo.org.

Other questionnaires

Other behavioral questionnaires are copyrighted and have to be ordered. Basically, any broadband, validated questionnaire with available norms can be used. The following are two of the most well-known and established questionnaires.

Child behavior checklist

The family of Achenbach questionnaires covers the age groups from 1 1/2 years to 30 years—with self-informant, parent, and teacher versions. The parental Child Behavior Checklist (CBCL) is one of the most widely used questionnaires world-wide with translations in many different languages and with national norms.

All Achenbach questionnaires (such as the CBCL), manuals and related materials can be ordered under: www.aseba.org

Behavior assessment system for children: Second edition (BASC-2)

The BASC questionnaires are in wide use in the United States, but not available in many other countries. They encompass the age range from 2 years to college age and come in self-, parent-, and teacher-report versions.

BASC questionnaires can be ordered under www.pearsonclinical.com

References

1 Feehan M, McGee R, Stanton W et al.: A 6 year follow-up of childhood enuresis: prevalence in adolescence and consequences for mental health. *J Paediatr Child Health* 1990; **26**: 75.
2 von Gontard A, and Nevéus T: *Management of Disorders of Bladder and Bowel Control in Childhood.* London: MacKeith Press 2006.
3 Baeyens D, Roeyers H, Vande Walle J et al.: Behavioural problems and attention-deficit hyper-activity disorder in children with enuresis: a literature review. *Eur J Pediatr* 2005; **164**: 665.
4 Butler R, Heron J and the Alspac Study Team: Exploring the differences between mono- and polysymptomatic nocturnal enuresis. *Scand J Urol Nephrol* 2006; **40**: 313.
5 American Psychiatric Association: *Diagnostic and Statistical Manual of Mental Disorders (DSM-5),* 5th ed. Washington, DC: American Psychiatric Publishing 2013.
6 Biederman J, Mick E, and Faraone SV: Age-related decline of symptoms of Attention Deficit Hyperactivity Disorder: Impact of Remission Definition and Symptom Type. *Am J Psychiatry* 2000; **157**: 816.

7 Polanczyk G, de Lima M, Horta B et al.: The worldwide prevalence of ADHD: A systematic review and metaregression analysis. *Am J Psychiatry* 2007;**164**: 942.

8 Baeyens D, Roeyers H, D'Haese L et al.: The prevalence of ADHD in children with enuresis: comparison between a tertiary and non-tertiary care sample. *Acta Paediatr* 2006; **95**: 347.

9 Baeyens D, Roeyers H, Demeyere I et al.: Attention-deficit/hyperactivity disorder (ADHD) as a risk factor for persistent nocturnal enuresis in children: a two-year follow-up study. *Acta Paediatr* 2005; **94**: 1619.

10 Baird G, Simonoff E, Pickles A, et al.: Prevalence of disorders of the autism spectrum in a population of children in South Thames: The Special Needs and Autism Project (SNAP). *Lancet* 2006; **368**: 210.

11 Gor RA, Fuhrer J, and Schober JM: A retrospective observational study of enuresis, daytime voiding symptoms, and response to medical therapy in children with attention deficit hyperactivity disorder and autism spectrum disorder. *J Pediatr Urol* 2012; **8**: 314.

12 Kroeger KA, Sorensen-Burnworth R: Toilet training individuals with autism and other developmental disabilities: a critical review. *Res Autism Spectr Disord* 2009; **3**: 607.

13 von Gontard A: Urinary and faecal incontinence in children with special needs. *Nat Rev Urol* 2013;**10**: 667.

14 Crimmins CR, Rathburn SR, and Husmann DA: Management of urinary incontinence and nocturnal enuresis in attention-deficit hyperactivity disorder. *J Urol* 2003;**170**:1347.

15 von Gontard A, Baeyens D, Van Hoecke E, et al.: Psychological and psychiatric issues in urinary and fecal incontinence. *J Urol* 2009; **185**: 1432.

16 Achenbach TM: *Manual for the Child Behavior Checklist/4–18 and 1991 profile*. Burlington: University of Vermont 1991.

17 Goodman R: The strengths and difficulties questionnaire: A research note. *J Child Psychol Psychiatry* 1997; **38**: 581.

18 Van Hoecke E, Baeyens D, Vanden Bossche H et al.: Early detection of psychological problems in a population of children with enuresis: construction and validation of the short screening instrument for psychological problems in enuresis. *J Urol* 2007; **178**: 2611.

19 National Institute for Health and Care Excellence. Nocturnal enuresis: the management of bedwetting in children and young people: CG111. 2010. https://www.nice.org.uk/guidance/cg111 [accessed on June 25, 2015].

20 Caldwell PHY, Deshpande AV, and von Gontard A: Management of nocturnal enuresis. BMJ 2013; doi: 10.1136/bmj.f6259

SECTION 6

Neurogenic bladder and bowel dysfunction

Stuart B. Bauer

Introduction

The last quarter century has seen an unparalleled advance in our understanding and management of children with neuropathic bladder dysfunction. With these advances came the realization that many affected children who were managed with urinary diversion as a means of controlling their incontinence in the past, could easily be improved upon currently. The advent of comprehensive physiologic testing with reproducible and meaningful results that predicted upper urinary tract deterioration, and the development of effective surgical therapies and a plethora of medicines that increased clinicians' armamentarium to fine tune outcomes have resulted in substantial gains in the quality of life in these children. This section of *Pediatric Incontinence* deals with the nuances of practical management of the child with a neuropathic bladder, based in part on the ICCS standardization committees' reports. This compendium gives the reader an opportunity to learn the most current facts on how to approach and provide therapy for these children.

Dr. Tom de Jong will introduce the topic and provide a detailed guide for evaluating a child with a suspected or known neurologic abnormality affecting the lower urinary tract. His discussion focuses on timing as well as appropriate testing, both noninvasive (imaging—ultrasonography, DMSA scanning, and spinal MRI) and invasive investigations (formal urodynamic testing and cystography), to assess potential dysfunctional conditions. He provides a cogent argument for early intervention in children at risk and then outlines a stepwise approach to these children as they grow into adults.

Drs. Bauer and Austin first describe the physiology of the lower urinary tract and then provide an analysis of the drugs (including their doses and adverse

Pediatric Incontinence: Evaluation and Clinical Management, First Edition. Edited by Israel Franco,
Paul F. Austin, Stuart B. Bauer, Alexander von Gontard and Yves Homsy.
© 2015 John Wiley & Sons, Ltd. Published 2015 by John Wiley & Sons, Ltd.

effects) that have been developed over the last 25 years to modulate abnormal function.

An important aspect in the management of lower urinary tract dysfunction involves a discussion on the medical management of insuring regular bowel emptying. Constipation and fecal incontinence are often overlooked by those interested in only the neuropathic bladder. However, treating the gastrointestinal tract helps reduce adverse events of drugs that affect bladder and bowel function. One side benefit when concentrating on both organ systems is that control over bowel function improves one's sociability as much as, if not more than just controlling urinary incontinence. Thus, Dr. Cain discusses the use of proper diet, laxatives, invasive therapies (cone enemas), and surgical options such as the cecostomy button and Malone antegrade continence enema (MACE), so as to provide the reader with an algorithm for therapy. His extensive clinical experience with the MACE procedure and the types of irrigating solutions to achieve success with effective elimination and continence is evident throughout the chapter.

Although labor intensive, stimulation therapy does have a role in the overall management of lower urinary tract function in children with neuropathic bladder dysfunction. As Drs. Yerkes and Kaplan assert, their own neuromodulation program (intravesical electrical stimulation or IVES) is not for everyone but by limiting its use to children who have a good chance of benefitting from it, the extra effort needed to make bladder stimulation an effective choice, is greatly improved. Furthermore, transcutaneous electrical nerve stimulation (TENS), posterior tibial nerve stimulation (PTNS), and sacral neuromodulation (SNM) are other modalities that have been promulgated for achieving improved continence and enhanced emptying ability in these children. Given the right conditions of function, very reasonable results have been obtained. When medical management fails, strong consideration should be given to employing these therapies before advancing to involved surgical alternatives. One benefit in almost everyone undergoing neuromodulation is that bowel function often improves, whether or not bladder function is altered for the better.

Prior to making the irreversible commitment for bladder replacement therapy, one final approach to lower urinary tract dysfunction has been the relatively new modality of botulinum toxin injections into the lower urinary tract. The ability of this compound to block the neurotransmitter, acetylcholine, has lead to an effective, albeit short-lived, means of paralyzing the detrusor muscle, leading to improved compliance and elimination of overactive contractions. When injected into the external urethral sphincter muscle, it lowers outlet resistance resulting in improved emptying, when continence is not an important issue. Drs. Austin and Franco provide a comprehensive discussion of the physiology of this "drug," the mechanics of its employment and the effectiveness of its outcome.

The progression to surgical intervention is a natural outcome when medicines or other less invasive therapies have not achieved their intended results. Dr. Khoury is a world expert on the nuances of surgery for this group of patients. From his vast experience, he and Dr. Wehbi provide logical arguments for which surgical technique will yield the best outcomes based on the neurourological function of the lower urinary tract, taking into consideration all aspects of an individual's well-being. Despite their surgical prowess, these authors strongly recommend taking all steps necessary with lesser therapies before embarking on any bladder replacement techniques. They espouse the latest information regarding the long-term effects and practical views of these various procedures. To their credit, they know that bladder replacement therapy is not ideal, but when indicated, it can be very effective. Reading their chapter puts all this in proper perspective.

Dr. Terry Buchmiller, a senior pediatric surgeon was asked to contribute her views on further options for managing the bowel in children who have lower urinary tract conditions that may not be just neurologically induced, but nonetheless affect the lower gastrointestinal tract. Often, these children will have urinary issues, and focusing on bowel dysfunction invariably helps their bladder. Her views as a pediatric surgeon provide a refreshing approach to managing the bowel. It gives the reader further insights into how to modify bowel dysfunction and hence improve bladder behavior.

Lastly, one would be remiss if there was no discussion about the neurological causes for lower urinary tract dysfunction and how the neurosurgeon views and manages these problems in a practical manner. Drs. Park and Tuite have a keen and long-term perspective on how various spinal conditions affect the lower urinary and the lower gastrointestinal tracts, how to assess these children and when to propose surgery. We have come to the rationale that most of these conditions are not static from birth but rather have a dynamic aspect to their evolution. Being vigilant about the possibility of progression, many a child may be saved from further deterioration that cannot be recovered when surgery is delayed too long. They are realistic when discussing outcomes from neurosurgical intervention. Their wisdom on surveillance is invaluable. Although last in this section and last in the book, this chapter is as important as the first. Taking heed from what can be learned will reward every reader. More importantly, patients and their families will benefit from the advanced knowledge their doctors and nurse practitioners gain from this tome, in regard to their care.

CHAPTER 26

Diagnostic evaluation in children with neurogenic bladder

Tom P.V.M. de Jong, Aart J. Klijn, Pieter Dik and Rafal Chrzan
University Children's Hospitals UMC Utrecht and AMC Amsterdam, Utrecht, The Netherlands

Introduction

This chapter stems from the recent (2012) standardization report: International Children's Continence Society's Recommendations for Initial Diagnostic Evaluation and Follow-Up in Congenital Neuropathic Bladder and Bowel Dysfunction in Children [1].

An important factor in children with open, or closed or occult spinal dysraphism (OSD) is the knowledge that most children are born with a normal upper urinary tract. Immediately after birth, when bladder sphincter dyssynergia (DSD) is present, it starts acting to create a hostile bladder with a subsequent risk of recurrent urinary tract infection (UTI), high intravesical pressure, and eventual kidney damage. Although the underlying mechanism of why rectal sphincter malfunction affects the lower colon is poorly understood, it is important to begin proper management of lower gastrointestinal function immediately after birth as well. This knowledge underscores the need to start the evaluation and treatment of children with a known risk for a neurogenic bladder dysfunction shortly after birth.

The vast majority of children with neurogenic bladder dysfunction arise from the spina bifida group with myelomeningocele (MMC), even though the incidence of this condition is declining due to prenatal ultrasound diagnosis and early termination of affected pregnancies. The second important group is a closed OSD with a tethered spinal cord and/or (partial) sacral agenesis, and thirdly, in 40% of children with anorectal malformations. Remarkably, the exact mechanism of the neurogenic bladder in partial or complete sacral agenesis is not well understood—why do some children exhibit evidence of a lesion above the sacral cord while others have the more likely effects of a sacral cord lesion and a small

Pediatric Incontinence: Evaluation and Clinical Management, First Edition. Edited by Israel Franco, Paul F. Austin, Stuart B. Bauer, Alexander von Gontard and Yves Homsy.
© 2015 John Wiley & Sons, Ltd. Published 2015 by John Wiley & Sons, Ltd.

number having no neurologic deficit at all. This is irrespective of the level of the bony abnormality; in some children with sacral agenesis sacral roots appear to be absent, whereas in others the cauda equina emerges out of the opening in L5.

Diagnosis and treatment of patients with neurogenic bladder dysfunction currently are focused on proactive management in order (i) to maintain a low pressure reservoir of adequate volume, (ii) to prevent the later need for bladder surgery, and (iii) to preserve the function of the kidneys. This chapter focuses on the situation where treatment is started proactively by clean intermittent catheterization (CIC) and antimuscarinic agents shortly after birth [2]. Those small number of children who need urinary diversion, that is, vesicostomy, will be managed along a different pathway.

Diagnostic modalities

Physical examination of the newborn with spina bifida begins with assessment of anal sphincter tone, as this is an important indicator of whether or not the patient will be in the 50% group of children who will develop detrusor/sphincter dyssynergia, a hostile bladder and subsequently have an increased risk for the upper urinary tract damage. In children with suspicion for an occult spinal dysraphism (OSD), up till the age of 4 months, US of the lumbosacral spine can give information regarding the level of the conus medullaris and the presence or absence of an intraspinal lipoma. Four channel urodynamic studies (UDS) are the cornerstone for assessing function of the lower urinary tract, although in situations where UDS are not available simple measurement of the water column with the bladder filled to 75% of expected volume for age may give sufficient information about the safety of the bladder pressures. For suspected secondary tethering at a later age, physical examination of the lumbosacral muscle function by a dedicated physical therapist, neurologist, or rehabilitation specialist is of greater value than UDS due to the fact that subtle changes in bladder and sphincter function will most likely be masked by antimuscarinic treatment of detrusor overactivity. At the present time, MRI gives adequate information on the anatomy of tethering but does not provide functional information of the spinal cord. In the near future, DTI MRI may allow for data on the function of the spinal cord under traction by tethering [3].

Evaluation of the neonate suspected for neuropathic bladder dysfunction

Apart from a complete examination by a pediatric neurologist who can accurately assess lower extremity function, inspection of the anal sphincter with a pinprick test to denote both sensation and presence of the anal reflex arc is done. When the anus is patulous and no residual urine is found by catheterization and/or on ultrasound, the child will probably have a paralyzed or completely denervated sphincter and low bladder filling pressure. In this instance, one can proceed with a wait-and-see policy with periodic reassessment or begin CIC twice a day to prevent UTI as well as monitor for changes in pelvic floor function during the first few months after birth. If the parents notice increasing amounts of urine with CIC, this implies that the pelvic floor musculature may be changing from being paralyzed to becoming a reactive muscle with DSD, and as a result additional treatment should be initiated. In those conditions with a closed anal sphincter and residual urine exceeding 5–10 mL on repeated US or catheterization, antimuscarinic treatment and CIC five times daily are started without UDS during those first few months. Rarely, when one or both kidneys are dilated in the neonatal period (5% or less), a VCUG should be performed to demonstrate vesicoureteric reflux (VUR). When present, CIC and antimuscarinic agents are begun to maintain lower detrusor filling pressures in order to reduce the effects of high pressure reflux on the kidneys. If upper urinary tract dilation is present in the absence of VUR, the same objective of lowering the intravesical pressure is sought with the same treatments.

In neonates with a suspicion for a closed or occult spinal dysraphism (cutaneous anomaly in the lower midline spine area, absence of the gluteal crease with flattened buttocks), or if anal atresia is present, ultrasound of the myelum (spinal cord) is done within the first 4 months of life to determine the anatomy and level of the conus medullaris, and the presence of an intraspinal lipoma or other abnormality. When the US does not give adequate information, an MRI can be performed to define the intraspinal anatomy.

In children with MMC, UDS is often delayed until the age of 3 months for the following reasons: (i) sphincter function may change during this critical period of growth; (ii) surgical closure of the MMC defect may lead to a phase of spinal shock that can last up to several weeks; and (iii) if the child is already on CIC and antimuscarinics, two UDS may be necessary, one on medication and one after antimuscarinics have been discontinued for 3 days. UDS without medication will prove the presence or absence of DSD and detrusor overactivity, whereas UDS on medication gives information as to the safety and efficacy of the treatment initiated.

During the first year of life, surveillance is advised every 3 months with a renal and bladder ultrasound. When UDS does not reveal a hostile bladder, the first follow-up can be undertaken at 1 year.

Toddler and school age

After the age of 1 year, reevaluation is done every 6 months by ultrasound. UDS is generally performed once a year, combined with a voiding or nuclear cystogram especially when there is dilation of the upper urinary tract due to known

VUR. Yearly UDS is done till the age of 5 years. After age 5, a repeat UDS is dictated by changes in clinical parameters such as upper urinary tract dilation, a change in the volume of urine obtained by the parents on catheterization, and by changes in the level of dryness of the child between catheterizations. Routine yearly ultrasound of the urinary tract is warranted but yearly UDS are not needed when the clinical situation is stable.

Puberty and adolescence

In general, puberty is a particularly critical time because rapid changes in somatic growth may affect lower extremity and lower urinary tract innervation due to additional spinal cord tethering. During later adolescence, no specific changes are expected in the behavior of the urinary tract and lower extremities since further somatic growth is limited. Thus, strict surveillance during puberty is warranted. Another factor comes into play during puberty and beyond; it is well known that children at this age tend to be less compliant with CIC and medication, which bring added risk for kidney damage. It is not unreasonable to double the frequency of US imaging of the urinary tract to every 6 months between 12 and 16 years of age in an attempt to impress the importance of maintaining current treatment regimens to these individuals.

The wet child with paralytic sphincter

Children with a paralytic or completely denervated urethral sphincter and an open bladder neck often need surgery to become dry. Timing of this surgery depends on parental and patient desires as well as preferences of the treating team. It is preferable to offer surgery to achieve dryness by the time the child is ready to start school. Before embarking on an operation information regarding reservoir function of the bladder is needed. This can be obtained by UDS with occlusion of the bladder neck by a balloon catheter. Often, repeat cystometry is needed, one without medication and one after several days of adequate dosing of oxybutynin or another anti-muscarinic agent. This provides clues as to how the bladder will react once outlet resistance has been raised and as well as helping determine if additional surgical procedures are needed to maintain adequate storage pressures.

UDS: Specific pitfalls

UTI during UDS may generate detrusor overactivity or hypertonicity in a bladder that is behaving normally when the urine is sterile. Therefore, routine culturing of the urine is needed several days before any UDS is undertaken. When a UTI is suspected or diagnosed, UDS should to be postponed until after the infection has been treated and the bladder returns to its usual state. Unfortunately, the exact timing of this "delay" has never been fully evaluated so there are no specific guidelines available to promote at this time.

EMG recording by surface electrodes may sometimes be insufficient to prove the presence or absence of DSD. In those cases where it is important to determine or if there is a question that spinal cord tethering has taken place, sphincter EMG using concentric needle electrodes placed into the sphincter is advisable to provide precise evaluation for innervation of the muscle.

When the rectum is distended with stool, as it often is in MMC children, UDS may show a gradual rise in rectal pressure during filling of the bladder. This is a normal phenomenon but one should bear in mind that this rise in rectal pressure may have a negative influence on the subtracted end filling or detrusor pressure, thus suggesting inappropriately good bladder compliance. Therefore, it is advisable to have parents get the rectal vault empty with a suppository or cathartic the day or night before the scheduled UDS in order to minimize this effect. If that is not possible, careful observation of both the intravesical and detrusor pressures is required. Further technical details can be found in the literature [4, 5]. The last review paper on spina bifida, from 2012, provides a comprehensive overview of all aspects of this condition [6].

Ultrasound, DMSA scan, and spinal MRI

Modern ultrasound imaging is perfectly suitable to follow growth, dilation, and possible scarring of the kidneys, in addition to giving information about the bladder contents and its wall, and the state of rectal distension. During puberty and beyond, ultrasound may not be able to provide accurate assessment of kidney growth and/ or the development of possible scarring in patients with severe spine deformities due to the inability to clearly view both kidneys. For those individuals, DMSA scan or MR urography may be a better option for imaging. Lastly, spinal MRI can provide exquisite details of the anatomy of the spinal cord but does not provide any information regarding function of the nerves that supply the lower urinary and gastrointestinal tracts and lower extremities. Therefore, the spinal cord may look tethered on MRI but UDS will accurately reveal if there has been any neurologic change involving innervation of the bladder and urinary and rectal sphincter muscles.

References

1 Bauer, S. B., Austin, P. F., Rawashdeh, Y. F., et al.: International Children's Continence Society's recommendations for initial diagnostic evaluation and follow-up in congenital neuropathic bladder and bowel dysfunction in children. *Neurourol Urodyn*, **31**: 610, 2012.

2 Dik, P., Klijn, A. J., van Gool, J. D., et al.: Early start to therapy preserves kidney function in spina bifida patients. *Eur Urol*, **49**: 908, 2006.

3 van der Jagt, P. K., Dik, P., Froeling, M., et al.: Architectural configuration and microstructural properties of the sacral plexus: a diffusion tensor MRI and fiber tractography study. *Neuroimage*, **62**: 1792, 2012.

4 Drzewiecki, B. A. and Bauer, S. B.: Urodynamic testing in children: indications, technique, interpretation and significance. *J Urol*, **186**: 1190, 2011.

5 de Jong, T. P. and Klijn, A. J.: Urodynamic studies in pediatric urology. *Nat Rev Urol*, **6**: 585, 2009.

6 Frimberger, D., Cheng, E., and Kropp, B. P.: The current management of the neurogenic bladder in children with spina bifida. *Pediatr Clin North Am*, **59**: 757, 2012.

CHAPTER 27

Medical management of the neurogenic bladder

Paul F. Austin[1] and Stuart B. Bauer[2]

[1] *Division of Urologic Surgery, St. Louis Children's Hospital, Washington University in St. Louis, School of Medicine, St. Louis, MO, USA*

[2] *Department of Urology, Boston Children's Hospital, Harvard University, Boston, MA, USA*

The last quarter century has seen an explosion of medications that modulate detrusor function. This has given clinicians a huge armamentarium of drugs to choose from, with the aim of improving continence, the degree of hydronephrosis, and the presence of reflux that often afflicts children with neurogenic bladder dysfunction. We now have a greater understanding of the physiology of detrusor muscle contractility, the distribution of receptors that influence this contractility, and the neuronal control of the lower urinary tract and neuropeptides that stimulate muscle cells to function in normal and abnormal ways [1–3]. From this knowledge base, pharmaceutical companies have responded with the development of a plethora of medications to influence the detrusor, bladder neck, and proximal urethral areas; unfortunately, no oral medicines have been developed that can effectively change the skeletal muscle component of the external urethral sphincter, which paradoxically has the greatest long-term impact on the lower and upper urinary tract. This chapter will provide a synopsis of lower urinary tract physiology as we currently understand it and then proceed to describe the various drugs available to change bladder function, their effect, dosing, and potential adverse events (AE), based on their specific characteristics.

Lower Urinary Tract Physiology

The lower urinary tract receives and sends messages of its state of distension and need to evacuate via the parasympathetic (pelvic nerves that course to and from the S2–S4 levels of the spinal cord), sympathetic (hypogastric nerves that course to and from T-10 to L2 areas of the spinal cord) and somatic (pudendal nerve

Pediatric Incontinence: Evaluation and Clinical Management, First Edition. Edited by Israel Franco, Paul F. Austin, Stuart B. Bauer, Alexander von Gontard and Yves Homsy.
© 2015 John Wiley & Sons, Ltd. Published 2015 by John Wiley & Sons, Ltd.

from S2 to S4 that course to and from the striated muscle component of the external urethral sphincter) nervous systems. There is also integration between Onuf's nucleus in the sacral cord and the thoracolumbar region and the pontine mesencephalic center (PMC) in the brain stem. This PMC coordinates these lower central nervous system connections with the cerebral cortex through several pathways to balance the need to empty the bladder with environmental and social customs.

Nerve endings release neuropeptides, acetylcholine, and norepinephrine, from the parasympathetic and sympathetic postganglionic neurons, respectively, that influence receptors in the detrusor, bladder neck, and proximal urethral muscles. Acetylcholine binds to muscarinic receptors whereas norepinephrine binds to adrenergic receptors. Five different subtypes of muscarinic receptors have been discovered throughout the body, but only two (labeled M2 and M3) play a significant role in the lower urinary tract physiology. They are located throughout the fundus, base of the bladder, and proximal urethra. Adrenergic receptors have been described and are divided into α- and β-types with several subtypes, but their exact functions have yet to be fully elucidated. These receptors are also located throughout the lower urinary tract with β3 receptors distributed throughout the fundus, whereas α1A receptors concentrated in the bladder neck region and proximal urethra—the importance of this distribution will become apparent later in the discussion.

M2 receptors help relax detrusor muscle cells by inhibiting cyclic AMP. This prevents release of calcium through adenylate cyclase from the sarcoplasmic reticulum, which in turn prevents contraction of the smooth muscle. Similarly, activation of β-adrenergic receptors reduces detrusor muscle contractility by inhibiting cAMP. In contrast, M3 stimulation activates phospholipase release, which enhances release of calcium to cause these muscle cells to contract. α1A receptors when stimulated increase the release of adenyl triphosphate (ATP) that has a direct effect on smooth muscle contractility. The striated muscle component of the external sphincter contracts in response to release of acetylcholine from postganglionic neurons emanating from the pudendal nerve.

The normal bladder functions like a balloon, accommodating the increasing volume by maintaining low pressure due to parasympathetic and sympathetic activity through activation of M2 and β3 receptors, while stimulation of α1 receptors tightens the bladder neck muscle mechanism and proximal urethra. The pudendal nerve is actively and progressively stimulating the striated external sphincter muscle as the bladder fills to its capacity. This allows the bladder to expand at low pressure, and the bladder neck region and the external urethral sphincter to tighten in an effort to maintain continence. When voiding is about to take place, M3 receptors are stimulated via the pelvic nerves causing the detrusor muscle to contract, while sympathetic stimulation becomes quiescent allowing the bladder neck region and posterior urethra to open. Pudendal nerve stimulation ceases as well, thus relaxing the external urethral sphincter. The resultant effect is a strong contraction of the fundus of the detrusor, relaxation of the bladder neck mechanism and total relaxation of the striated external sphincter so the bladder empties completely in an unimpeded manner with physiologically normal pressures until it is fully empty.

In individuals with varying degrees of neurologic dysfunction and other conditions that might influence neural pathways, this coordinated innervation goes awry, leading to overactive contractions of the detrusor before capacity is reached, diminution of bladder neck stimulation leading to a reduction in resistance at the bladder neck/proximal urethra, and failure of the striated external sphincter to fully relax throughout the voiding phase.

These pathophysiologic changes lead to incontinence, elevated detrusor storage pressures, detrusor overactivity, emptying at nonphysiologic pressures, hydronephrosis, vesicoureteral reflux, incomplete emptying with residual urine, and urinary infection. The remainder of this chapter will focus on medicines that have been developed which attempt to return the lower urinary tract back to its normal physiologic state.

Medical management of the overactive bladder

Antimuscarinics

Antimuscarinic drugs are the first-line treatment for detrusor overactivity [4]. Use of antimuscarinics in children with an overactive bladder results in increased capacity, a greater volume to first detrusor contraction, and diminished number of incontinence episodes during the day and night (for non-monosymptomatic enuresis). Common AE include dry mouth, constipation, blurred vision, facial flushing, dizziness, and headache due to their affinity for other M receptors that are found in other organ systems throughout the body, that is, the salivary glands, GI tract, iris, peripheral vasculature system, heart, and brain. There have been some concerns about potential cognitive effects of antimuscarinics, but a prospective, randomized, double-blind trial showed no negative effect of anticholinergic medications on attention or memory [5]. Additionally, there does not appear to be any long-term behavioral impact from antimuscarinics usage in patients with spinal dysraphism [6].

The second oldest and now most commonly used antimuscarinic agent in children is *oxybutynin*. It is a tertiary amine that has primary affinity for M3 receptors in the bladder but also for M1 receptors in the brain; however, claims that it causes problems with cognition, memory, and behavioral issues have been refuted [5–7]. It may be delivered orally in liquid form and in short- and long-acting tablets, transcutaneously [8], or intravesically [9]. Oral preparations include syrup, tablets, and extended-release tablets. Oral dosing is usually done at 0.2 mg/kg/dose for the liquid and short-acting tablet forms, usually administered twice but can be given as much as three times daily, as its $T \frac{1}{2}$ is only 2 h.

The liquid formulation is very convenient for titration based on the child's weight. All three have been shown to be safe and effective in children [10]. In one study evaluating the short-term oral preparation effectiveness in 81 children with symptoms of OAB, 38% became dry but 42% reported varying degrees of side effects [11]. In another study assessing the extended-release preparation in 27 children treated for 20 months, 44% became dry with another 11% having improvement, but again, almost 50% had side effects [12].

Alternative routes of delivery of oxybutynin have the benefit of avoiding the first-pass metabolism through the hepatic portal system. The metabolite desethyloxybutynin is responsible for many of the attributed side effects through its affinity for other muscarinic receptors and is avoided with transdermal and intravesical modes of delivery. Transdermal dosing ranges from 1.3, 2.9, or 3.9 mg patches administered twice a week [8]. The transdermal route has been shown to be a well tolerated and an effective alternative to the oral route in children with neurogenic detrusor overactivity. Skin irritation has been noted in some patients [8]. A recent systematic review noted a low level of evidence for the intravesical use of oxybutynin in children with neurogenic dysfunction requiring intermittent catheterization to empty. It did increase maximum bladder capacity and decrease bladder pressure with fewer side effects than oral dosing; however, 9% of children discontinued its use due to side effects and 22% because other issues arose that made it inconvenient to administer, such as crushing pills to prepare the solution [9, 13].

Tolterodine was the next antimuscarinic agent to be developed for use in adults and children. It too is a tertiary amine that selectively inhibits nonvoiding bladder activity, as well as the amplitude of voiding contractions due to its affinity for M3 receptors [14]. It is well tolerated in children with minimal treatment-related AE such as dry mouth, constipation, and central nervous system side effects as it does not cross the blood–brain barrier. Its $T\frac{1}{2}$ is 4 h so dosing is twice daily, 1–2 mg/dose for the short-acting form and once per day for the extended-release preparation. It increases functional bladder capacity in children less than 10 years of age with a decrease in the mean number of incontinence episodes with long-term (1 year) use [15]. When the dysfunctional voiding symptom score (DVSS) was used to quantify its efficacy, there was a statistically significant decrease in the score with fewer side effects (mostly dry mouth, 31%, and headache, 4%) than oxybutynin [16].

Trospium HCl is a quaternary amine with quite selective affinity for M3 receptors. Although it crosses the blood–brain barrier, it has a low affinity for M1 receptors so CNS effects are very limited. It has a long $T\frac{1}{2}$ of 20 h, resulting in once-a-day dosing, but it can be given twice daily in doses from 10 up to 20 mg to improve its effectiveness. In one placebo-controlled study of 50 children with OAB, the response was excellent in 32% and markedly improved in another 42%; urodynamic parameters in these children pre- and post-drug trial were better, with detrusor overactivity curtailed, volume at first contraction increased, and maximum pressure at capacity diminished, with just 8% showing some increase in residual urine and only 8% experiencing any AE [17].

Fesoterodine is another oral antimuscarinic that is closely related to tolterodine as both agents are metabolized into the same active metabolite, 5-hydroxy-methyltolterodine (5-HMT) [18]. Fesoterodine, however, has less pharmacokinetic variability because the formation of 5-HMT is not dependent on the cytochrome oxidase enzymes (CYP2D6) as it is with tolterodine. Instead, the formation of 5-HMT from fesoterodine is independent of CYP2D6 and occurs via ubiquitous esterases. In a randomized, crossover, open-label, multiple-dose study in CYP2D6 extensive metabolizers and poor metabolizers, there is less variability in the pharmacokinetics with fesoterodine than tolterodine [19]. In a multicenter, randomized, double-blind, placebo- and active-controlled trial with tolterodine extended release, the efficacy of fesoterodine was more pronounced compared with tolterodine [20]. Fesoterodine has been shown to be safe and tolerable in children with daily doses of 4 and 8 mg [21].

Solifenacin is a once-daily antimuscarinic that has been shown to increase urodynamic bladder capacity, decrease overactive contractions, and improve continence with acceptable tolerability and safety in an open-label study of children with neurogenic and nonneurogenic detrusor overactivity in those who were recalcitrant to oxybutynin or tolterodine therapy [22]. In this study, urodynamic findings were impressively improved with almost a doubling of capacity, two-thirds reduction in the height of the detrusor contractions, and a 90% reduction in incontinence episodes per week. Overall, 92% had either 100 or 90% improvement in dryness. Conversely, 21% had mild and 4% had moderate side effects, whereas 5% withdrew due to intolerable AE. In a long-term extension of this study, high subjective and objective success rates were maintained and the tolerability and safety profile with solifenacin was also deemed acceptable with long-term usage [23].

Currently there is a randomized controlled study evaluating the effectiveness and safety of solifenacin in children of varying ages from 5 to 15 years with overactive bladder symptoms or neurogenic dysfunction.

Propiverine hydrochloride is an alternative antimuscarinic agent that diminishes bladder muscle contractions through the inhibition of calcium influx and modulation of intracellular calcium. Additionally, propiverine binds to M3 receptors to produce a direct effect on the smooth muscle [24]. Even though it binds to M1 receptors, it does not cross the blood–brain barrier, resulting in few CNS and cardiac side effects, but its most troubling effect is dry mouth due to the M1 receptor affinity and concentration of M1 receptors in the parotid gland. In children, its recommended dose is 0.8 mg/kg/day, generally given twice a day, as its $T\frac{1}{2}$ is 8 h. Both urodynamic parameters and continence are improved with short- and long-term use [25, 26]. In a comparison study of propiverine to oxybutynin in 621 children with OAB, the efficacy on the number of voids per day, incontinence episodes/week, and overall continence was similar in both cohorts, but patients taking propiverine had a fourth less AE [27].

β3 Receptors

Recent advances in our understanding about the physiology of bladder and urethral function yield evidence for three β-adrenergic receptors, labeled β1, β2, and β3. β3 receptors are thought to be the main bladder subtype, accounting for 97% of the β receptors and when stimulated elicit relaxation of the detrusor muscle by activating adenylate cyclase causing increases in the intracellular levels of cyclic AMP and calcium. *Mirabegron* is the first β3 agonist developed and entered into clinical practice. Currently, it is approved for adult use in OAB in several countries, including the United States at a dose of 25 mg/day. Its $T\frac{1}{2}$ is approximately 40 h, so it is a once-a-day drug. It has a very high affinity for β3 with minimal activity for β1 and β2 receptors. It is rapidly absorbed in an unchanged state from the GI tract, metabolized by the liver by cytochrome P450 (CYP) 3A4 with 55% recovery in the urine and 34% in the feces. Due to its cytochrome pharmacokinetics, caution must be taken for it might interact with other drugs metabolized by these enzymes. In addition, one must carefully consider its use in patients with renal insufficiency due to its urinary excretion.

There have been numerous randomized placebo-controlled studies evaluating its efficacy; none have been reported in children less than 18 years of age. In placebo-controlled trials, mirabegron significantly increases voided volumes and reduces incontinence episodes, urgency incontinence, nocturia, and the mean number of micturitions/24 h in patients with OAB. This was true even when adult patients failed prior antimuscarinic agents, and when compared in different arms in randomized controlled studies [28]. Although few cystometric studies have been done to date, mirabegron appears to lower or even abolish overactive bladder contractions without affecting the ability to empty during voluntary voiding.

The side effects associated with mirabegron are few. Cardiac side effects are a concern because $\beta3$ receptors are also found in the heart. No significant EKG changes and only a slight increase (from baseline) in heart rate, that was dose dependent, have been reported in bladder efficacy trials [28, 29]. Maximum blood pressures increases of 4 mmHg (systolic) were noted, but no patients have been cited with a substantial cardiovascular AE. Other reported effects noted by patients included dry mouth, constipation, and headache, but the incidence of these effects is less than 3% and much lower than that reported when mirabegron was compared to other antimuscarinic medications. Residual urine was not statistically increased nor was urinary retention reported in anyone, even in adult males with symptoms of bladder outlet obstruction. The drug is well tolerated with very low rates of AE (2–5%) or discontinuation (4–5%). Thus, it appears to be safe in adults but no studies yet exist for children [29, 30].

α-Adrenergic antagonists (α-blockers)

The rationale of utilizing α-blocker therapy in the neurogenic bladder population was established over 40 years ago when Krane and Olsson demonstrated that bladder emptying can be significantly improved in neurogenic bladders treated with the nonselective α-blocker phenoxybenzamine [31]. Further reports of nonselective α-blockers in neurogenic bladders with myelodysplasia noted improved emptying, decreased post-void residuals, lowered urethral profile pressures, and lowered detrusor pressures [32–36]. Resolution of upper tract changes was also noted in some of these reports with improved vesicoureteral reflux and hydronephrosis. The utilization of nonselective α-blockers is however limited in clinical practice because they antagonize both the α-1 and α-2 adrenergic receptors, which can produce a profound hypotensive effect.

The reemergence of α-blockers in the clinical management of pediatric neurogenic bladders developed with the advent of "selective" α-blockers that target the preponderance of the α-1 adrenergic receptors at the bladder outlet and along the proximal urethra. The clinical treatment of pediatric neurogenic bladder with selective α-blockers has been reported using doxazosin [37], alfuzosin [38], and tamsulosin [39]. These reports focus on lowering the detrusor leak point pressures and improvement of detrusor muscle compliance. In an uncontrolled, selected group of 17 children with neurogenic bladder, treatment with alfuzosin resulted in a significant decrease in the detrusor leak point pressure and an increase in the detrusor wall compliance values [38]. In contrast, no efficacy was seen using tamsulosin in a double-blind, randomized, placebo-controlled trial in children with neurogenic bladders and detrusor leak point pressure of $40\,cm\,H_2O$ or greater [39]. Given the limitations and the paucity of overall data in the literature, α-blockers are considered investigational in the pediatric neurogenic population.

References

1 Franco I. Overactive bladder in children. Part 1: Pathophysiology. *The Journal of Urology*. 2007;**178**:761–8.

2 Kitta T, Chancellor MB, de Groat WC, Kuno S, Nonomura K, Yoshimura N. Roles of adenosine A1 and A2A receptors in the control of micturition in rats. *Neurourology and Urodynamics*. 2014;**33**:1259–65.

3 Elbadawi A, Schenk EA. A new theory of the innervation of bladder musculature. 4 Innervation of the vesicourethral junction and external urethral sphincter. *The Journal of Urology*. 1974;**111**:613–5.

4 Hood B, Andersson KE. Common theme for drugs effective in overactive bladder treatment: inhibition of afferent signaling from the bladder. *International Journal of Urology*. 2013;**20**(1):21–7.

5 Giramonti KM, Kogan BA, Halpern LF. The effects of anticholinergic drugs on attention span and short-term memory skills in children. *Neurourology and Urodynamics*. 2008;**27**(4): 315–8.

6 Veenboer PW, Huisman J, Chrzan RJ, Kuijper CF, Dik P, de Kort LM, et al. Behavioral effects of long-term antimuscarinic use in patients with spinal dysraphism: a case control study. *The Journal of Urology*. 2013;**190**(6):2228–32.

7 Sommer BR, O'Hara R, Askari N, Kraemer HC, Kennedy WA, 2nd. The effect of oxybutynin treatment on cognition in children with diurnal incontinence. *The Journal of Urology*. 2005;**173**(6):2125–7.

8 Cartwright PC, Coplen DE, Kogan BA, Volinn W, Finan E, Hoel G. Efficacy and safety of transdermal and oral oxybutynin in children with neurogenic detrusor overactivity. *The Journal of Urology*. 2009;**182**(4):1548–54.

9 Guerra LA, Moher D, Sampson M, Barrowman N, Pike J, Leonard M. Intravesical oxybutynin for children with poorly compliant neurogenic bladder: a systematic review. *The Journal of Urology*. 2008;**180**(3):1091–7.

10 Franco I, Horowitz M, Grady R, Adams RC, de Jong TP, Lindert K, et al. Efficacy and safety of oxybutynin in children with detrusor hyperreflexia secondary to neurogenic bladder dysfunction. *The Journal of Urology*. 2005;**173**(1):221–5.

11 Van Arendonk KJ, Austin JC, Boyt MA, Cooper CS. Frequency of wetting is predictive of response to anticholinergic treatment in children with overactive bladder. *Urology*. 2006;**67**(5):1049–53; discussion 53–4.

12 Van Arendonk KJ, Knudson MJ, Austin JC, Cooper CS. Improved efficacy of extended release oxybutynin in children with persistent daytime urinary incontinence converted from regular oxybutynin. *Urology*. 2006;**68**(4):862–5.

13 Wan J, Rickman C. The durability of intravesical oxybutynin solutions over time. *The Journal of Urology*. 2007;**178**(4 Pt 2):1768–70.

14 Gillespie JI, Palea S, Guilloteau V, Guerard M, Lluel P, Korstanje C. Modulation of non-voiding activity by the muscarinergic antagonist tolterodine and the beta(3)-adrenoceptor agonist mirabegron in conscious rats with partial outflow obstruction. *BJU International*. 2012;**110**(2 Pt 2):E132–42.

15 Reddy PP, Borgstein NG, Nijman RJ, Ellsworth PI. Long-term efficacy and safety of tolterodine in children with neurogenic detrusor overactivity. *Journal of Pediatric Urology*. 2008;**4**(6):428–33.

16 Ayan S, Kaya K, Topsakal K, Kilicarslan H, Gokce G, Gultekin Y. Efficacy of tolterodine as a first-line treatment for non-neurogenic voiding dysfunction in children. *BJU International*. 2005;**96**(3):411–4.

17 Lopez Pereira P, Miguelez C, Caffarati J, Estornell F, Anguera A. Trospium chloride for the treatment of detrusor instability in children. *The Journal of Urology*. 2003;**170**(5):1978–81.

18 Malhotra B, Guan Z, Wood N, Gandelman K. Pharmacokinetic profile of fesoterodine. *International Journal of Clinical Pharmacology and Therapeutics*. 2008;**46**(11):556–63.

19 Malhotra B, Darsey E, Crownover P, Fang J, Glue P. Comparison of pharmacokinetic variability of fesoterodine vs. tolterodine extended release in cytochrome P450 2D6 extensive and poor metabolizers. *British Journal of Clinical Pharmacology*. 2011;**72**(2):226–34.

20 Chapple C, Van Kerrebroeck P, Tubaro A, Haag-Molkenteller C, Forst HT, Massow U, et al. Clinical efficacy, safety, and tolerability of once-daily fesoterodine in subjects with overactive bladder. *European Urology*. 2007;**52**(4):1204–12.

21 Malhotra B, El-Tahtawy A, Wang EQ, Darekar A, Cossons N, Crook TJ, et al. Dose-escalating study of the pharmacokinetics and tolerability of fesoterodine in children with overactive bladder. *Journal of Pediatric Urology*. 2012;**8**(4):336–42.

22 Bolduc S, Moore K, Nadeau G, Lebel S, Lamontagne P, Hamel M. Prospective open label study of solifenacin for overactive bladder in children. *The Journal of Urology*. 2010;**184** (4 Suppl):1668–73.

23 Nadeau G, Schroder A, Moore K, Genois L, Lamontagne P, Hamel M, et al. Long-term use of solifenacin in pediatric patients with overactive bladder: Extension of a prospective open-label study. *Canadian Urological Association Journal*. 2014;**8**(3–4):118–23.

24 Madersbacher H, Murtz G. Efficacy, tolerability and safety profile of propiverine in the treatment of the overactive bladder (non-neurogenic and neurogenic). *World Journal of Urology*. 2001;**19**(5):324–35.

25 Schulte-Baukloh H, Murtz G, Heine G, Austin P, Miller K, Michael T, et al. Urodynamic effects of propiverine in children and adolescents with neurogenic bladder: results of a prospective long-term study. *Journal of Pediatric Urology*. 2012;**8**(4):386–92.

26 Schulte-Baukloh H, Murtz G, Henne T, Michael T, Miller K, Knispel HH. Urodynamic effects of propiverine hydrochloride in children with neurogenic detrusor overactivity: a prospective analysis. *BJU International*. 2006;**97**(2):355–8.

27 Alloussi S, Murtz G, Braun R, Gerhardt U, Heinrich M, Hellmis E, et al. Efficacy, tolerability and safety of propiverine hydrochloride in comparison to oxybutynin in children with urge incontinence due to overactive bladder: Results of a multicentre observational cohort study. *BJU International*. 2010;**106**(4):550–6.

28 Andersson KE, Martin N, Nitti V. Selective beta(3)-adrenoceptor agonists for the treatment of overactive bladder. *The Journal of Urology*. 2013;**190**(4):1173–80.

29 Chapple CR, Cardozo L, Nitti VW, Siddiqui E, Michel MC. Mirabegron in overactive bladder: a review of efficacy, safety, and tolerability. *Neurourology and Urodynamics*. 2014;**33**(1):17–30.

30 Yamaguchi O, Marui E, Kakizaki H, Homma Y, Igawa Y, Takeda M, et al. Phase III, randomised, double-blind, placebo-controlled study of the beta-adrenoceptor agonist mirabegron, 50 mg once daily, in Japanese patients with overactive bladder. *BJU International*. 2014;**113**(6):951–60.

31 Krane RJ, Olsson CA. Phenoxybenzamine in neurogenic bladder dysfunction. II. Clinical considerations. *The Journal of Urology* 1973;**110**(6):653–6.

32 Amark P, Nergardh A. Influence of adrenergic agonists and antagonists on urethral pressure, bladder pressure and detrusor hyperactivity in children with myelodysplasia. *Acta Paediatrica Scandinavica*. 1991;**80**(8–9):824–32.

33 de Voogt HJ, van der Sluis C. Preliminary evaluation of alpha-adrenergic blocking agents in children with neurogenic bladder due to myelomeningocele. *Developmental Medicine and Child Neurology. Supplement* 1976(**37**):82–8.

34 Harrison NW, Whitfield HN, Williams DI. The place of alpha-blocking drugs in the treatment of children with neuropathic bladders. *Urologia Internationalis*. 1977;**32**(2–3):224–31.

35 Seiferth J. Types of neurogenic bladder in children with spina bifida, and response to treatment with phenoxybenzamine. *Developmental Medicine and Child Neurology. Supplement*. 1976(**37**):94–6.

36 Stockamp K, Herrmann H, Schreiter F. Conservative bladder treatment in myelodysplasia. Differentiation of patients by cystomanometry. *Urologia Internationalis*. 1976;**31**(1–2):93–9.

37 Austin PF, Homsy YL, Masel JL, Cain MP, Casale AJ, Rink RC. Alpha-Adrenergic blockade in children with neuropathic and nonneuropathic voiding dysfunction. *The Journal of Urology*. 1999;**162**(3 Pt 2):1064–7.

38 Schulte-Baukloh H, Michael T, Miller K, Knispel HH. Alfuzosin in the treatment of high leak-point pressure in children with neurogenic bladder. *BJU International*. 2002;**90**(7):716–20.

39 Homsy Y, Arnold P, Zhang W. Phase IIb/III dose ranging study of tamsulosin as treatment for children with neuropathic bladder. *The Journal of Urology*. 2011;**186**(5):2033–9.

CHAPTER 28

Treatment of constipation and fecal incontinence: Neuropathic

Mark P. Cain

Department of Pediatric Urology, Riley Hospital for Children at IU Health, Indiana University School of Medicine, Indianapolis, IN, USA

Managing the patient with neuropathic bowel disease is often frustrating for both the patient/family and medical caregiver. The bowel problems can lead to both constipation and incontinence due to a combination of slow colonic transit, limited physical mobility, reduced anal sphincter tone, and reduced sensation. In addition, many of these patients require anticholinergic or antimuscarinic medication for neuropathic bladder that compounds the underlying bowel problems. This creates the difficult situation of extremes from severe constipation and obstipation to liquid stool incontinence sometimes in the same patient. Management requires very individualized plans with constant adjustment to achieve satisfactory toileting habits and social fecal continence.

Medical management

The first step in treatment for neuropathic bowel is to optimize medical management. This is reviewed earlier in the text, but it cannot be emphasized enough that despite all the surgical options for these patients, managing the constipation and fecal incontinence with a surgically created colon channel still require *medical management*.

In the pretoilet-trained child, the goals are to avoid chronic overdilation of the colon and obstipation with daily regimens of dietary additives, stool softeners, and enemas. For children with persistent incontinence as they approach school age, most centers will introduce more aggressive therapy in an attempt to achieve continence. This will usually entail a regimen of timed toileting, retrograde enemas with or without manual disimpaction [1, 2]. The cornerstones of medical management are listed in Table 28.1.

Pediatric Incontinence: Evaluation and Clinical Management, First Edition. Edited by Israel Franco,
Paul F. Austin, Stuart B. Bauer, Alexander von Gontard and Yves Homsy.
© 2015 John Wiley & Sons, Ltd. Published 2015 by John Wiley & Sons, Ltd.

Table 28.1 Medical management of neuropathic bowel.

High fiber and fluid intake
Oral stool lubricants (mineral oil) or osmotic laxatives (polyethylene glycol)
Oral stimulants (senna and lactulose)
Oral bulk laxatives
Rectal suppositories (docusate and bisacodyl)
Digital stimulation/disimpaction
Retrograde enema (tap water, saline, soap, glycerin, and phosphates)

Since many of the patients with neuropathic bowel disease can have associated poor muscular control of the anal sphincter, the enema program will frequently require use of either a cone enema or the Peristeen® anal irrigation system (Coloplast), both of which allow high-volume enemas to be given with occlusion of the lax anal sphincter.

Surgical options

The Malone Antegrade Continence Enema (MACE) was a tremendous addition for patients with neuropathic bladder and bowel, as it offered the potential for complete continence in the patient refractory to medical management. Malone first introduced this procedure in 1990 [3], and there have since been multiple variations described to create the continent catheterizable colon channel.

The most common surgical technique used to create the MACE channel is the *in situ* appendicocecostomy. As with any of the other major genitourinary reconstructive procedures, careful patient and family selection and preoperative counseling are major factors in determining the success of the procedure. Patients must demonstrate compliance with a daily routine, and be able to sit for the required 30–45 min for bowel cleansing. At our institution, we will introduce the potential options of medical and surgical management for fecal incontinence early in the patient's life, but as they get close to the time of decision to pursue a surgical procedure, we will have them meet our surgical and nursing team for an in-depth discussion including videos of the procedure and management protocols after surgery.

Surgical technique: *In situ* appendicocecostomy

We have found that most patients can undergo an outpatient bowel preparation with oral polyethylene glycol and clear liquids starting 36–48 h prior to the procedure. All patients are given perioperative intravenous antibiotics for 24 h.

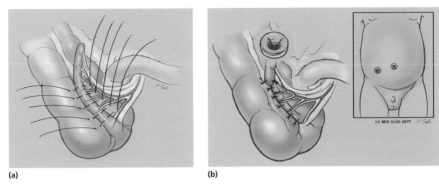

(a)   (b)

Figure 28.1 *In situ* appendicocecostomy. **(a)** Mesenteric windows are created in the mesentery of the appendix, and the appendix is positioned against the tenia. One or two 4-0 silk sutures are placed through each of the mesenteric windows to create a cecal wrap. **(b)** Completed *in situ* appendicocecostomy. Note that the appendix is secured to the cecum at the distal hiatus. Skin stomal site is chosen based on where the cecum and mesoappendix can reach in a tension-free fashion. Source: Sharon Teal, The Office of Visual Media, Indiana University. Reproduced with permission of The Trustees of Indiana University.

When the MACE procedure is being done as an isolated procedure, we will frequently use a laparoscopic-assisted approach, utilizing three ports to mobilize the appendix and cecum to the hepatic flexure, avoiding the need for a larger abdominal incision. A small infraumbilical incision is then made, and the appendix and cecum further mobilized, taking care to not injure the appendiceal mesentery. The appendix is then opened distally, and a 12–14 Fr catheter is secured to the tip of the appendix with a catheter plug placed to avoid contamination. Windows are then created in the mesoappendix to allow cecoplication (Figure 28.1). If the appendix has a good length, the proximal end is intussuscepted and secured with 2-3 silk sutures. Cecoplication is carried out with 4-0 silk sutures, placing 1-2 plication sutures through each mesenteric window. The appendix is secured at the distal end of the cecum to secure the continence wrap. The stomal site is selected either in the lower abdomen or the umbilicus, which is dictated by the mobility of the cecum and also the need to select a site for a potential urinary channel. A "U"- or "V"-shaped skin incision is then created at the stomal site, and a cruciate incision is made in the fascia. The appendix is brought through the fascial incision with the catheter intact. Once the abdominal incision is completely closed, the catheter is removed, the appendix spatulated and secured to the skin with 4-0 absorbable sutures. The catheter is left in place for 3–4 weeks before intermittent catheterization is initiated. Several studies have demonstrated improved outcomes using a temporary stent across the skin stoma for the first 6 months after surgery [4].

MACE options when the appendix is absent

In situations where the appendix is either nonusable or absent, there are two options for creating a MACE channel. The simplest to construct is the cecal flap MACE, first described by Kiely et al. [5], utilizing a nonimbricated lateral flap. This technique was later modified by Hanna and others [6], using a medially based colon flap to preserve the blood supply to the flap, and in addition, the continence mechanism was reinforced with colon plication as described for the *in situ* appendix. A 2×5 cm rectangular flap is outlined based on the medial ileocolic blood supply. The cecal flap is raised, and the donor site is closed in two layers. The cecal flap is then closed in two layers over a 12 Fr catheter. The colon tube is then positioned against the closed cecal donor site, and a cecal wrap is created, securing the cecum over the tube with 4-0 nonabsorbable sutures, creating approximately a 2.5–3 cm continence wrap. The neoappendix is secured to the cecum at the distal hiatus, and the cecum is secured to posterior fascial wall at the site of the stoma. The stoma is matured at the skin level using a wide V flap of skin.

The other alternative for creating a neoappendix is to utilize a retubularized small or large bowel channel, using the Monti principal [7, 8]. The Monti channel is harvested and reconfigured as described for use as a bladder channel. The right colon is mobilized, and the anterior tenia is opened to the level of the mucosa for 3–4 cm. The serosal flaps are sharply mobilized lateral to the mucosal incision. A small incision is made in the bowel mucosa, and the Monti channel is secured circumferentially with absorbable suture. The serosa is then secured anterior to the Monti channel using 3-0 absorbable sutures to create the continence mechanism, with occasional bites of the channel to fix it within the tunnel. The channel is secured at the hiatus, and the cecum is then secured with nonabsorbable sutures to the posterior fascia at the site of the stoma. We have also found it helpful to secure the serosal closure along the continence channel to the posterior fascia to prevent disruption of the continence mechanism with colonic distension.

Minimally invasive MACE procedures

The MACE procedure can easily be performed with either laparoscopic or robotic techniques. There is still a lack of consensus as to the need to plicate the appendix to achieve stomal continence, but a recent single institutional report demonstrated a 10% increases risk of stomal leakage in the absence of plication [9]. The greatest advantage of laparoscopy is the minimal morbidity by avoiding a large abdominal incision to mobilize the colon in the older patient, especially when performed utilizing a single-port system (Figure 28.2). The procedure can be carried out with or without appendiceal plication depending on the technical

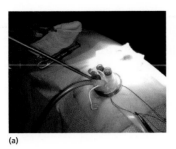 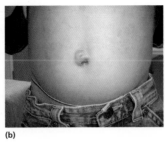 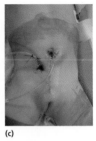

(a)   (b)   (c)

Figure 28.2 Single-port laparoscopic-assisted appendicocecostomy with extracorporeal plication. **(a)** The single-port site can be placed at the umbilicus and converted to an umbilical stoma. The cecum and appendix are mobilized and then delivered through the fascial incision at the port site for extracorporeal plication. **(b)** Postoperative stomal site after single-port MACE procedure. **(c)** Comparison of incision required for Mitrofanoff and MACE procedure with extension of abdominal incision to allow mobilization of colon.

ability of the laparoscopic surgeon. Alternatively, the cecum can be delivered through an extension of one of the laparoscopic port sites, allowing for extracorporeal plication through a small abdominal incision.

Left colon MACE procedure

One of the patient complaints of the MACE procedure is duration of time required to flush the colon, especially in patients with a chronically distended right colon, where large volume enemas are frequently required. The left colon MACE provides a good alternative, and can be constructed either using the Monti-MACE or colon flap technique. Results have been similar to right colon procedures using the same channels, but have demonstrated a significant reduction in irrigation times [10].

Minimally invasive percutaneous cecostomy tube

For patients who are either poor operative candidates or wish to avoid major abdominal surgery, Shandling and Chait described a technique for placing a percutaneous low-profile cecostomy button [11, 12], available as the Chait Percutaneous Cecostomy Catheter® (Cook Medical). This has minimized the patient dissatisfaction with a larger external appliance, and minimized peristomal leakage. The catheter can be placed percutaneously under radiographic guidance with general anesthesia or sedation but still requires a short hospital stay for periprocedure antibiotics. An initial tube is usually placed for several weeks to allow the tract to mature, then later replaced with the Chait catheter. Alternatively, the cecostomy tube can be placed under vision in the operating room with laparoscopic guidance, with the advantage of securing the cecum at the cecostomy site, and the ability to place the Chait tube at the initial procedure [13]. The disadvantage of the external tube is granulation tissue developing around the exit site, and what is usually described as minor leakage around the tube. One clear advantage is to allow a trial to determine if the MACE is helpful in individual patient, and in those that severe constipation may improve over time. In these patients, the tube can be removed in the clinic, and the fistula will close spontaneously.

Enema protocols for MACE

Because of reports of complications associated with saline and phosphate enemas, our standard has been to begin all patients on MACE irrigations utilizing tap water, which have been shown to be safe [14]. Our initial approach is to initiate MACE flushes after bowel function has returned and the patient is still in the hospital. The protocol begins with low volume irrigation starting at 50 mL of tap water, and increasing by 50 mL every 3 days until satisfactory results are obtained, usually taking up to a month after surgery. In a review of 236 patients at our institution, Bani Hani found that the average irrigation volume was 600 mL but ranged from 100 to 1000 mL [15]. Eighty-three percent of patients were completely continent with tap water enemas alone; the remainder of the patients required some type of additives or adjustment of their schedule. For patients with immediate or overnight accidents we recommend increasing MACE flush volumes and/or sitting longer on the commode. For persistent incontinence, we would then recommend adding 30 mL of mineral oil or 17 g of polyethylene glycol in 250 mL water given 15–30 min prior to the routine enema. For patients having accidents the following day we evaluate the stool burden with an abdominal radiograph, then perform a bowel clean out through the MACE with one liter of Golytely® over an hour, repeating it the following day if necessary. Polyethylene glycol is added to the daily enema routine as outlined earlier. For patients with high rectal tone, they will frequently respond to bisacodyl suppositories with digital rectal stimulation prior to the enema. For patients that fail all these measures, we change irrigation solution to glycerin 60 mL in 60 mL of water. With this aggressive program, we have achieved a 94% success rate for fecal continence. Other investigators have reported similar good results with glycerin enemas, but it can increase the cost of the MACE program considerably [16].

Outcomes and complications of the MACE procedure

Several reports have confirmed the significant improvement in quality of life for spina bifida patients following a MACE procedure [17, 18]. Despite improved quality of life and improved independence in bowel management, up to 18%

at 5 years and 40% at 10 years will stop routinely using their MACE [19]. Explanations for this "failure" may be due to poorer surgical results in the earlier series, lack of effectiveness over time, and lack of transition care into the adult clinic setting. Despite the continued late dropout of patients, the satisfaction rate remained high for those still using their MACE channel.

The common surgical complications following a MACE procedure include stomal stenosis, stomal incontinence, traumatic injury/obliteration, difficulty catheterizing, and channel prolapse. Early experience with the MACE channel demonstrated a high complication rate of stomal stenosis in 55% and channel obliteration in 6% [20]. Significant refinements in the technique have improved outcomes dramatically. Two large contemporary reviews have reported stomal continence rates of 94–97% and overall need for surgical revision rate of 17–25% [21, 22]. VanderBrink reported the largest series, with 282 patients undergoing a MACE procedure. The complication rate was 17%, with 1/3 of these patients requiring more than one revision. Stomal stenosis or endoscopic procedures accounted for over 75% of the revisions, usually accomplished in an outpatient setting. Although the experience was heavily weighted to the *in situ* appendix technique, there was a significant difference in complication rate between the different procedures: *in situ* appendix (16%), split appendix (21%), Monti-MACE (16%), and cecal flap (30%). Mean time to first revision was 19 months, but complications occurred as late as 9 years.

References

1 Vande Velde, S, Van Biervliet, S, Van Renterghem, K, et al.: Achieving fecal continence in patients with spina bifida: a descriptive cohort study. *J Urol* 2007: **178**; 2640–4.

2 Bischoff, A, Levitt, MA, Bauer, C, et al.: Treatment of fecal incontinence with a comprehensive bowel management program. *J Pediatr Surg* 2009: **44**; 1278–84.

3 Malone, PS, Ransley, PG, Kiely, EM. Preliminary report: the antegrade continence enema. *Lancet* 1990: **336**; 1217–8.

4 Subramaniam, R, Taylor, C. The use of an antegrade continence enema stopper in catheterizable channels virtually eliminates the incidence of stomal stenosis; preliminary experience. *J Urol* 2009: **181**; 299–301.

5 Kiely, EM, Ade-Ajayi, N, Wheeler, RA. Caecal flap conduit for antegrade continence enemas. *Br J Surg* 1994: **81**; 1215.

6 Weiser, AC, Stock, JA, Hanna, MK. Modified cecal flap neoappendix for the Malone antegrade continence enema procedure: a novel technique. *J Urol* 2003: **169**; 2321–4.

7 Monti PR, Lara RC, Dutra MA, et al. New techniques for construction of efferent conduits based on the Mitrofanoff principle. *Urology* 1997: **49**; 112–5.

8 Yerkes, EB, Rink, RC, Cain, MP, Casale, AJ: Use of monti channel for administration of antegrade continence enemas. *J Urol* 2002: **168**; 1883–5.

9 Henrichon, S, Hu, B, Kurzrock, EA. Detailed assessment of stomal incontinence after Malone antegrade continence enema: development of a new grading scale. *J Urol* 2012: **187**; 652–5.

10 Churchill, BM, De Ugarte, DA, Atkinson, JB. Left-colon antegrade continence enema (LACE) procedure for fecal incontinence. *J Pediatr Surg* 2003: **38**; 1778–80.

11 Shandling, B, Chait, PG, Richards, HF. Percutaneous cecostomy: a new technique in the management of fecal incontinence. *J Pediatr Surg* 1996: **31**; 534–7.

12 Chait, PG, Shandling, B, Richards, HF. The cecostomy button. *J Pediatr Surg* 1997: **32**; 849–51.

13 Becmeur, F, Demarch, M, Lacreuse, I, et al. Cecostomy button for antegrade enemas; survey of 29 patients. *J Pediatr Surg* 2008: **43**; 1853–7.

14 Yerkes, EB, Rink, RC, King, S, Cain, MP, Kaefer, M, Casale, AJ. Tap water and the Malone antegrade continence enema: a safe combination? *J Urol* 2001: **166**: 1476–8.

15 Bani-Hani, AH, Cain, MP, King, S, Rink, RC: Tap water irrigation and the use of additives to optimize success with the Malone Antegrade Continence Enema (MACE) – The Indiana University Algorithm. *J Urol* 2008: **180**; 1757–60.

16 Chu, DI, Balsara, ZR, Routh, JC, et al. Experience with glycerin for antegrade continence enema in patients with neurogenic bowel. *J Urol* 2013: **189**; 690–3.

17 Yerkes, EB, Cain, MP, King, S, et al. The Malone antegrade continence enema procedure: quality of life and family perspective. *J Urol* 2003: **169**; 320–3.

18 Ok, J, Kurzrock, EA. Objective measurement of quality of life changes after ACE Malone using the FICQOL survey. *J Pediatr Urol* 2011: **7**; 389–93.

19 Yardley, IE, Pauniaho, SL, Baillie, CT, et al. After the honeymoon comes the divorce: long-term use of the antegrade continence enema procedure. *J Pediatr Surg* 2009: **44**; 1274–7.

20 Curry, JI, Osborne, A, Malone, PSJ. How to achieve a successful Malone antegrade continence enema. *J Pediatr Surg* 1998: **33**; 138–41.

21 Rangel, SJ, Lawal, TA, Bischoff, A, et al. The appendix as a conduit for antegrade continence enemas in patients with anorectal malformations: Lessons learned from 163 cases treated over 18 years. *J Pediatr Surg* 2011: **46**; 1236–42.

22 VanderBrink, BA, Cain, MP, Kaefer, M, et al. Outcomes following Malone antegrade continence enema and their surgical revisions. *J Pediatr Surg* 2013: **48**; 2134–9.

CHAPTER 29

Neuromodulation for neurogenic bladder in pediatric spinal dysraphism

Elizabeth B. Yerkes and William E. Kaplan

Division of Pediatric Urology, Northwestern University Feinberg School of Medicine, Ann and Robert H. Lurie Children's Hospital of Chicago, Chicago, IL, USA

Clean intermittent catheterization (CIC) and antimuscarinic agents have positively redirected the urologic outcomes for children with neurogenic bladder secondary to spinal dysraphism. Coordinated voiding and intact sensation for volitional continence occur only in the minority of individuals with spinal dysraphism. In the absence of sensation of bladder fullness, timed CIC results is the best opportunity for urinary continence. When maximum medical therapy fails to achieve or maintain a natural reservoir that is protective of the renal units, surgical intervention becomes the reliable standard for renal protection. While augmenting the bladder capacity with enterocystoplasty is highly effective at achieving safe storage pressure and an adequately sized reservoir, it comes at a steep price over the long term, and even the most prolific reconstructive surgeons recognize the value of avoiding augmentation cystoplasty. Consequently, various less invasive second-tier strategies have been and will be investigated and employed to avoid this successful but burdensome (for the individual and caregivers) surgical approach. Among these alternative strategies is neuromodulation therapy. As with many new but intriguing therapeutic options, the pediatric community often proceeds with caution and lags behind the experience in adult medicine. Neuromodulation is no exception, in part due to the reluctance of governmental regulatory bodies to permit use of unapproved devices in children but also in part due to a need to have a better understanding of potential irreversible complications for young patients with a long life ahead.

The actual neural mechanisms to explain the successes (and failures) of neuromodulation are incompletely understood. It can be viewed simply as reeducating the nervous system to enhance bladder and sphincter function. Why—in the majority of cases—it appears to either have the desired effect or have little effect, rather than causing detrimental changes, is not yet clear.

Pediatric Incontinence: Evaluation and Clinical Management, First Edition. Edited by Israel Franco, Paul F. Austin, Stuart B. Bauer, Alexander von Gontard and Yves Homsy.
© 2015 John Wiley & Sons, Ltd. Published 2015 by John Wiley & Sons, Ltd.

Despite acknowledging the incomplete understanding of neuromodulation, [1] very nicely summarized the known neurophysiologic supportive evidence for management of detrusor overactivity and urinary retention. Stimulation of peripheral afferent fibers modulates urinary reflex pathways in the central nervous system (CNS). Dormant sensory pathways activated by inflammation or noxious stimuli can lead to overactivity if not overridden by other sensory signals reaching the spinal cord. Neuromodulation for neurogenic detrusor overactivity (NDO) may be successful by restoring the balance between inhibitory and excitatory messages. Detrusor underactivity can be addressed by awakening dormant efferent pathways [1]. Improving our understanding of the neural mechanisms will help improve patient selection and treatment parameters for neuromodulation techniques.

While the focus on quality of research calls for more prospective randomized controlled trials, even the adult experience with neuromodulation techniques for neurogenic and nonneurogenic bladder conditions has a paucity of high-quality data [2]. Promising individual outcomes and group trends with reasonable safety profiles will continue to push the pediatric community to fine-tune stimulation protocols and to develop high-quality prospective trials to determine the best young candidates for neuromodulation [3].

The primary focus of this chapter is the international experience with transurethral intravesical electrical stimulation (IVES) in children with spinal dysraphism, but the chapter will also include discussion of the most current published experience with transcutaneous electrical nerve stimulation (TENS), posterior tibial nerve stimulation (PTNS), and implantation of sacral neuromodulation (SNM) devices in children.

IVES (Intravesical Electrical Stimulation)

In theory, IVES progressively recruits afferent fibers in the bladder mucosa and submucosa in individuals in whom efferent stimulation of the bladder was disrupted by a spinal cord condition. Through repeated treatments, the spinal cord and higher centers are engaged to result in recognition of the detrusor contraction and volitional voiding. Engaging the patient in visual experience of bladder contractility may help with acquisition of volitional voiding and ultimate control [4].

The initial experience came from Hungary in 1975 by Katona and Berenyi [5]. Their initial work was directed at the underactive detrusor, and over 70% of patients achieved spontaneous voiding with daytime continence. The experience was subsequently confirmed by Madersbacher [6].

The largest reported experience comes from Kaplan and Richards at Children's Memorial Hospital in Chicago, with over 400 patients treated over 22 years [7]. They are to be credited for introducing the European method for IVES to the United States. In 1986, they published an initial very encouraging experience of 10 patients in which sustained therapy created sensation and spontaneous voiding with continence in a young man with myelomeningocele [4]. This work was initially designed with the goal of "normalizing" the neurogenic bladder in myelomeningocele by improving sensation of filling and by generating an effective voiding contraction. Secondarily the child would learn to control micturition through visual biofeedback. Although the initial results were very encouraging, albeit after extensive labor- and time-intensive therapeutic courses, the longer experience revealed that this remarkable response was achievable in no more than 20% of those treated. In those who did achieve volitional control over elimination, the results were durable and valuable. Additional benefits included improved capacity, compliance, and sensation that enhanced continence via awareness of the need for CIC. Importantly, the results appeared to be durable [4, 7–9].

Reports from other US institutions, each with somewhat different protocols and objectives, showed variable results, and none have ongoing programs currently [10–13]. A large multi-institutional experience published in 1996, however, included children treated on the same protocol as that espoused at Children's Memorial Hospital [8]. There was adequate pre- and posttreatment data on 335 children, nearly half of whom were treated at Children's Memorial Hospital and the balance treated at 10 other institutions (including three of the aforementioned series). More than 50% had an increase in bladder capacity of 20% or greater over an average of 1.9 years of IVES. Those who did not respond had normal capacity prior to IVES. Of those with increased capacity, storage pressures were decreased to or remained below 40 cm water in 90% of children. When the Chicago results were compared to the other 10 institutions, there were no appreciable differences. The length of therapy required to achieve the desired result, however, can be extensive.

Cheng et al also reported the Children's Memorial Hospital's experience with the subgroup of seven children who had a high-risk urodynamic profile with a percent expected capacity of 60% or less and terminal storage pressure of 50 cm water or greater [9]. All seven had improved compliance that averted a need for enterocystoplasty, and four patients had a statistically significant increase in percent of expected capacity for age. These results were durable.

Two important points were emphasized that may help guide future success with neuromodulation. First, it was emphasized that the specific stimulation parameters were individualized and adjusted during the course of treatment based upon the observed response of the bladder during each session. This was felt to be critical to the success of IVES. The second pearl was that a "staircase" response was noted from one IVES series to the next in the children with high-risk bladders, meaning that they may take a step backward in terms of bladder capacity at times but then subsequently have an even more favorable response [9].

In 2007, Hagerty et al published the 22-year Children's Memorial Hospital experience with IVES for neurogenic bladder dysfunction in children [7]. There was reportable data for 372 patients, treated for a median of 29 sessions (2–197). The mean age at treatment was 5.5 years and the mean follow-up was 6.6 years. Essentially three-quarters of the patients had a 20% or greater increase in bladder capacity, and of that group, three-quarters had storage pressures less than 40 cm water. Of those who had no change in bladder capacity, more than 80% had storage pressures less than 40 cm water after treatment. Sensation was acquired and sustained in over 60%. In a reply to an editorial comment for this experience, the authors shared observations that the best responders are young children with a small poorly compliant bladder, with improvement in sensation most likely in those under 6 years of age. Poor candidates, based upon this experience, were those with a large hypotonic bladder, severe NDO with frequent strong contractions, unstable lesions, complete cord transections, prior bladder augmentation, and low outlet resistance.

A more recent long-term experience comes from Sang Won Han and associates [14]. This report involved a series of 88 children with spina bifida who received at least four cycles of IVES and with pre- and posttreatment urodynamic evaluation, so all had at least 1 year follow-up. As in the Children's Memorial Hospital series, improvement in bladder capacity was reported as percent bladder capacity for age to take current age of the patient into account. The majority had neurogenic detrusor overactivity ($n=60$); a smaller group had acontractile detrusor ($n=25$) and three had underactive detrusor. Also as in the Children's Memorial Hospital series, oral anticholinergic therapy was discontinued for at least several days prior to each treatment cycle and prior to urodynamic evaluation. Forty-one percent of those with NDO became synergic and 16.7% developed normal detrusor function. In the acontractile group, the majority remained acontractile but 48% developed some contractions and only one developed normal function. In the underactive detrusor group, only one of the three patients showed a change and that child developed normal detrusor activity. Of those who developed normal function, most had NDO and none had poor compliance or upper urinary tract damage at the start; nearly all had lipomyelomeningocele and only two used CIC.

In the series by Han, predictive factors were also noted for bladder capacity. The percent bladder capacity increased in 45% of children. When stratified by detrusor function and compliance at outset of treatment, two important differences were noted. Of those with NDO and normal compliance, there was a statistically significant increase in capacity from a mean of 65% of expected capacity to 97% of expected capacity. In the group with poor compliance, however, the capacity decreased from 89 to 68.5% of expected, also statistically significant. Both of the acontractile groups had a decrease in percent expected capacity, but this was only significant in the group with impaired compliance. In the group with NDO, bladder capacity increased significantly in the subgroup who had their first IVES cycle prior to 18 months of age but a significant decrease in those first treated after 18 months of age.

Voiding function improved in many, with resolution of detrusor sphincter dyssynergia in 55% of children. Sensation developed and was sustained in over 80%. Improvement in continence was also noted. Of the 48 children using CIC, 18.7% acquired volitional voiding without CIC and half of those were continent. Forty-eight percent had improved continence on CIC, while three children had increased wetting on CIC [14]. Improvement in fecal continence also reached statistical significance, with a greater than 50% improvement in incontinence episodes in 75% of children as a result of IVES [15].

Protection of the upper urinary tracts is obviously critical when considering any manipulation of the lower urinary tract. When looking at vesicoureteral reflux and evidence of upper urinary tract defects, those with resolution of reflux during therapy had no new defects. There were however seven children with new reflux after IVES, and one had an upper urinary tract defect. Hydronephrosis was not specifically described so the upper urinary tract defect is interpreted as a parenchymal defect related to reflux [14].

When looking at the specific successes of both large series, it is clear that success requires not only meticulous dedication, but also careful patient selection. The therapy involves such a large commitment for all, that IVES is not advised for every child with neurogenic bladder dysfunction. When synthesizing the data of both series, it appears that IVES treatment at a younger age is more likely to be successful. Acontractile bladders are not likely to see clinically relevant improvement. Treatment in the setting of a small poorly compliant bladder may be successful but deterioration may also be seen. Close follow-up is advisable to verify whether additional more aggressive surgical intervention will be required.

In 2014, intravesical bladder stimulation programs are active around the globe, but updated published series other than the aforementioned are lacking. The IVES program at the authors' institution, the former Children's Memorial Hospital, closed 7 years ago due to unavailability of the specialized electrical stimulation catheters. This technology is again potentially available on a protocol basis in the United States, pending demonstration of safety and efficacy of the acquired equipment by federal regulatory agencies.

Although results differ somewhat from institution to institution, the cumulative experience suggests benefit of one form or another that is sufficient to continue to promulgate the investigation and use of forms of neuromodulation for children with spinal dysraphism. Given the invasiveness of intravesical bladder stimulation for children who do not participate in CIC and given the time-intensive nature of the program, it makes perfect sense to investigate other less invasive forms of neuromodulation or home programs of IVES to rehabilitate the bladder and pelvic floor. In order of the least invasive to the most invasive approaches, we will now review the results of these neuromodulation techniques in children with neurogenic bladder dysfunction, with correlation to the adult experience and the experience with pediatric nonneurogenic dysfunction, where potentially relevant.

TENS

The concept of therapeutic transcutaneous electrical stimulation is to encourage atrophied muscle to become useful, first by strengthening the muscle body with subsequent work with biofeedback to learn control [16]. In children with myelomeningocele, this stimulation may benefit the atrophic pelvic floor complex related to the spinal cord lesion.

Balcom and associates reported initial experience with a home program of overnight long-duration, low-intensity transcutaneous electrical stimulation [17]. That institution had previous experience with the time and labor intensity but successes of IVES and saw the value in a less invasive home therapy. Based upon impact seen by McLorie and associates [18] with enhanced urethral pressure profile in children with myelomeningocele, they investigated the impact of this home program on bladder and bowel continence. Electrodes were paired on the trunk and gluteal region. Eleven children with lumbar and sacral myelomeningocele were treated, with a statistically significant increase in bladder capacity but less apparent strengthening of the pelvic floor. In nearly half the children previously treated with IVES, there was a less notable increase in bladder capacity, suggesting similar benefit with this noninvasive therapy. A subjective improvement in sensation was noted in nearly all, but this was not confirmed by cystometry [17].

The first randomized clinical trial of parasacral TENS in pediatric nonneuropathic overactive bladder was published in 2010 by Barroso and associates. Statistically significant improvement was seen in bladder symptom scores, voided volumes, and voiding frequency in the treatment group versus shams (superficial scapular), with 61% reporting a cure. A high success rate was also seen with crossover treatment of the sham group [19].

In a 2010 pilot study of 12 children with lumbosacral myelomeningocele, aged 3 years or greater with moderate to severe urinary incontinence on CIC and pharmacotherapy, transcutaneous functional electrical stimulation was performed via suprapubic and perineal leads. The therapy was based on the theory that stimulation of afferent fibers of the pudendal nerve results in an efferent contraction of the external sphincter with inhibition of NDO, both of which could facilitate continence. Daytime incontinence resolved in two of twelve patients, improved in five and failed to change in the remaining three patients. Detrusor leak point pressure increased significantly, as did bladder capacity. Long-term follow-up was not described but the short-term results were encouraging [20]. The transcutaneous approach is appealing for children in that it is less invasive than intravaginal or intra-anal leads used in adult women with neurogenic and nonneurogenic urge incontinence [21].

PTNS

The principle for neuromodulation via the posterior tibial nerve was based on traditional Chinese acupuncture over the posterior tibial nerves to inhibit the irritable bladder [22]. The posterior tibial nerve is a mixed sensory and motor peripheral nerve related to the L4 through S3 nerve roots; thereby it contributes to the sensory and motor aspects of the bladder and pelvic floor [1]. Published experience in children with neurogenic bladder dysfunction is very limited. In 2009, Capitanucci and associates reported on PTNS in 44 children with a variety of lower urinary tract dysfunction. Only seven in the series had neurogenic bladder dysfunction. They saw 78% response in the nonneurogenic group versus only 14% in the neurogenic group, suggesting that this approach is amenable to primarily the former group [23].

Sacral nerve stimulation

The mechanism of action of SNM is not well understood but appears to have a stabilizing effect on the networks via afferents rather than a direct stimulation of motor neurons to the detrusor or external urethral sphincter. Decreased bladder and sphincter instability by stimulation of the pelvic floor may increase sphincter tone and result in more coordinated voiding via reflex pathways [2, 24].

SNM was initially approved for use for nonneurogenic bladder dysfunction, so the bulk of experience is with these conditions in adults. A high satisfaction and patient experience has been reported for a variety of nonneuropathic voiding concerns. There was variable benefit for secondary pelvic disorders such as bowel function, abdominal pain, or sexual dysfunction. Despite satisfaction with this treatment, 40% expressed concerns about perceived quality of life interference or concerns with its long-term use: pain at the site during stimulation, difficulties with reimbursement, trouble with commercial or airport metal detectors, inability to have an MRI, concerns regarding pregnancy, a need for batter exchange procedure, and decreased efficacy over time [25]. Concerns regarding MRI with an implantable device include dislocation of the leads with nerve injury, excessive thermal impact on the nerves, reprogramming, and damage to the unit [1]. These concerns were not supported by a small series of patients undergoing MRI with the unit turned off, but the body site imaged during the MRI was remote from the device [26].

In one series of SNM in 27 adults with neurogenic bladder, none of whom had a congenital anomaly of the lumbosacral region such as spina bifida or sacral agenesis, all but two reported moderate to severe pain during acute stimulation. Some noted involuntary activation or deactivation in strong electrical fields such as the subway or microwave devices. In terms of success in those with neurogenic bladder dysfunction, they saw no improvement in those with complete or near-complete lesions. Overall, these researchers felt the technique to be of value but only as a temporary reprieve for refractory neurogenic bladder in individuals who otherwise would have required bladder augmentation [27].

When retrospectively assessing utility of SNM in adults with neurogenic bladder, none of whom had spina bifida, Game and associates demonstrated clinical and urodynamic benefit during the test phase in 66% of a large heterogeneous series. After implantation the benefit was sustained in 75% at a mean of 4.3 years. They noted that the long-term outcome was related to the underlying neurologic condition, with progressive conditions such as multiple sclerosis having less likelihood of a sustained result [28]. This may indicate that if a positive response were obtained in children with spina bifida, these results may likely be more durable.

While we cannot be certain how the results in adults with neurogenic bladders apply to children with spinal dysraphism or sacral agenesis or how much of an impact these concerns or potential complications will have during long-term assessment, we will certainly need to be mindful of potential complications and nuisances when considering implantation of a chronic stimulation device in children.

The question has to be raised whether a trial of SNM prior to the bladder becoming truly refractory to medical management could be more beneficial. SNM for neurogenic bladder dysfunction in children was reported by Guys and associates in 2004 [24]. Permanent electrical stimulation of S3 nerve roots with an implantable pulse generator (InterStim System, Medtronic France SAS) in a prospective randomized trial of 42 patients with a predominant diagnosis of spina bifida at a mean age 11.9 years, children were randomized to conventional medical management versus SNM implantation. Anticholinergic medications were discontinued prior to treatment in the SNM group but not in the control group. Additionally, a bulking agent at the bladder neck was permitted in the control group, with the authors anticipating that a greater than 30% difference in outcomes would be a significant response due to the expected 30% success rate with conventional therapy alone. They noted an S3 root response in 70% but presumed that the ability to respond was related to the variability of intact sensory afferents and motor efferents in these individuals. They found improvements in bladder compliance and functional capacity at 6 and 9 months, and the total capacity increased substantially. Other improvements included intestinal transit times, reduction in urinary tract infection, and improved sensation of a full bladder. No improvements were observed in the control group, while improvements in the treated group did not reach statistical significance. Revision was required in three cases: mechanical issues developed in two and wound infection in one. Despite a commendable effort in creating a randomized trial, the study is limited by heterogeneity in terms of medical and minimally invasive therapies in the control group, as well as inconsistent use of CIC in both groups.

A subsequent trial including Guys' group was a multicenter, open-label randomized crossover study for children with urinary and fecal incontinence. Many of the patients had nonneurogenic dysfunction, but 18 of the 33 patients did have spinal dysraphism. Clinical improvement in urinary continence did not always correlate with urodynamic parameters. Statistically significant improvements in cystometric capacity were noted with SNM. Improved urinary (81%) and fecal (78%) incontinence was noted [29], similar to a study by Roth and colleagues in children with nonneurogenic dysfunction [30], suggesting that outcomes for spina bifida and nonneurogenic dysfunction may be similar. The implantation procedure and treatments were well tolerated, and the rate of explantation or revision for mechanical issues was low [29].

While not all children with neurogenic bladder dysfunction will have an excellent response and while it is not clear yet who will be a responder, the observation that some children will benefit from this technique makes it a therapeutic option to consider prior to major irreversible surgical procedures.

Summary

Neuromodulation techniques are intriguing and mysterious. From the published experience with the spectrum of current techniques, it seems that there is real potential for benefit on an individual basis. Parents are savvy about seeking progressive therapies, and this should be encouraged as long as these therapies are safe, do not burn therapeutic bridges, and could potentially avert the need for aggressive surgical interventions such as enterocystoplasty. If we continue to examine prior results and develop sound prospective trials, we may be able to offer even more exciting results in the future. Being able to demonstrate reliable therapeutic value from these expensive and intensive modalities will also be important in the changing healthcare landscape here in the United States.

References

1 Burks FN, Bui DT, Peters KM. Neuromodulation and the neurogenic bladder. *Urol Clin N Am* 2010; **37**:559–565.
2 Kessler TM, La Framboise D, Trelle S, Fowler CJ, Kiss G, Pannek J, Schurch B, Sievert K-D, Engeler DS. Sacral neuromodulation for neurogenic lower urinary tract dysfunction: systematic review and meta-analysis. *Eur Urol* 2010; **58**:865–874.
3 De Gennaro M, Capitanucci ML, Mosiello G, Zaccara A. Current state of nerve stimulation technique for lower urinary tract dysfunction in children. *J Urol* 2011; **185**:1571–1577.

4 Kaplan WE, Richards I. Intravesical transurethral electrotherapy for the neurogenic bladder. *J Urol* 1986; **136**:243–246.

5 Katona F, Berenyi M. Intravesical transurethral electrotherapy in meningomyelocele patients. *Acta Paediatr Acad Sci Hung* 1975; **16**:363.

6 Madersbacher H, Pauer W, Reiner E. Rehabilitation of micturition by transurethral electrostimulation of the bladder in patients with incomplete spinal cord lesions. *Paraplegia* 1982; **20**:191.

7 Hagerty JA, Richards I, Kaplan WE. Intravesical electrotherapy for neurogenic bladder dysfunction: a 22-year experience. *J Urol* 2007; **178**:1680–1683.

8 Cheng EY, Richards I, Balcom A, Steinhardt G, Diamond M, Rich M, Donovan JM, Carr MC, Reinberg Y, Hurt G, Chandra M, Bauer SB, Kaplan WE. Bladder stimulation therapy improves bladder compliance: results from a multi-institutional trial. *J Urol* 1996; **156**:761–764.

9 Cheng EY, Richards I, Kaplan WE. Use of bladder stimulation in high risk patients. *J Urol* 1996; **156**:749–752.

10 Boone TB, Roehrborn CG, Hurt G. Transurethral intravesical electrotherapy for neurogenic bladder dysfunction in children with myelodysplasia: a prospective, randomized clinical trial. *J Urol* 1992; **148**:550–554.

11 Decter RM, Snyder P, Laudermilch C. Transurethral electrical bladder stimulation: a follow-up report. *J Urol* 1994; **152**:812.

12 Pugach JL, Salvin L, Steinhardt GF. Intravesical electrostimulation in pediatric patients with spinal cord defects. *J Urol* 2000; **164**:965–968.

13 Gladh G, Mattsson S, Lindstrom S. Intravesical electrical stimulation in the treatment of micturition dysfunction in children. *Neurourol Urodyn* 2003; **22**:233–242.

14 Choi EK, Hong CH, Kim MJ, Im YJ, Jung HJ, Han SW. Effects of intravesical electrical stimulation therapy on urodynamic patterns for children with spina bifida: a 10-year experience. *J Pediatr Urol* 2013; **9**:798–803.

15 Han SW, Kim MJ, Kim JH, Hong CH, Kim JW, Noh JY. Intravesical electrical stimulation improves neurogenic bowel dysfunction in children with spina bifida. *J Urol* 2004; **171**:2648–2650.

16 Gould N, Donnermeyer D, Pope M, Ashikaga T. Transcutaneous muscle stimulation as a method to retard disuse atrophy. *Clin Orthop Relat Res* 1982; **164**:215.

17 Balcom AH, Wiatrak M, Biefeld T, Rauen K, Langenstroer P. Initial experience with home therapeutic electrical stimulation for continence in the myelomeningocele population. *J Urol* 1997; **158**:1272–1276.

18 McLorie GA, Kirsch SA, Chabot J, Gilmour RF, Pape KE. A non-invasive electro-stimulation technique with measurable effects on bladder function in children with myelomeningocele. Presented at American Academy of Pediatrics, Section on Urology, San Francisco, California, October 11, 1992.

19 Lordelo P, Teles A, Veiga, ML, Correia LC, Barroso U. Transcutaneous electrical nerve stimulation in children with overactive bladder: a randomized clinical trial. *J Urol* 2010; **184**:683–689.

20 Kajbafzadeh A-M, Sharifi-Rad L, Dianat SS. Efficacy of transcutaneous functional electrical stimulation of urinary incontinence in myelomeningocele: results of a pilot study. *Int Braz J Urol* 2010; **36**(5):614–620.

21 Primus G, Kramer G. Maximal external electrical stimulation for treatment of neurogenic or non-neurogenic urgency and/or urge incontinence. *Neurourol Urodyn* 1996; **15**:187–194.

22 Geirsson G, Wang YH, Lindstrom S, et al. Traditional acupuncture and electrical stimulation of the posterior tibial nerve: a trial in chronic interstitial cystitis. *Scand J Urol Nephrol* 1993; **27**:67.

23 Capitanucci ML, Camanni D, Demelas F, Mosiello G, Zaccara A, DeGennaro M. Long-term efficacy of percutaneous tibial nerve stimulation for different types of lower urinary tract dysfunction in children. *J Urol* 2009; **182**:2056–2061.

24 Guys JM, Haddad M, Planche D, Torre M, Louis-Borrione C, Breaud J. Sacral neuromodulation for neurogenic bladder dysfunction in children. *J Urol* 2004; **172**:1673–1676.

25 Leong RK, Marcelissen TA, Nieman FH, DeBie RA, Vankerrebroeck PE, De Wachter SG. Satisfaction and patient experience with sacral neuromodulation: results of a single center sample survey. *J Urol* 2011; **185**:588–592.

26 Elkelinin MS, Hassouna MM. Safety of MRI at 1.5 Tesla in patients with implanted sacral nerve neurostimulator. *Eur Urol* 2006; **50**:311–316.

27 Hohenfellner M, Humke J, Hampel C, Dahms S, Matzel K, Roth S, Thuroff JW, Schultz-Lampel D. Chronic sacral neuromodulation for treatment of neurogenic bladder dysfunction: long-term results with unilateral implants. *Urology* 2001; **58**(6):887–892.

28 Chaabane W, Guillotreau J, Castel-lacanal E, Abu-Anz S, De Boissezon X, Malavaud B, Marque P, Sarramon J-P, Rischmann P, Game X. Sacral neuromodulation for treating neurogenic bladder dysfunction: clinical and urodynamic study. *Neurourol Urodyn* 2011; **30**:547–550.

29 Haddad M, Besson R, Aubert D, Ravasse P, Lemelle J, El Ghoneimi A, Moscovici J, Hameury F, Baumstark-Barrau K, Hery G, Guys JM. Sacral neuromodulation in children with urinary and fecal incontinence: a multicenter, open label, randomized, crossover study. *J Urol* 2010; **184**:696–701.

30 Roth TJ, Vandersteen DV, Hollatz P, et al. Sacral neuromodulation for dysfunctional elimination syndrome: a single center experience with 20 children. *J Urol* 2008; **180**:206.

CHAPTER 30

Botulinum toxin in the treatment of neuropathic lower urinary tract dysfunction

Paul F. Austin[1] and Israel Franco[2]

[1]*Division of Urologic Surgery, Washington University in St. Louis, School of Medicine, St. Louis Children's Hospital, St. Louis, MO, USA*

[2]*Maria Fareri Children's Hospital, Valhalla, NY, USA*

Pharmacology

Botulinum toxin

Botulinum toxin (BTX) is a neurotoxin protein produced by the gram-positive bacterium *Clostridium botulinum*. BTX acts by inhibiting acetylcholine release at the presynaptic neuromuscular junction, resulting in muscle paralysis. BTX has also been found to modulate both sensory and motor pathways by inhibiting the release of other neurotransmitters including adenosine triphosphate and neuropeptides such as substance P and downregulating the expression of purinergic and capsaicin receptors on afferent neurons within the bladder [1, 2]. These mechanisms of action have subsequently provided opportunities to modulate the lower urinary tract (LUT).

An extensive review of the history and the pathophysiology of BTX A is outlined in Chapter 22 in this textbook.

BTX has different formulations with different degrees of efficacy at the neuromuscular junction. (Table 30.1) The pharmacological and clinical details of the selected BTX formulation are important in the clinical application of the LUT. For this chapter, we will refer to the formulation of onabotulinumtoxinA unless stated otherwise.

Clinical application

Bladder

Clinically, BTX injections have been used safely for the treatment of focal dystonias, muscle spasm, and spasticity [3]. The application in the LUT has followed similar applications to diminish muscle spasticity and tone. BTX may be injected

Pediatric Incontinence: Evaluation and Clinical Management, First Edition. Edited by Israel Franco, Paul F. Austin, Stuart B. Bauer, Alexander von Gontard and Yves Homsy.

© 2015 John Wiley & Sons, Ltd. Published 2015 by John Wiley & Sons, Ltd.

Table 30.1 Botulinum toxin preparations and properties.

Botulinum toxin type	Generic name	Product name	Molecular size (kDa)	Units/vial (U)
Type A	OnabotulinumtoxinA	Botox®	900	100/200
Type A	AbobotulinumtoxinA	Dysport®	>300	300/500
Type A	IncobotulinumtoxinA	Xeomin®	150	100

into the detrusor muscle to reduce overactivity as well as improve detrusor compliance. This application can be used in either neuropathic or nonneuropathic bladders.

Presently, BTX is used after exhaustion of other medical treatments. Detrusor overactivity and low detrusor compliance are typically treated with anticholinergic therapy as outlined in Chapter 29. The indications for BTX subsequently include a lack of efficacy with anticholinergics, synergy with present anticholinergics, or intolerance toward anticholinergics.

Neuropathic bladder

Intravesical injection with BTX is considered an alternative treatment to improve continence and urodynamic parameters of neurogenic bladder in children. Although the FDA and the European Medicines Agency (EMA) have approved the usage of BTX for the treatment of adult patients for neuropathic bladder, BTX usage in children with neuropathic bladder is off-label and requires informed consent. There is a current pediatric trial that examines the use of onabotulinumtoxinA for urinary incontinence due to neurogenic detrusor overactivity in pediatric patients (*ClinicalTrials.gov Identifier: NCT01852045*).

A literature review summarizing the efficacy and safety profile of BTX in children with neuropathic bladder has been performed [4]. In this literature review, there is a significant improvement in clinical and urodynamic parameters as evidenced by complete continence in approximately 65–87% of patients, a reduction in the maximum detrusor pressure, and an increase in detrusor compliance in the majority of children treated with BTX. The minimal age for treatment in these small, uncontrolled studies was 2 years old, which corresponds to the minimal age that has been approved by the FDA and the EMEA for the treatment of spasticity from cerebral palsy. In most published studies, the dose of BTX of 8–10 U/kg is injected into the detrusor muscle with a maximal dose ranging from 100 to 300 U. It is noteworthy that the maximum FDA-approved total dosage for BTX injected into neuropathic bladder is 200 U. BTX reaches significant efficacy levels at 2 weeks and maximum effects within 4–6 weeks. Interestingly, the duration of the BTX effect ranges from 3 to 8 months depending on short-term versus long-term repeated injections [4]. In the authors' experiences, the duration is approximately 6–9 months.

Neuropathic sphincteric dysfunction

Another potential application of BTX in children with neurogenic bladder besides targeting the detrusor muscle includes treatment of the external urethral sphincter (EUS). This would be beneficial in the setting of detrusor–external sphincter dyssynergia (DSD). In a comparison study of the efficacy of BTX intravesical injections with and without injections into the EUS, there was a significant improvement in postvoiding residual volume only among patients with BTX injected at the EUS [5]. Both treatment methods resulted in a significant reduction in daily incontinence grade, constipation, and vesicoureteral reflux, but there were better outcomes for patients treated with concomitant BTX injections of the EUS in relation to incontinency, constipation, vesicoureteral reflux, and creatinine level.

Autonomic dysreflexia

The problem of autonomic dysreflexia in patients with thoracic and cervical lesions can be a difficult one to manage. It is a potentially fatal complication of such injuries and merits aggressive management. In some patients, they can be overly sensitive to stimuli from the bladder and be at risk for autonomic dysreflexia regularly, which is very disturbing to the patient and their caretakers. The authors (IF) have used it to manage this problem with excellent results in several patients utilizing the same dosing schedule as for neurogenic bladder detrusor overactivity. There is evidence in rats that it is an effective treatment for this problem as well and it appears that its mode of action is likely sensory, acting through a reduction in nerve growth factor. This reduction in NGF leads to afferent pathway desensitization and eventual reduction in autonomic dysreflexia in the patients [6].

BTX injection technique

The injection of BTX is performed under endoscopic guidance. The technical approaches are identical in children with neuropathic or nonneuropathic LUT dysfunction. BTX is generally reconstituted in 10 mL of injectable saline and injected intramuscularly or submucosally. Some people use 20 mL of saline to dilute the BTX for bladder injections so a larger area can be covered with the injections. There is insufficient data to suggest superiority of one technique over another.

Bladder injection

Patients are given perioperative antibiotics. The bladder is drained and refilled with a small amount of irrigation fluid to partially distend the bladder. The bladder volume for the procedure is approximately 25–50% of the expected bladder capacity. Optimal bladder distension volume is important to establish adequate visualization but not too much volume that would over distend and result in compression and thinning of the detrusor muscle resulting in an increased risk for BTX injection outside the bladder wall. Once the bladder filling is optimized for visualization, the BTX is injected in the posterior bladder wall 1 cm above the trigone. The injection is distributed over two rows along the posterior bladder wall and spaced approximately 0.5–1.0 cm apart. One author (PA) prefers to inject 8 U of BTX/kg up to a maximum of 200 U of BTX, while the other author (IF) prefers to inject 300 U of BTX up to 12 U/kg. The exact dose is a matter open to interpretation since there is some evidence that the larger dose does have a longer duration effect than the lower 200 U dose. We use a 9.5 FR offset cystoscope and a Williams needle that consists of a flexible shaft and a 8 mm needle tip or a needle that is available for the injection of Deflux, which is rigid. There are numerous other needles available for cystoscopic injection, which are user dependent. After the last injection, a 1.0 mL flush of normal saline is used to inject the remaining BTX from the needle system. The bladder is drained afterward and viscous lidocaine is placed into the urethra and bladder.

EUS injection

Unlike the bladder injection technique, the BTX injection approach into the EUS is different in males and females. The injection technique in males, however, is similar to the approach for bladder injections. Both occur transurethrally and employ the passage of a 23 gauge needle through the working channel of a 9.5 FR offset cystoscope. The EUS is visualized and injected at the 3, 6, 9, and 12 o'clock positions. In females, the cystoscope is placed into the urethra, but the injection is not done transurethrally but periurethrally. A 23 gauge spinal needle or a 25 gauge 2 in. needle is inserted periurethrally and under direct vision with the cystoscope right at the bladder neck. In this position, the needle can be seen if it protrudes past the bladder neck, and the BTX is injected at the midurethra at four quadrants at the 3, 6, 9, and 12 o'clock positions. The dose injected differs between authors. Either 100 U (PA) in 4 cc of saline or 200 U (IF) in 10 cc of saline can be injected.

Conclusion

In summary, the current pediatric trials investigating the treatment of children with neurogenic bladder and dysfunctional voiding are promising. Further clarification and optimization of BTX will elucidate the ultimate role of BTX in the management of pediatric LUT dysfunction. Furthermore, collection of detailed safety data in children will be necessary to support the reported excellent tolerability of BTX.

References

1 Apostolidis A, Dasgupta P, Fowler CJ. Proposed mechanism for the efficacy of injected botulinum toxin in the treatment of human detrusor overactivity. *Eur Urol.* 2006;**49**(4):644–50.

2 Chapple C, Patel A. Botulinum toxin—new mechanisms, new therapeutic directions? *Eur Urol.* 2006;**49**(4):606–8.

3 Grazko MA, Polo KB, Jabbari B. Botulinum toxin A for spasticity, muscle spasms, and rigidity. *Neurology.* 1995;**45**(4):712–7.

4 Game X, Mouracade P, Chartier-Kastler E, Viehweger E, Moog R, Amarenco G, et al. Botulinum toxin-A (Botox) intradetrusor injections in children with neurogenic detrusor overactivity/neurogenic overactive bladder: a systematic literature review. *J Pediatr Urol.* 2009;**5**(3):156–64.

5 Safari S, Jamali S, Habibollahi P, Arshadi H, Nejat F, Kajbafzadeh AM. Intravesical injections of botulinum toxin type A for management of neuropathic bladder: a comparison of two methods. *Urology.* 2010;**76**(1):225–30.

6 Elkelini MS, Bagli DJ, Fehlings M, Hassouna M. Effects of intravesical onabotulinumtoxinA on bladder dysfunction and autonomic dysreflexia after spinal cord injury: role of nerve growth factor. *BJU Int.* 2012;**109**(3):402–7.

CHAPTER 31

The surgical management of the neurogenic bladder

Elias Wehbi and Antoine E. Khoury

Department of Urology, Children's Hospital of Orange County, University of California in Irvine, Irvine, CA, USA

Introduction

The surgical management of the child with a neurogenic bladder (NGB) can oftentimes pose a challenge to the inexperienced surgeon. Not only does the accurate assessment of the severity of the condition pose a diagnostic dilemma for many physicians, but the surgical approach is frequently complex.

Treating these children should be consistent, regardless of the severity of the condition or variation in presentation. The goal of surgical management is to protect the upper urinary tract, create an ideal reservoir that provides low-pressure storage, avoid reservoir–ureteral reflux, and allow facile and complete emptying with a reliable continence mechanism that prevents the development of urinary tract infections.

It is also imperative to appreciate that the management of the urinary tract should not be undertaken in isolation. If the child is also incontinent of stool, embarking on a large reconstructive procedure to treat urinary incontinence without addressing the possibly even more troublesome stool incontinence, would not be in the best interests of the patient. The treatment of stool incontinence, although important, will not be discussed further in this chapter.

To achieve safe continence, it is imperative that the surgeon appreciates the overall balance between storage pressures and outlet resistance. Increasing outlet resistance without addressing the presence of elevated storage pressures, although may be safe in the short term, eventually will fail and ultimately prove detrimental to renal function.

Finally, bladder augmentation should be considered as a last resort. Bladder augmentation carries with it significant and lifelong consequences. There are

Pediatric Incontinence: Evaluation and Clinical Management, First Edition. Edited by Israel Franco,
Paul F. Austin, Stuart B. Bauer, Alexander von Gontard and Yves Homsy.
© 2015 John Wiley & Sons, Ltd. Published 2015 by John Wiley & Sons, Ltd.

established metabolic considerations and potential surgical complications that should not be underestimated. It is the surgeon's responsibility to ensure that all avenues of conservative treatment are exhausted, by maximizing anticholinergic use and by optimizing bladder emptying through clean intermittent catheterization (CIC). Overnight catheterization and injectables, such as onabotulinum toxin (Botox), are also worthwhile attempting [1].

Patients may present across the spectrum of disease severity; however, if one uses the aforementioned principles to guide their surgical approach, the patient can have the greatest chance of being infection-free, with healthy upper tracts and dry for life.

Evaluation of the patient with NGB

The mainstay of diagnostic investigations used to evaluate the child with a NGB who is being considered as a surgical candidate include ultrasound, VCUG, urodynamics, with or without the video component, and cystoscopy in select cases. When renal function is in question, blood work can be helpful, although with normal upper tracts on ultrasound, renal function is unlikely to be abnormal.

In those children with a significant leak, which can make the urodynamics evaluation of their bladder capacity and compliance difficult, the use of a Foley catheter can be helpful. This is a simple, yet extremely practical strategy to help identify those children with difficult to diagnose poor compliance and reduced capacity. In these children with low outlet resistance, spuriously low-pressure readings may be observed due to the low outlet resistance. With the Foley catheter occluding the outlet, any sudden rise in bladder cystometric pressure, which would not have been perceived on normal filling due to leak, should raise the clinician's suspicion of poor compliance, reduced storage capacity, and high cystometric pressures at low volumes. A negative test should be interpreted with caution and these children should nonetheless be monitored closely if an outlet resistance increasing procedure is considered as the long-term effects that may result in myogenic hypertrophy cannot be predicted. In this situation, a reconstructive procedure to correct the incontinence in isolation may place the child's upper tracts at risk.

Ensuring that a child has optimized their emptying schedule is critical before being considered a candidate for surgery. If a child maintains an elevated postvoid residual, due to incomplete catheterization or sporadic spontaneous voiding, their functional capacity is reduced and consequently complete bladder emptying improves storage capacity. Only when bladders are drained completely will storage occur in the low-pressure range. In those patients with hydronephrosis and hydroureter, overnight catheterization may be of significant benefit.

Patients who, despite optimal medical management with anticholinergic therapy, and bladder drainage regimens with regular CIC, continue to have incontinence, or in those where high pressures are seen at low volumes, surgical intervention should be considered.

In the case of newborns after closure of the spinal defect, urologic management should always include a predilection for initiation of CIC and can be initiated in hospital. This has several benefits, mainly that this approach is well tolerated and ensures safe management of upper tracts [2]. Once residuals are established to be at a safe volume, CIC can be tapered appropriately.

Surgical reconstruction: General principles

Principles of surgical reconstruction encompass preservation of the upper urinary tract, ensuring a safe reservoir for storage and preventing unwanted incontinence. Achieving this balance, while at the same time safeguarding the upper urinary tracts, should always be weighted toward establishing adequate storage capacity instead of increasing outlet resistance. When the patient presents with significant trabeculation, this provides evidence for the presence of outlet resistance. Often times patients may achieve a favorable result with regard to continence with a storage-improving procedure alone. This was well demonstrated in a cohort of patients where a significant proportion of those who had an augmentation cystoplasty alone were able to achieve continence, regardless of the appearance of the bladder neck on cystography [3].

Many patients may also present with vesicoureteral reflux, which is almost always secondary in nature. Treatment of the reflux without addressing the underlying primary bladder or outlet pathology will inevitably fail. Not only will injection with bulking agents, such as Deflux, or ureteric reimplantation be highly unsuccessful, but particularly in the case of reimplantation, the surgery itself can be quite challenging, even to the most experienced reconstructive surgeon. Some studies have also shown resolution of secondary reflux in children with optimal CIC regimens, although this may not be as predictable in children with the highest grades of reflux [4, 5].

Regardless of presentation, concomitant genitourinary anomalies or comorbidities, there is no standard approach for surgical management. Each child is unique and requires a tailored approach to ensure optimal care.

Components of surgical management for children with neuropathic bladders

There is a great deal of nuance to treating children with NGBs and thorough adherence to core principles of surgery by ensuring that stents are secured in place, adequate drainage is provided, and optimal postoperative pain control is established, keeping in mind that many patients have a decreased level of sensation, is crucial.

Unless ureteric reimplantation is performed, ureteric stents are rarely used. Latex allergies can be a serious issue and primary preventative programs can be of benefit, as well as the usage of nonlatex products throughout surgical care of all patients who frequently catheterize [6, 7]. Drains can also be of benefit; however, they are rarely required with good drainage per urethra. We prefer to leave a nonlatex Jackson-Pratt drain as a suprapubic tube. Many patients have ventriculoperitoneal shunts, and therefore, transperitoneal drains should be used with caution.

Approach to treating the bladder
Injectables to improve storage

Recent literature has shown an emerging role for Botox injections in the detrusor muscle for the treatment of children with NGBs [1, 8, 9]. Its durability is limited and for most patients, there is a need for repeat injections every 3–6 months. Several of the referenced studies have shown an improvement in capacity and compliance and also an improvement in urinary incontinence. There has also been an associated high satisfaction rate in some studies [1]. Botox may have an emerging role for the treatment of NGBs, delaying and possibly preventing the need for augmentation cystoplasty in select cases. Its long-term role is yet to be definitively established.

Augmentation cystoplasty

The incidence of augmentation cystoplasty appears to have been decreasing in recent years [10]. Reasons for this occurrence may be multifactorial and reflect changing national practice patterns. Ultimately, the recommendation for augmentation cystoplasty should only be made in select patients who have failed all other less invasive treatments, as this major surgery carries with it established surgical and metabolic risk factors. Compliance and partnership by the patients and their families are critical for a successful surgery and to establish long-term efficacy.

Contraindications to the surgery will only be mentioned, as we will focus on aspects of surgical care and technique. Contraindications include intrinsic bowel disease, such as Crohn's disease, congenital anomalies, previously resected bowel where further resection will place the child at risk for short bowel syndromes and in the context of previously irradiated bowel. Reduced manual dexterity, renal impairment, and limited cognitive function with inability to perform CIC are other relative contraindications [11]. Anticipated poor compliance by family or adolescent patients should also be considered a relative contraindication.

The two most commonly used segments of bowel are detubularized ileum or colon. Ileum appears to have less contractions and produces less mucous; however, one drawback is its higher metabolically active properties with regard to absorption, when compared to large intestine [12]. Although the colon has been shown to have more contractions and produce more mucous, it is less metabolically active than small bowel [11].

Oftentimes, a guiding approach when deciding on the segment of bowel to use during augmentation is the length of associated mesentery. In children with NGBs and bowels, there may be a large redundant sigmoid on a robust and mobile mesentery that can facilitate mobility of the bowel segment for tension-free anastomosis. In other cases, use of ileum for its previously described properties is preferred.

Regardless of the harvested portion or bowel, several configurations have been described for preparation of the bowel segment prior to augmentation [13]. Depending on the length of the segment, configuration can be fashioned appropriately. For short segments, a "U" configuration can be used, whereas as an "S" or "W" can be used for intermediate and longer segments, respectively. When choosing the type of bowel configuration and the type of bowel to be used, each has its own advantages and disadvantages and the surgeon should choose carefully, taking into account history of previous surgeries, concomitant endocrine and metabolic disturbances, as well as surgeon experience and preference.

In select patients where there is a nonfunctioning kidney with hydronephrosis and hydroureter, a unique opportunity may arise allowing augmentation of the bladder with the nonfunctioning collecting system, thereby eliminating the risk of metabolic disturbances associated with using intestine [14–16]. The surgeon should be vigilant of problems, which can arise when a suboptimal augmentation is performed if there is a deficiency of ureter or renal pelvis, or if the vascular pedicle is compromised.

Gastrocystoplasty has been largely abandoned as it is usually associated with significant metabolic disturbances, such as metabolic alkalosis and aciduria, despite oral treatment with oral proton pump inhibitors [17].

Similarly, the autoaugmentation, originally described in 1989 by Cartwright and Snow, has been shown to be an unfavorable surgical approach to children with NGBs [18–20]. Creation of a diverticulum to increase storage capacity is not a suitable long-term option as its durability is limited by the tendency to scar; contraction and gains in compliance, capacity, and contractility are limited at best. Modifications to the autoaugmentation have likewise failed to achieve results similar to the enterocystoplasty with regard to maximal storage potential and improve compliance [21].

Bladder incision

The classic clamshell cystoplasty was originally described by Bramble and later popularized by several others [13, 22–24]. This type of incision in the bladder can reduce the incidence of mucus trapping and stone formation in the augment by reducing the tendency to form an hourglass shape.

When the bladder is small, a clamshell incision may increase the risk of developing a configuration consistent with an hourglass shape. To avoid this, a star-type incision can be made in the bladder to widen the body of the augmented bladder. That technique has been shown to have comparable outcomes with the traditional incision and possibly further defunctionalize the bladder and increase the length of bladder edge available for the anastomosis [25].

Finally, should the need for creation of a catheterizable channel arise in a small bladder, an anterior bladder wall flap can be elevated as part of the cystoplasty to decrease the distance to the umbilicus. This is also helpful when the appendix is short.

Creation of a catheterizable channel

As a principle, the surgeon should have a low threshold for creation of a catheterizable channel at time of surgery to serve as a safety mechanism if spontaneous, complete voiding may not be possible, or if catheterization of the native urethra is difficult. Catheterizable channels such as an appendicovesicostomy, or a Monti, utilizing a segment of suitable bowel, are two of many, effective surgical options that the surgeon should have readily accessible in their armamentarium [26, 27]. As a general rule, it is useful to prevent redundancies in length and diameter of the catheterizable channel to lessen potential complications and promote easy and effective catheterization. If the need to reimplant the appendix or catheterizable channel into bowel arises, it is preferable to use the serous-lined extramural reimplant [28].

Catheterization can be challenging at first for some families and it is always advisable not to preceed with augmentation until the family is comfortable with CIC.

Procedures to increase outlet resistance

The mainstay of current surgical techniques for bladder outlet reconstruction, essentially, all involve increasing the resistance with the creation of a nondynamic outlet with increased yet fixed outlet resistance. The object should be to instill as many of the dynamic properties inherent to the native sphincter complex.

Increasing this outlet resistance can either be done with injection of bulking agents, bladder neck constriction by narrowing the lumen, lengthening the lumen, or by external compression, usually through a sling or with an artificial urinary sphincter. Ideally, the goal of all these approaches is to create a balanced obstruction, where safe storage can occur until a threshold volume and pressure is reached, where leakage through the continence mechanism will act as a popoff mechanism, reducing the likelihood of renal injury.

In select cases, closure of the bladder neck may be useful if reconstruction with a catheterizable urethra is not possible; however, it is not elaborated on in great detail here [29, 30].

We will focus on the approach of bladder neck reconstruction as a primary means to achieve continence, and provide a few pearls for those that use bulking agents in those children with mild incontinence, or in the setting postbladder neck reconstruction where there is persistent incontinence.

Bulking agents

Several materials have been used to bulk the bladder neck in an attempt to optimize continence. Durability has been studied extensively with no clear long-term efficacy [31, 32]. Our approach generally utilizes bulking agents as supplement to partially successful surgery or when incontinence is mild, with the knowledge that there is no universally acceptable grading system for incontinence in children.

Both transurethral (retrograde) and antegrade, usually through a suprapubic tract, approaches have been described. Our preference is to perform an antegrade injection, with simultaneous endoscopic views through the urethra and through a suprapubic tract. Injecting in a transurethral retrograde fashion alone can be misleading with regard to deposition of the bulking agent bolus. Typically, we use Macroplastique as the bulking agent, injecting in the 5 and 7 o'clock locations. Others have described injecting in males at the bladder neck and below the verumontanum in males, and along the urethra in females [33].

Bladder neck surgery

There have been several approaches to achieve continence in the child with an incompetent bladder neck. Notable are the Young–Dees–Leadbetter (YDL) procedure, the Kropp procedure, and the Pippi Salle bladder neck reconstruction [34–40]. Several variations of these have been described, some with suspensions and slings; however, we will not focus on these techniques beyond their mention. The Mitchell modification of the YDL

In 1993, Jones, Mitchell, and Rink described a modification of the existing YDL procedure that is worth mentioning and is our preferred approach for reconstruction of the bladder neck [41]. This modification bares notable importance as it narrows the bladder neck without sacrificing vital bladder capacity, effectively increasing the length of the resistant, narrow portion of the bladder neck. Some studies have shown a less than optimal rate of success with the modification of the YDL in children with NGBs, and so we carefully assess the need for additional support with an autologous fascial sling to maximize the child's chance at achieving complete dryness [39, 42, 43]. In males, we place the sling proximal to the prostate, which improves its efficacy.

Fascial slings

The use of a fascial sling can be quite helpful in optimizing a bladder neck procedure to give the child the best chance at complete dryness. Several authors have used the addition of a fascial sling with good continence results in patients who have and have not undergone augmentation [44, 45].

The dissection for passage of the sling, described by Lottmann et al., usually involves passing the sling between the bladder and rectum in boys and bladder and vagina in girls. This reduces the injury to the urethra by establishing the plane of dissection for passage of the sling from above [46].

Artificial urinary sphincter

The artificial urinary sphincter (AUS) remains an attractive option for those with incontinence as it is the only surgical intervention that can replicate the normal sphincteric mechanism. It has been used in children who void spontaneously and those that require catheterization [47]. The need for revision occurs in at least 50% of children, and in some large series, removal in up to 20% [48]. More contemporary mechanical devices have reduced the need for reoperation; however, regardless of the device used, all children with an AUS should be followed lifelong.

Summary

The approach to surgical treatment of the child with urinary incontinence due to a NGB can pose a difficult diagnostic and surgical dilemma. Although children may present with the same signs of incontinence, the successful approach to each may be drastically different and should be tailored, based on the underlying issues they have with regard to storage capacity, bladder compliance, and outlet resistance.

Approaching the child in a systematic way, evaluating the capacity of the bladder and its compliance, critically examining the quality of their outlet and continence mechanism, and taking great care to ensure that secondary conditions such as reflux are addressed in a thoughtful way will allow for the best possible outcome in the greatest number of patients. Without minimizing its impact on a child's quality of life, ultimately incontinence is an extremely troublesome social issue. A guiding principle should be that no surgical intervention should ever lead to damage of the upper urinary tracts and transform a social issue into a serious medical one.

References

1 Figueroa V, Romao R, Pippi-Salle JL, Koyle MA, Braga LHP, Bagli DJ, et al. Single-center experience with botulinum toxin endoscopic detrusor injection for the treatment of congenital neuropathic bladder in children: effect of dose adjustment, multiple injections, and avoidance of reconstructive procedures. *J Pediatr Urol*. 2013 Nov;**10**(2):368–73.

2 Pohl HG, Bauer SB, Borer JG, Diamond DA, Kelly MD, Grant R, et al. The outcome of voiding dysfunction managed with clean intermittent catheterization in neurologically and anatomically normal children. *BJU Int*. 2002 Jun;**89**(9):923–7.

3 Khoury AE, Dave S, Peralta-Del Valle MH, Braga LHP, Lorenzo AJ, Bagli D. Severe bladder trabeculation obviates the need for bladder outlet procedures during augmentation cystoplasty in incontinent patients with neurogenic bladder. *BJU Int*. 2008 Jan;**101**(2):223–6.

4 Agarwal SK, McLorie GA, Grewal D, Joyner BD, Bagli DJ, Khoury AE. Urodynamic correlates of resolution of reflux in meningomyelocele patients. *J Urol*. 1997 Aug;**158**(2):580–2.

5 Agarwal SK, Khoury AE, Abramson RP, Churchill BM, Argiropoulos G, McLorie GA. Outcome analysis of vesicoureteral reflux in children with myelodysplasia. *J Urol*. 1997 Mar;**157**(3):980–2.

6 Cremer R, Kleine-Diepenbruck U, Hering F, Holschneider AM. Reduction of latex sensitisation in spina bifida patients by a primary prophylaxis programme (five years experience). *Eur J Pediatr Surg*. 2002 Dec;**12**(Suppl. 1):S19–21.

7 Martínez-Lage JF, Moltó MA, Pagán JA. Latex allergy in patients with spina bifida: prevention and treatment. *Neurocirugia (Astur)*. 2001;**12**(1):36–42.

8 Marte A. Onabotulinumtoxin A for treating overactive/poor compliant bladders in children and adolescents with neurogenic bladder secondary to myelomeningocele. *Toxins (Basel)*. 2013 Jan;**5**(1):16–24.

9 Sager C, Burek C, Bortagaray J, Corbetta JP, Weller S, Durán V, et al. Repeated injections of intradetrusor onabotulinumtoxinA as adjunctive treatment of children with neurogenic bladder. *Pediatr Surg Int*. 2014 Jan;**30**(1): 79–85.

10 Schlomer BJ, Saperston K, Baskin L. National trends in augmentation cystoplasty in the 2000s and factors associated with patient outcomes. *J Urol*. 2013 Oct;**190**(4):1352–7.

11 Biers SM, Venn SN, Greenwell TJ. The past, present and future of augmentation cystoplasty. *BJU Int*. 2012 May;**109**(9):1280–93.

12 Smith GL, Kobashi KC. Augmentation cystoplasty. *Curr Bladder Dysfunct Rep*. 2011 Mar;**6**(1):31–6.

13 Mast P, Hoebeke P, Wyndaele JJ, Oosterlinck W, Everaert K. Experience with augmentation cystoplasty. *A review. Paraplegia*. 1995 Oct;**33**(10):560–4.

14 MF Bellinger. Ureterocystoplasty: a unique method for vesical augmentation in children. *J Urol*. 1993 Apr;**149**(4):811–3.

15 Churchill BM, Aliabadi H, Landau EH, McLorie GA, Steckler RE, McKenna PH, et al. Ureteral bladder augmentation. *J Urol*. 1993 Aug;**150**(2 Pt 2):716–20.

16 Landau EH, Jayanthi VR, Khoury AE, Churchill BM, Gilmour RF, Steckler RE, et al. Bladder augmentation: ureterocystoplasty versus ileocystoplasty. *J Urol*. 1994 Aug;**152**(2 Pt 2):716–9.

17 Kinahan TJ, Khoury AE, McLorie GA, Churchill BM. Omeprazole in post-gastrocystoplasty metabolic alkalosis and aciduria. *J Urol*. 1992 Feb;**147**(2):435–7.

18 Stothers L, Johnson H, Arnold W, Coleman G, Tearle H. Bladder autoaugmentation byvesicomyotomy in the pediatric neurogenic bladder. *Urology*. 1994 Jul;**44**(1):110–3.

19 MacNeily AE, Afshar K, Coleman GU, Johnson HW. Autoaugmentation by detrusor myotomy: its lack of effectiveness in the management of congenital neuropathic bladder. *J Urol*. 2003 Oct;**170**(4 Pt 2):1643–6; discussion, 1646.

20 Cartwright PC, Snow BW. Bladder autoaugmentation: early clinical experience. *J Urol*. 1989 Aug;**142**(2 pt 2):505–8; discussion 520–521.

21 Buson H, Manivel JC, Dayanç M, Long R. Seromuscular colocystoplasty lined with urothelium: experimental study. *Urology*. 1994 Nov;**44**(5):743–8.

22 BRAMBLE FJ. The clam cystoplasty. *Br J Urol*. 1990 Oct;**66**(4):337–41.

23 BRAMBLE FJ. The treatment of adult enuresis and urge incontinence by enterocystoplasty. *Br J Urol*. 1982 Dec;**54**(6):693–6.

24 Eltahawy EA, Virasoro R, Schlossberg SM, McCammon KA, Jordan GH. Long-term followup for excision and primary anastomosis for anterior urethral strictures. *J Urol*. 2007 May;**177**(5):1803–6.

25 Keating MA, Ludlow JK, Rich MA. Enterocystoplasty: the star modification. *J Urol*. 1996 May;**155**(5):1723–5.

26 Leslie B, Lorenzo AJ, Moore K, Farhat WA, Bagli DJ, Pippi Salle JL. Long-term followup and time to event outcome analysis of continent catheterizable channels. *J Urol*. 2011 Jun;**185**(6):2298–302.

27 Monti PR, Lara RC, Dutra MA, de Carvalho JR. New techniques for construction of efferent conduits based on the Mitrofanoff principle. *Urology*. 1997 Jan;**49**(1):112–5.

28 Abol-Enein H, Ghoneim MA. Functional results of orthotopic ileal neobladder with serouslined extramural ureteral reimplantation: experience with 450 patients. *J Urol*. 2001 May;**165**(5):1427–32.

29 Nguyen HT, Baskin LS. The outcome of bladder neck closure in children with severe urinary incontinence. *J Urol*. 2003 Mar;**169**(3):1114–6; discussion 1116.

30 Bergman J, Lerman SE, Kristo B, Chen A, Boechat MI, Churchill BM. Outcomes of bladder neck closure for intractable urinary incontinence in patients with neurogenic bladders. *J Pediatr Urol*. 2006 Dec;**2**(6):528–33.

31 Lottmann HB, Margaryan M, Bernuy M, Rouffet M-J, Bau M-O, El-Ghoneimi A, et al. The effect of endoscopic injections of dextranomer based implants on continence and bladder capacity: a prospective study of 31 patients. *J Urol*. 2002 Oct;**168**(4 Pt 2):1863–7; discussion 1867.

32 Ramseyer P, Meagher-Villemure K, Burki M, Frey P. (Poly)acrylonitrile-based hydrogel as a therapeutic bulking agent in urology. *Biomaterials*. 2007 Feb;**28**(6):1185–90.

33 Lottmann HB, Margaryan M, Lortat-Jacob S. Long-term effects of dextranomer endoscopic injections for the treatment of urinary incontinence: an update of a prospective study of 61 patients. *J Urol*. 2006 Oct;**176**(4):1762–6.

34 Kropp KA, Angwafo FF. Urethral lengthening and reimplantation for neurogenic incontinence in children. *J Urol*. 1986 Mar;**135**(3):533–6.

35 Mollard P, Mouriquand P, Joubert P. Urethral lengthening for neurogenic urinary incontinence (Kropp's procedure): results of 16 cases. *J Urol*. 1990 Jan;**143**(1):95–7.

36 Dave S, Salle JLP. Current status of bladder neck reconstruction. *Curr Opin Urol*. 2008 Jul;**18**(4):419–24.

37 Salle JL, McLorie GA, Bagli DJ, Khoury AE. Modifications of and extended indications for the Pippi Salle procedure. *World J Urol*. 1998;**16**(4):279–84.

38 Kryger JV, González R, Barthold JS. Surgical management of urinary incontinence in children with neurogenic sphincteric incompetence. *J Urol*. 2000 Jan;**163**(1):256–63.

39 Leadbetter GW. Surgical reconstruction for complete urinary incontinence: a 10 to 22-year followup. *J Urol*. 1985 Feb;**133**(2):205–6.

40 Young HH. An operation for the cure of incontinence of urine. *Surg Gynecol Obstet*. 1919;**28**:84–90.

41 Jones JA, Mitchell ME, Rink RC. Improved results using a modification of the Young–Dees–Leadbetter Bladder neck repair. *Br J Urol*. 1993 May;**71**(5):555–61.

42 Sidi AA, Reinberg Y, Gonzalez R. Comparison of artificial sphincter implantation and bladder neck reconstruction in patients with neurogenic urinary incontinence. *J Urol*. 1987 Oct;**138**(4 Pt 2):1120–2.

43 Tanagho EA. Bladder neck reconstruction for total urinary incontinence: 10 years experience. *J Urol*. 1981 Mar;**125**(3):321–6.

44 Snodgrass W, Barber T, Cost N. Detrusor compliance changes after bladder neck sling without augmentation in children with neurogenic urinary incontinence. *J Urol*. 2010 Jun;**183**(6):2361–6.

45 Castellan M, Gosalbez R, Labbie A, Ibrahim E, Disandro M. Bladder neck sling for treatment of neurogenic incontinence in children with augmentation cystoplasty: long-term follow-up. *J Urol*. 2005 Jun;**173**(6):2128–31; discussion 2131.

46 Lottmann H, Traxer O, Aigrain Y, Melin Y. Posterior approach to the bladder for implantation of the 800 AMS artificial sphincter in children and adolescents: techniques and results in eight patients. *Ann Urol (Paris)*. 1999;**33**(5):357–63.

47 Catti M, Lortat-Jacob S, Morineau M, Lottmann H. Artificial urinary sphincter in children—voiding or emptying? An evaluation of functional results in 44 patients. *J Urol*. 2008 Aug;**180**(2):690–3.

48 Herndon CDA, Rink RC, Shaw MBK, Simmons GR, Cain MP, Kaefer M, et al. The Indiana experience with artificial urinary sphincters in children and young adults. *J Urol*. 2003 Feb;**169**(2):650–4; discussion 654.

CHAPTER 32

Surgery for bowel dysfunction

Terry L. Buchmiller

Department of Surgery, Boston Children's Hospital, Harvard Medical School, Boston, MA, USA

Introduction

Severe intractable constipation, often in combination with fecal incontinence, is a rare but disabling condition in the pediatric population. This may be idiopathic, or occur in the setting of complicated disease processes such as congenital anorectal malformations, genetic conditions, and spinal cord dysfunction from myelodysplasia, tethering, or injury. If maximal medical therapy does not provide an effective solution, surgical intervention can provide additional management options to achieve social continence. The reader is referred to previous chapters that detail the evaluation of colonic motility disorders.

The surgeon should confirm thorough medical, pathologic, and motility evaluation prior to intervention. Full-thickness rectal biopsies, an examination under anesthesia, and contrast studies may be recommended as the individual situation dictates.

This chapter will review the most common surgical procedures used to manage severe intractable constipation, and provide an overview of the principles underlying their application. Benefits, risks, and long-term expectations are briefly discussed. Many of these surgical procedures have been studied in great detail in diverse patient populations, and an exhaustive review is beyond the scope of this chapter. Multidisciplinary management teams, including gastroenterologists, urologists, and psychiatric support providers are instrumental to long-term patient success.

Pediatric Incontinence: Evaluation and Clinical Management, First Edition. Edited by Israel Franco, Paul F. Austin, Stuart B. Bauer, Alexander von Gontard and Yves Homsy.
© 2015 John Wiley & Sons, Ltd. Published 2015 by John Wiley & Sons, Ltd.

Antegrade continence enemas

Malone first introduced the concept of providing access to the cecum to administer antegrade colonic enemas [1] through the native appendix as a conduit in 1990. Providing access to the most proximal part of the colon allows the lavage to be administered antegrade in concert with the native intrinsic contractions and promotes complete colonic evacuation. Additionally, in children where rectal enema administration is no longer tolerated, or if greater independence is desired, antegrade administration is a preferable alternative. There are several decades of experience with this technique that has improved the quality of life in many pediatric patients. Surgeons managing children with the aforementioned disorders should avoid the "incidental appendectomy" to allow a full spectrum of options in potential surgical management.

The conduit is constructed utilizing the native *in situ* appendix. The appendiceal tip is removed to provide access through the appendix to the lumen of cecum. Many surgeons will try to construct an "antireflux" mechanism that renders the channel continent to minimize the leakage of mucous, and prevent the leakage of stool or flatus. The appendix can be imbricated in the cecal wall providing an intussusception type valve, imbricated into the cecal wall with a Witzel-type closure, or placed in a seromuscular channel within the cecal wall, similar in concept to a ureteral reimplantation (Figure 32.1).

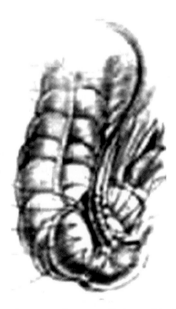

Figure 32.1 Appendicostomy schematic. The appendix is used *in situ* as a conduit for the administration of antegrade flushes. The appendix is imbricated into the cecal wall to minimize leaking.

Depending on the type of construction the surgeon prefers, this is often done by an open surgical technique, although the laparoscopic approach is amenable to the more simple configurations. The appendiceal opening is usually located in a lower umbilical fold for greatest cosmesis. It can also be located in the RLQ above the scar if preferred by the patient or if the umbilicus is being utilized for a Mitrofanoff for urinary catheterization. The initial catheter is typically left in place the first several weeks while the channel heals. The catheter is then removed in the office and intermittent catheterization is taught to the patient and family. Antegrade enema administration is typically begun daily utilizing 15 cc/kg of normal saline to minimize cramping. Eventual transition to a polyethylene glycol solution is often undertaken. A log to monitor efficacy is encouraged, and adjustment of the enema solution over time to achieve social continence should be anticipated. The channel should be catheterized daily to prevent stenosis of the opening. The patient and family must consider acceptance of this daily intubation of a tract from a psychological and practical standpoint versus the presence of an indwelling medical device (see "Cecostomy"). Indeed, noncompliance with the antegrade continence enema (ACE) has been shown to be a predictor of failure [2].

Successful management of constipation and fecal incontinence occurs in 73–96% in diverse populations using an ACE [3]. Children with structural issues, such as anorectal malformations tend to demonstrate better outcomes. Those with idiopathic constipation are a diverse group including those with severe total colonic neuropathy. These patients are a particular challenge that may not respond as predictably to an ACE [4].

The overall incidence of complications can range from 25 to 63% in most series [5] and includes stricture, leakage, prolapse, and intestinal obstruction.

The appendiceal opening at the skin level may become stenotic in 10–30% over time due to local trauma, ischemia, or the natural tendency toward scar contraction. Therefore, it is typically created in a V–V or V–Y fashion to minimize this risk. If becoming snug, the patient can leave the catheter taped *in situ* for several days or the surgeon can perform dilations. If refractory, most stenosis can be managed by surgical revision of the skin/subcutaneous channel on an outpatient basis.

Leakage from the tract is uncommon. One should ensure efficacy of the flushes to minimize the stool burden. If persistent, the submucosa of the tract may be injected with a bulking agent such as Deflux® (Salix Pharmaceuticals, Inc., Raleigh, NC). In refractory situations, revision of the tract may be required. The creation of a false passage and tract perforation are very rare events. Contrast studies may be judiciously used to query channels that have become difficult to reliably cannulate.

In some cases, conduits for urinary and colonic catheterization can be created at the same surgical setting. Occasionally, the appendix is of sufficient length to be split to construct both conduits. However, this is never assured until the operation is underway. Close coordination to discuss a contingency plan within the operative team in accordance with the patient's preferences should be delineated preoperatively, and optimally, recorded in the surgical consent or medical record.

Kiely described the creation of a catheterizable conduit if the appendix is surgically absent or previously utilized as a urinary conduit [6]. A "neoappendicostomy" using a cecal flap can be constructed if a catheterizable channel is still desired. Chatoorgoon reported a significant experience in 80 patients with an overall rate of stricture in only 11% and leakage in 9% [7]. This improved to an even lower rate within the series as experience accrued. Though more technically demanding, particularly in obese patients, this is a reasonable alternative.

Some authors have preferred an ACE created with a tubularized bowel conduit into the left or sigmoid colon to decrease symptoms of bloating and discomfort during flush administration [8]. However, the excellent results of most series with the classic ACE would not uniformly support this approach.

In cases where the etiology of the colonic dysfunction is expected to be permanent such as myelodysplasia, an ACE may be utilized long-term. In situations such as idiopathic constipation, where colonic recovery may be anticipated in the majority, a several-year period of colonic "rest" is recommended. The baseline colonic manometry has not been shown to be predictive of success [9]. Repeat colonic manometry testing at one-year post-ACE has shown significant improvement in most [2]. The restoration of normal HAPC's on repeat testing was associated with ACE decrease and may be predictive of ultimate outcome [9]. Flushes may be tapered and spontaneous bowel movements recorded. If the ACE is no longer needed, the tract may be allowed to stenose and close down, or the tract may be surgically closed by a modified appendectomy.

Cecostomy

If catheterization of a tract is not desirable, access to the cecum for ACE flushes may be provided by placement of an indwelling medical device located in the right lower quadrant. Products such as the MIC-Key® (Kimberly-Clark Worldwide, Inc.) or MINI-One® (Applied Medical Technology, Inc.) buttons allow for a skin level device if the abdominal wall is not too thick. These are secured by an intraluminal water filled balloon. Anchoring Stamm-type sutures are encouraged at initial placement to prevent tract disruption if accidental dislodgement occurs during the healing phase. We prefer to place our cecostomy tubes under laparoscopic and endoscopic guidance (LAPEC, laparoscopic assisted, percutaneous endoscopic cecostomy) to maximize safety as reported by Rodriguez [10]. Conversion to an open procedure occurs in approximately 2%, and intraoperative complications are rare.

In obese patients, a longer PEG-type tube must be first utilized. Placement of a percutaneous endoscopic cecostomy (PEC) should utilize a full bowel preparation to minimize fecal contamination of the abdominal wall as a pull-technique is used. Laparoscopic visualization is also encouraged, although Stamm sutures are not mandatory as the intraluminal disc is quite secure. A custom length skin level device may be later ordered, or the tube changed to a more pliable product once healing of the tract has occurred. Cecostomy tubes may also be placed by an open technique, laparoscopic, or in interventional radiology. The Chait Trapdoor system® (Cook Medical, Inc.) provides another alternative skin level device.

Complications of a cecostomy include the development of granulation tissue and the rare tube dislodgement. Granulation tissue may be treated with topical agents as needed, and if recalcitrant, surgical excision may be warranted. The balloon should be checked weekly to ensure proper function. We do not recommend changing the device at mandated time intervals. Rather, the device can be changed electively when mechanical issues arise such as balloon leakage, or the fit needs to be adjusted due to weight changes. One may instruct the family how to change the cecostomy button, similar to routine gastrostomy changes. If the change is atraumatic, and stool contents are verified, a contrast study is not mandated.

When a cecostomy is no longer needed, surgical closure of the tract is preferred as spontaneous closure of the remaining colocutaneous fistula, though possible, is typically gradual and the ensuing drainage of stool undesirable.

Diversion

Temporary

Patients suffering from severe constipation that has been refractory to medical management are candidates for complete diversion of the fecal stream by placing an ileostomy. This is the most aggressive way to "rest" the colon to allow for relief of dilation and recovery of function. Many have undergone attempts at enema therapy, either per rectum or by placement of an ACE or cecostomy. Patients with significant total colonic dysfunction on motility testing are a subset more prone to failure of lavage therapy. If the colon is markedly dilated (Figure 32.2), proceeding directly to ileostomy placement as a primary surgical procedure should be considered. In these circumstances, formal colonic motility testing may be bypassed as it will uniformly be markedly abnormal.

Most surgeons choose an end ileostomy as the incidence of prolapse is lessened versus a loop stoma [11]. Some will perform stomapexy at the primary operation to minimize this risk, but must be cognizant that intra-abdominal tethering, particularly if the small bowel is dilated may predispose to obstruction. One is fortunate to create the "perfect" stoma in cases of bowel dysmotility, as stomas tend to prolapse, stenose, or retract.

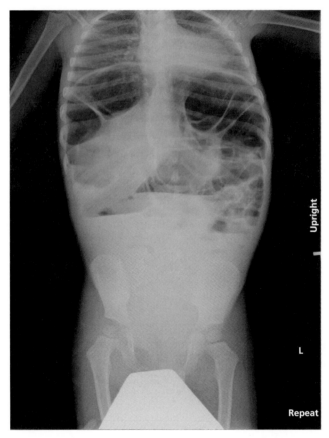

Figure 32.2 Massive colonic dilation. This KUB shows massive colonic distension with elevation of the diaphragms and resultant atelectasis. Such children failing medical management may proceed directly to diverting ileostomy.

Families are asked to plan on diversion for several years to allow for potential recovery of colonic function [2]. If colonic recovery is documented, simple stoma reversal is undertaken. If the colon is still dysfunctional after prolonged diversion, the stoma may be left, or reversal combined with an ACE, cecostomy, or colonic resection based on preoperative manometry testing. Subtotal colectomy may be preferred as segmental resections may not provide sustained results.

Permanent

Permanent diversion by placement of an end ileostomy or colostomy may be considered in patients suffering from neurogenic bowel with severe incontinence, typically in combination with refractory constipation in whom medical management and an antegrade conduit (MACE/cecostomy) has not been successful in managing soiling. This is quite uncommon, but could be chosen to promote quality of life for the patient and their caregiver.

Colonic resection

Colonic motility testing will often reveal a segmental portion of the colon that is significantly more dysfunctional versus severe total colonic involvement. This is typically the sigmoid or left colon in the majority. It is logical to assume that removal of the offending segment with end-to-end restoration of continuity could provide a "cure." Unfortunately, numerous studies have not given support to sustainable success [2]. The performance of a total colectomy with ileoanal anastomosis would certainly eliminate constipation and has been applied with success with very low complication rates in the adult population [12]. However, this aggressive treatment has not been embraced in the pediatric population.

One exception may be when a portion of the colon, typically the rectosigmoid, has developed massive dilation, the so-called megarectum/megasigmoid. These areas can harbor massive impactions of stool that are refractory to medical and lavage therapy (Figure 32.3). Primary colonic resection back to normal caliber bowel and restoration of continuity has provided longer term satisfactory outcomes [13].

Colonic resection has a significant role as a secondary procedure in those patients who have failed to respond to an ACE or diversion. Colonic resection, either segmental or total, has led to improvement or resolution of symptoms in the majority of patients who failed cecostomy [4]. However, this is a complex and

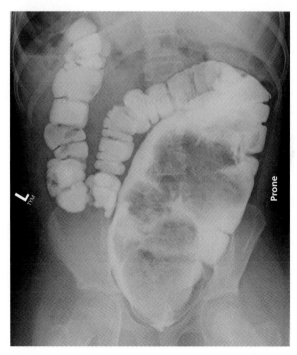

Figure 32.3 Megarectum. The contrast enema shows massive segmental chronic dilation of the rectum or "megarectum" with fecal impaction.

heterogeneous group and some will have continued issues. A conduit for antegrade flushes may be considered in combination with resection as a safeguard.

Conclusion

Numerous surgical options exist for assistance in the management of severe refractory constipation and/ or fecal incontinence. The surgeon should confirm a complete preoperative evaluation and carefully review all applicable options with the patient and family. A full discussion about the range of outcomes, risks, and expectations should be carefully reviewed. Surgeon involvement should be expected to be long-term to ensure the greatest chance of individual success, while providing long-term outcome data for continuous quality assessment.

References

1 Malone PS, Ransley PG, Kiely EM. Preliminary report: the antegrade continence enema. *Lancet*. 1990 Nov;**336**(8725):1217–8.

2 Christison-Lagay ER, Rodriguez L, Kurtz M, St Pierre K, Doody DP, Goldstein AM. Antegrade colonic enemas and intestinal diversion are highly effective in the management of children with intractable constipation. *J Pediatr Surg*. 2010 Jan;**45**(1):213–9; discussion 219.

3 Siddiqui AA, Fishman SJ, Bauer SB, Nurko S. Long-term follow-up of patients after antegrade continence enema procedure. *J Pediatr Gastroenterol Nutr*. 2011 May;**52**(5):574–80.

4 Bonilla SF, Flores A, Jackson CC, Chwals WJ, Orkin BA. Management of pediatric patients with refractory constipation who fail cecostomy. *J Pediatr Surg*. 2013 Sep;**48**(9):1931–5.

5 Rangel SJ, Lawal TA, Bischoff A, Chatoorgoon K, Louden E, Peña A, Levitt MA. The appendix as a conduit for antegrade continence enemas in patients with anorectal malformations: lessons learned from 163 cases treated over 18 years. *J Pediatr Surg*. 2011 Jun;**46**(6):1236–42.

6 Kiely EM, Ade-Ajayi N, Wheeler RA. Caecal flap conduit for antegrade continence enemas. *Br J Surg*. 1994 Aug;**81**(8):1215.

7 Chatoorgoon K, Pena A, Lawal T, Hamrick M, Louden E, Levitt MA. Neoappendicostomy in the management of pediatric fecal incontinence. *J Pediatr Surg*. 2011 Jun;**46**(6):1243–9.

8 Kim SM, Han SW, Choi SH. Left colonic antegrade continence enema: experience gained from 19 cases. *J Pediatr Surg*. 2006 Oct;**41**(10):1750–4.

9 Rodriguez L, Nurko S, Flores A. Factors associated with successful decrease and discontinuation of antegrade continence enemas (ACE) in children with defecation disorders: a study evaluating the effect of ACE on colon motility. *Neurogastroenterol Motil*. 2013 Feb;**25**(2):140–e81.

10 Rodriguez L, Flores A, Gilchrist BF, Goldstein AM. Laparoscopic-assisted percutaneous endoscopic cecostomy in children with defecation disorders (with video). *Gastrointest Endosc*. 2011 Jan;**73**(1):98–102.

11 Fonkalsrud EW, Thakur A, Roof L. Comparison of loop versus end ileostomy for fecal diversion after restorative proctocolectomy for ulcerative colitis. *J Am Coll Surg*. 2000 Apr;**190**(4):418–22.

12 Thakur A, Fonkalsrud EW, Buchmiller T, French S. Surgical treatment of severe colonic inertia with restorative proctocolectomy. *Am Surg*. 2001 Jan;**67**(1):36–40.

13 Eradi B, Hamrick M, Bischoff A, Frischer JS, Helmrath M, Hall J, Peña A, Levitt MA. The role of a colon resection in combination with a Malone appendicostomy as part of a bowel management program for the treatment of fecal incontinence. *J Pediatr Surg*. 2013 Nov;**48**(11):2296–300.

CHAPTER 33

Neurological surgery for neurogenic bladder dysfunction

Michael S. Park[1] and Gerald F. Tuite[1,2]

[1] Department of Neurosurgery & Brain Repair, Morsani College of Medicine, University of South Florida, Tampa, FL, USA

[2] Neuroscience Institute, All Children's Hospital/Johns Hopkins Medicine, St. Petersburg, FL, USA

Introduction

Pediatric neurosurgeons often work in close collaboration with their urological counterparts to diagnose and treat abnormalities of the central and peripheral nervous system that lead to neurogenic bladder dysfunction (NBD). These collaborations have strengthened over the past 25 years as MRI has allowed markedly improved diagnostic ability. Tethered spinal cord (TSC) is the most common condition, but there are numerous developmental, structural, and neoplastic abnormalities that tie the two specialties. Improved diagnostic accuracy and availability, coupled with improvements in microsurgical technique and intraoperative neurophysiologic monitoring, have also led to an increase in the frequency of neurosurgical operations for NBD. In addition to tethered cord release (TCR), other nerve sectioning, stimulation, and rerouting techniques have been explored as potential solutions to NBD. We review the most common conditions, their diagnosis, evaluation, treatment, outcomes, and complications in this chapter.

Tethered spinal cord

Tethered spinal cord can result from either open spinal defects (OSD), such as myelomeningocele (MMC), or closed (skin covered) spinal defects (CSD). CSD may or may not be associated with a subcutaneous mass (Figure 33.1), and include abnormalities associated with imperforate anus, thickened or fatty infiltration of the filum (Figure 33.2), split cord malformations (diastematomyelia and diplomyelia), anterior meningocele, sacrococcygeal teratoma, and spinal cord syrinx.

Pediatric Incontinence: Evaluation and Clinical Management, First Edition. Edited by Israel Franco, Paul F. Austin, Stuart B. Bauer, Alexander von Gontard and Yves Homsy.

© 2015 John Wiley & Sons, Ltd. Published 2015 by John Wiley & Sons, Ltd.

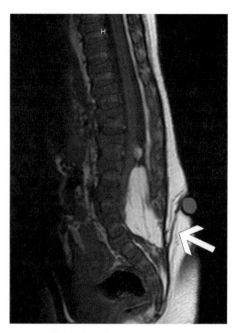

Figure 33.1 T1 sagittal lumbosacral spine MRI of patient with spinal cord lipoma and tethered cord. Note the low-lying spinal cord with a large fatty mass (white). A vitamin E capsule was taped to skin over the lipoma, corresponding to an area of a small skin dimple, which is associated with a dermal sinus tract (arrow).

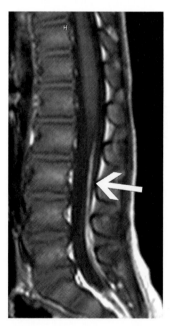

Figure 33.2 T1 sagittal lumbosacral spine MRI of patient with fatty infiltration of the filum (arrow). The conus terminates at L2.

Typical neurologic presenting signs and symptoms of TSC include back and leg pain, foot deformities, scoliosis, and motor disturbances, which can manifest with subtle decrements in gait, coordination, and endurance. Sensory changes can occur but they are relatively rarely seen in isolation. Urologic symptoms of TSC are also common, including incontinence (especially worsening incontinence in patients with prior TSC release) and urinary tract infections. On occasion, there may be issues with constipation and bowel incontinence in addition to urinary dysfunction. Patients with occult spinal dysraphism will also frequently have one or more orthopedic deformities, usually involving the foot or hip [1].

Imaging, nearly always MRI, should be obtained as part of the work up for TSC, especially if neurologic signs and symptoms are present. In any patient who is shunt dependent, it is necessary to thoroughly evaluate the shunt and exclude it as a cause of the TSC symptoms [2]. It is also necessary to determine the presence of any scoliosis and progression of deformity, as this can occur in many MMC patients, with 43% of these ultimately requiring spinal fusion in one series [3].

Indications for neurosurgical intervention for TSC are most dependent on the underlying pathology and the presence of associated symptoms. In the setting of OSD, MMC defects have typically been repaired within the first 48 hours of life. Over the last 20 years, however, there has been an increasing enthusiasm for *in utero* repair; this was investigated in the National Institutes of Health-sponsored, decade-long prospective randomized controlled multi-center MOMS trial, which revealed lower rates of Chiari malformation (i.e., hindbrain herniation, 25% vs. 67%) and CSF shunting (40% vs. 82%), as well as better mean lower extremity motor function as compared to traditional postnatal repair [4]. Urologic outcomes from the MOMS trial have not yet been published, but preliminary results have not shown significant improvements in urologic function with *in utero* versus postnatal MMC repair [5].

Regardless of when the MMC is repaired, the vast majority of patients with open MMC will have lifelong neurogenic bowel and bladder dysfunction. Close monitoring of bladder dysfunction is particularly important during childhood because retethering at some point during childhood is very common for children with MMC. In one series with 25-year follow-up, 32% of MMC patients required surgical detethering during childhood [4].

For CSD, indications for neurosurgical intervention vary. Patients with neurogenic bladder dysfunction associated with caudal regression syndrome, which is often associated with sacral dysgenesis, are not typically candidates for TCR (Figure 33.3). Conversely, in patients with CSD and signs and symptoms of TCS, the decision to operate is straightforward. However, the decision to perform a TCR in asymptomatic patients diagnosed with TSC is more controversial. Natural history studies suggest prophylactic surgery for many of these conditions carries a better long-term prognosis, as patients frequently develop urologic, neurologic, and orthopedic difficulties in the long term if these abnormalities are left

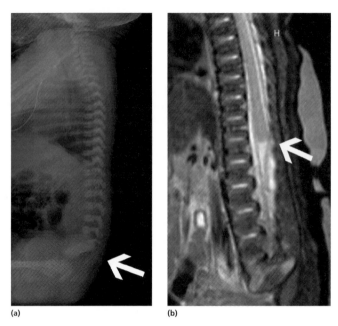

(a)   (b)

Figure 33.3 Images of a child with caudal regression syndrome. **(a)** Plain radiographs of lower spine and pelvis illustrate sacral dysgenesis (arrow). **(b)** T2 sagittal lumbosacral spine MRI shows the characteristic truncated conus (arrow) typical in caudal regression syndrome.

untreated [6, 7]. Urologic symptoms, in particular, are often irreversible once they occur. There is evidence that the relatively low risk of prophylactic detethering of straightforward TSC lesions is less than the long-term risk of waiting for symptoms, which are thought to be irreversible once they do occur. La Marca, in a series of 213 children with spinal lipomas, demonstrated superior outcomes and a decreased rate of worsening symptoms in those undergoing prophylactic surgery, as opposed to those undergoing surgery after onset of symptoms [8]. Phuong *et al.* estimate that 60% with a symptomatic TSC will experience continued urologic and orthopedic decline within 5 years without a TCR [9].

The primary surgical objective of the TCR is detachment of the spinal cord from its surrounding attachments, including the dura and soft tissues, which usually result from abnormal embryological development. TCR is nearly always performed in the lumbosacral spine, and rarely in the cervical or thoracic cord. The simplest of the spinal cord detethering procedures is the filum terminale section, which can be performed for thickened or fatty filum [10], but has also been reported for tight filum syndrome (see subsequent discussions), in which case the filum has a normal diameter on direct visual inspection as well as on preoperative imaging. Filum terminale sectioning, as for all spinal cord detethering procedures, is frequently performed with neuromonitoring. Detethering in the setting of a spinal cord lipoma is similar to filum sectioning, although the tethering element is obviously different, and additional care must be taken to perform neurophysiologic stimulation prior to division of the lipoma [11]. Lipomyelomeningoceles (LMMs) are classically described as dorsal, transitional, or caudal, depending on the anatomic relationship of the lipoma and the neural elements [12], although other classification schema have been proposed [13, 14]. Significant controversy exists as to whether all lesions can be safety detethered in their entirety; as such, this controversy extends to the role of TCR in asymptomatic lipomyelomeningocele patients, although detethering in asymptomatic patients is generally advocated given superior outcomes in asymptomatic patients and poor rates of return of function in symptomatic patients.

Data regarding the effectiveness of neurosurgical procedures in treating NBD with TCR are mixed and vary by underlying pathology. Bowman *et al.* reviewed their series of 502 children undergoing MMC closure, with 114 cases of subsequent TSC. Rerelease was required in 33 (29%) patients. TCR was performed in 37 cases for worsening urologic function in this series, 64% of who experienced improvement postoperatively, while the remaining 36% remained stable. In all cases, pain was improved following TCR [15], which is consistent with results by Rinaldi [16] and Hoffman [10], the latter series investigating filum sectioning. Fone, in a smaller series comparing TCR for lipoma versus retethering following MMC repair found that 75% of the patients undergoing primary TCR experienced improved urinary symptoms but only 30% in the retethered group, with another 48% in the latter group with worsening of symptoms [17]. For lipomyelomeningocele repair, postoperative functional status is largely dependent on preoperative functioning; in most series, the majority of patients remain stable or obtain some degree of functional improvement, but most children with little bladder or bowel function fail to regain any significant function postoperatively [13, 18, 19].

Complication rates following TCR for lipomyelomeningocele range from 5 to 30% [13, 20]. Complications, reported to be 5.8% in one series [13], can include wound infection, CSF leak, and worsening urologic or neurologic function. Urologic manifestations after TCR include premature or spastic bladder emptying, increasing incontinence, and bowel and erectile dysfunction. In the long-term, retethering of the spinal cord can occur, and present with signs and symptoms discussed previously. Younger patients undergoing TCR, particularly preadolescent children, are most likely to experience recurrent TSC during growth spurts [19–21]. Retethering has been described in 10–20% [18, 22] and can be delayed, ranging from 3 to 8 years postoperatively [13, 18]. The incidence of recurrent TSC also varies by underlying pathology, with patient with MMC and lipomyelomeningoceles much more likely to retether as compared to patients who have undergone fatty filum sectioning. The long-term management of TSC requires vigilant neurosurgical and urologic follow-up, although the frequency of visits and urodynamic studies will vary from case to case.

Tight filum syndrome

Tight filum syndrome, also known as occult tethered (spinal) cord syndrome (OTCS), is a relatively new diagnostic entity initially described by Khoury [23]. The diagnosis and management of OTCS are controversial [24, 25]. Patients present with typical urologic symptoms of neurogenic bladder dysfunction with a completely normal MRI of the neuraxis, including normal conus position. In some cases, there is urodynamic confirmation of the bladder dysfunction. Motor or sensory changes, musculoskeletal abnormalities, or fecal incontinence are much less commonly the presenting symptom(s). The pathophysiologic substrate for this has been attributed to either increased fibrous tissue within [26] or an otherwise thicker than normal filum [27]. Surgical criteria are not universally agreed upon, but generally include progressive bladder instability when there is no other definable etiology. In Wehby's early report of 60 children undergoing occult tight filum untethering, 52% demonstrated complete resolution of urinary incontinence or retention, greater than 95% resolution in another 35%, moderate (>75%) improvement in 6%, and minimal or no improvement in 8%. Fecal incontinence completely resolved in 56% and improved in another 41%. All patients experienced improvement in motor weakness, sensory deficit, and pain [28]. Similarly favorable outcomes were found in additional series of OTCS [23, 28–31]. Further studies are ongoing to better define the role of surgery in this rare condition [32]. Until further studies are completed, only a minority of children with neurogenic bladder dysfunction and a normal spinal MRI are candidates for filum sectioning.

Sacral (or selective dorsal) rhizotomy

Selective sacral dorsal rhizotomy has been described in children without findings of ongoing TSC for pharmacologically resistant overactive bladder [33]. In order to avoid complete bladder deinnervation and the sexual dysfunction associated with motor (ventral) sacral root rhizotomy, the ventral and dorsal roots were separated intradurally and only portions of the sensory (dorsal) roots were sectioned. Patients who underwent this procedure were found to have improved bladder capacity and an overall improvement in urinary incontinence. However, this procedure has not gained widespread acceptance in the treatment of such children because the results have been inconsistent and the durability of the effect has been questioned. Until more consistent long-term results can be demonstrated, many patients with this sort of hostile bladder undergo augmentation procedures.

Xiao procedure and other nerve transfer techniques

Neurosurgeons and urologists continue to explore creative experimental options for rerouting functional peripheral nerves to connect to dysfunctional sacral nerves, in hopes of creating new voluntary voiding mechanisms for patients with NBD. Most recently described is the Xiao procedure, which involves the intradural transfer of portions of a functional motor (ventral) root to ventral sacral roots. By maintaining a functional dorsal (sensory) root at the donor nerve level, a new reflex arc is created that allows patients to voluntarily void when they scratch themselves in the sensory root distribution. Xiao and other Chinese investigators have reported high success rates in animal studies and clinical trials [34–37]. Limited studies outside of China have produced less consistent and convincing results [38], but further studies are ongoing. At this time, the Xiao procedure remains experimental.

Brain anomalies

Hydrocephalus, which can result from multiple etiologies, can present with signs and symptoms of NBD, especially in post-MMC closure patients. The most common signs and symptoms of hydrocephalus in the pediatric population include headache, nausea, vomiting, lethargy, and somnolence; in newborns increased tension of the fontanelles and enlarging head circumference crossing percentiles can be found. Papilledema can be found on fundoscopic examination in the setting of chronic hydrocephalus, and Parinaud's syndrome, which includes palsy of upward gaze and eyelid retraction (Collier's sign), can be present. The treatment for hydrocephalus is CSF diversion, most commonly by ventriculoperitoneal shunting, although this can also be accomplished through other types of shunts (e.g., ventriculoatrial, ventriculopleural) or endoscopic third ventriculostomy [39]. As for many neurologic causes of bladder dysfunction, in the setting of acute hydrocephalus, the urologic symptoms will usually resolve with successful drainage of CSF.

Additional intracranial pathologies that can present with urologic dysfunction include brain tumors and cysts, particularly involving the frontal lobe or brainstem [40]. Fowler cites a range of 32–70% of urinary dysfunction in patients with posterior fossa tumors [41]. A detailed discussion of these pathologies is outside the scope of this chapter, but in many cases, as for acute hydrocephalus, treatment and resection of the tumor or cyst generally results in improvement, and in many cases, complete resolution, of the urologic disturbance.

Cerebral palsy (CP) and other forms of brain injury can also manifest with a urologic component [42, 43]. Unlike the other intracranial pathologies discussed here, effective neurosurgical options are not available at this time. While selective dorsal rhizotomy can have a profoundly positive effect on lower extremity spasticity and mobility in this patient population, lumbar and/or sacral rhizotomy has not been associated with an improvement in bladder dysfunction in children with CP.

Other spinal cord lesions and vertebral anomalies

These can include masses and tumors of the spinal cord, which are classified as intramedullary, intradural-extramedullary, or extradural; spinal cord cysts; spinal cord injury; as well as vertebral anomalies such as hemivertebra and sacral agenesis. Conditions more often associated with degeneration can also appear in the pediatric population, such as disc herniation and spinal stenosis. Signs and symptoms will vary by size, degree, and location, but it is important to evaluate for motor and sensory function, as well as reflexes. As for hydrocephalus and most other intracranial lesions, urologic symptoms accompanying cord compression or intrinsic cord pathology such as tumors and cysts will often resolve once the underlying brain or spinal cord lesion is treated by decompression, resection, or drainage, respectively.

Conclusions

Neurogenic bladder dysfunction has traditionally been associated with mye-lomeningocele, but neurosurgeons and urologists work collaboratively on the care of children with many types of NBD. Greater access to safe and highly sensitive MRI scanning has increased the diagnosis and neurosurgical treat-ment of abnormalities of the brain and spinal cord. Patients with TSC are often followed by pediatric urologists and neurosurgeons until adulthood because of a propensity of the spinal cord to retether. When signs of tethering are present, surgical treatment is recommended. However, prophylactic surgery is recom-mended for many types of TSC because long-term natural history studies sug-gest the risk of operating is often less than the risk associated with long-term monitoring, which has been associated with irreversible neurologic and uro-logic decline. Additional research focusing on further defining the indications for surgery, refining surgical technique, and developing novel techniques for spinal cord or nerve regeneration and/or rerouting can lead to improvement in clinical outcomes for children with NBD.

References

1 McLone DG, La Marca F. The tethered spinal cord: Diagnosis, significance, and manage-ment. *Semin Pediatr Neurol* 1997; **4** (3): 192–208.

2 Dias MS, McLone DG. Hydrocephalus in the child with dysraphism. *Neurosurg Clin N Am* 1993; **4**: 715–726.

3 Bowman RM, McLone DG, Grant JA, Tomita T, Ito JA. Spina bifida outcome: A 25-year perspective. *Pediatr Neurosurg* 2001; **34**: 114–120.

4 Adzick NS, Thom EA, Spong CY, Brock JW III, Burrows PK, Johnson MP, et al. A rand-omized trial of prenatal versus postnatal repair of myelomeningocele. *NEJM* 2011; **364** (11): 993–1004.

5 Clayton DB, Tanaka ST, Trusler L, Thomas JC, Pope JC IV, Adams MC, et al. Long-term urological impact of fetal myelomeningocele closure. *J Urology* 2011; **186** (4 Suppl): 1581–1585.

6 Cochrane DD, Finley C, Kestle J, Steinbok P. The patterns of late deterioration in patients with transitional lipomyelomeningocele. *Eur J Pediatr Surg* 2000; **10** (Suppl 1): 13–17.

7 Kulkarni AV, Pierre-Kahn A, Zerah M. Conservative management of asymptomatic spinal lipomas of the conus. *Neurosurgery* 2004; **54**: 868–875.

8 La Marca F, Grant JA, Tomita T, McLone DG. Spinal lipomas in children: Outcome of 270 procedures. *Pediatr Neurosurg* 1997; **26**: 8–16.

9 Phuong LK, Schoeberl KA, Raffel C. Natural history of tethered cord in patients with menin-gomyelocele. *Neurosurgery* 2002; **50**: 989–993.

10 Hoffman HJ, Hendrick EB, Humphreys RP. The tethered spinal cord: Its protean manifestations, diagnosis and surgical correction. *Childs Brain* 1976; **2**: 145–155.

11 Sarris CE, Tomei KL, Carmel PW, Gandhi CD. Lipomyelomeningocele: Pathology, treatment, and outcomes: A review. *Neurosurg Focus* 2012; **33** (4): e3.

12 Chapman PH. Congenital intraspinal lipomas. Anatomic considerations and surgical treatment. *Childs Brain* 1982; **9**: 37–47.

13 Arai H, Sato K, Okuda O, Miyajima M, Hishii M, Nakanishi H, Ishii H. Surgical experience of 120 patients with lumbosacral lipomas. *Acta Neurochir* 2001; **143**: 857–864.

14 Hakuba A, Fujitani K, Hoda K, Inoue Y, Nishimura Y. Lumbo-sacral lipoma, the timing of the operation and morphological classification. *Neuro Orthopedics* 1986; **2**: 34–42.

15 Bowman RM, Mohan A, Ito J, Seibly JM, McLone DG. Tethered cord release: A long-term study in 114 patients. *J Neurosurg Pediatrics* 2009; **3**: 181–187.

16 Rinaldi F, Cioffi FA, Columbano L, Krasagakis G, Bernini FP. Tethered cord syndrome. *J Neurosurg Sci* 2005; **49**: 131–135.

17 Fone PD, Vapnek JM, Litwiller SE, Couillard DR, McDonald CM, Boggan JE, Stone AR. Urodynamic findings in the tethered spinal cord syndrome: Does surgical release improve bladder dysfunction? *J Urology* 1997; **157**: 604–609.

18 Kanev PM, Lemire RJ, Loeser JD, Berger MS. Management and long-term follow-up review of children with lipomyelomeningocele, 1952–1987. *J Neurosurg* 1990; **73**: 48–52.

19 Hoffman HJ, Taecholam C, Hendrick EB, Humphreys RP. Management of lipomyelomeningoceles. Experience at the hospital for sick children, Toronto. *J Neurosurgery* 1985; **62**: 1–8.

20 Kanev PM, Bierbrauer KS. Reflections on the natural history of lipomyelomeningocele. *Pediatr Neurosurg* 1995; **22**: 137–140.

21 Ohe N, Futamura A, Kawada R, Minatsu H, Kohmura H, Hayashi K, et al. Secondary tethered cord syndrome in spinal dysraphism. *Childs Nerv Syst* 2000; **16**: 457–461.

22 Colak A, Pollack IF, Albright AL. Recurrent tethering: A common long-term problem after lipomyelomeningocele repair. *Pediatr Neurosurg* 1998; **29**: 184–190.

23 Khoury AE, Hendrick EB, McLorie GA, Kulkarni A, Churchill BM. Occult spinal dysraphism: Clinical and urodynamic outcome after division of the filum terminale. *J Urol* 1990; **144**: 426–429.

24 Steinbok P, Garton HJL, Gupta N. Occult tethered cord syndrome: A survey of practice patterns. *J Neurosurg Pediatr* 2006; **104** (5 Suppl): 309–313.

25 Drake JM. Occult tethered cord syndrome: Not an indication for surgery. *J Neurosurg Pediatr* 2006; **104** (5 Suppl): 305–308.

26 Selçuki M, Vatansever S, Inan S, Erdemli E, Bagdatolu C, Polat A. Is a filum terminale with a normal appearance really normal? *Childs Nerv Syst* 2003; **19**: 3–10.

27 Selden NR, Nixon RR, Skoog SR, Lashley DB. Minimal tethered cord syndrome associated with thickening of the terminal filum. *J Neurosurg* 2006; **105** (3 Suppl): 214–218.

28 Wehby MC, O'Hollaren PS, Abtin K, Hume JL, Richards BJ. Occult tight filum terminale syndrome: Results of surgical untethering. *Pediatr Neurosurg* 2004; **40**: 51–57.

29 Warder DE, Oakes WJ. Tethered cord syndrome and the conus in a normal position. *Neurosurgery* 1993; **33**: 374–378.

30 Nazar GB, Casale AJ, Roberts JG, Linden RD. Occult filum terminale syndrome. *Pediatr Neurosurg* 1995; **23**: 228–235.

31 Selçuki M, Ünlü A, Çaglar Ugur H, Soygür T, Arikan N, Selçuki D. Patients with urinary incontinence often benefit from surgical detethering of tight filum terminale. *Childs Nerv Syst* 2000; **16**: 150–154.

32 Steinbok P. Treatment of persistent urinary incontinence in children. ClinicalTrials.gov Identifier: NCT00124046. https://www.clinicaltrials.gov/ct2/show/NCT00124046?term= steinbok&rank=1, accessed March 17, 2015.

33 Franco I, Storrs B, Firlit CF, Zebold K, Richards I, Kaplan WE. Selective sacral rhizotomy in children with high pressure neurogenic bladders: Preliminary results. *J Urol* 1992; **148**: 648–650.

34 Xiao CG. Reinnervation for neurogenic bladder: Historic review and introduction of a somatic-autonomic reflex pathway procedure for patients with spinal cord injury or spina bifida. *Eur Urol* 2006; **49**: 22–29.

35 Xiao CG, Du MX, Dai C, Li B, Nitti VW, de Groat WC. An artificial somatic-central nervous system pathway for controllable micturition after spinal cord injury: Preliminary results in 15 patients. *J Urol* 2003; **170**: 1237–1241.

36 Xiao CG. Xiao procedure for neurogenic bladder in spinal cord injury and spina bifida. *Curr Bladder Dysfunct Rep* 2012; **7**: 83–87.

37 Lin H, Hou C, Zhen X, Xu Z. Clinical study of reconstructed bladder innervation below the level of spinal cord injury to produce urination by Achilles tendon-to-bladder reflex contractions. *J Neurosurg Spine* 2009; **10**: 452–457.

38 Tuite GF, Storrs BS, Homsy YL, Gaskill SJ, Polsky EG, Reilly MA, et al. Attempted bladder reinnervation and creation of a scratch reflex for bladder emptying through a somatic-to-autonomic intradural anastomosis. *J Neurosurg Pediatr* 2013; **12**: 80–86.

39 Anderson RCE, Garton HJL, Kestle JRW. Treatment of hydrocephalus with shunts. In: Albright AL, Pollack IF, Adelson PD, eds. *Principles and Practice of Pediatric Neurosurgery*, 2nd ed. New York: Thieme Medical Publishers, Inc.; 2008.

40 Lang EW, Chesnut RM, Hennerici M. Urinary retention and space-occupying lesions of the frontal cortex. *Eur Neurol* 1996; **36** (1): 43–47.

41 Fowler C. Neurological disorders of micturition and their treatment. *Brain* 1999; **122**: 1213–1231.

42 Roijen LE, Postema K, Limbeek VJ, et al. Development of bladder control in children and adolescents with cerebral palsy. *Dev Med Child Neurol* 2001; **43** (2): 103–107.

43 Wyndaele JJ, Castro D, Madersbacher H, et al. Neurogenic urinary and faecal incontinence. In: Abrams P, Cardozo L, Khoury S, Wein A, eds. *Incontinence*, 4th ed. Paris: Health Publications Ltd.; 2009.

Index

Page numbers in *italic* refer to figures.
Page numbers in **bold** refer to tables.

Pediatric Incontinence: Evaluation and Clinical Management, First Edition. Edited by Israel Franco,
Paul F. Austin, Stuart B. Bauer, Alexander von Gontard and Yves Homsy.
© 2015 John Wiley & Sons, Ltd. Published 2015 by John Wiley & Sons, Ltd.